COGNITIVE APPROACHES TO CULTURE

Frederick Luis Aldama, Patrick Colm Hogan,
Lalita Pandit Hogan, and Sue Kim, Series Editors

A PASSION FOR SPECIFICITY

Confronting Inner Experience in Literature and Science

MARCO CARACCIOLO
and RUSSELL T. HURLBURT

With a Foreword by Eric Schwitzgebel

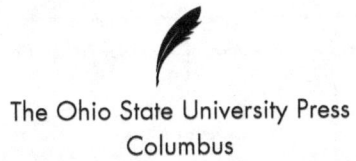

The Ohio State University Press
Columbus

Copyright © 2016 by Marco Caracciolo and Russell T. Hurlburt.
All rights reserved.

Library of Congress Cataloging-in-Publication Data
Names: Caracciolo, Marco, author. | Hurlburt, Russell T., author. | Schwitzgebel, Eric, writer of foreword.
Title: A passion for specificity : confronting inner experience in literature and science / Marco Caracciolo and Russell T. Hurlburt ; with a foreword by Eric Schwitzgebel.
Other titles: Cognitive approaches to culture.
Description: Columbus : The Ohio State University Press, [2016] | Series: Cognitive approaches to culture | Includes bibliographical references and index.
Identifiers: LCCN 2016032780 | ISBN 9780814213209 (printed case ; alk. paper) | ISBN 0814213200 (printed case ; alk. paper)
Subjects: LCSH: Psychology and literature. | Literature—Philosophy. | Experience in literature. | Literature and science. | Introspection. | Philosophy of mind.
Classification: LCC PN56.P93 C37 2016 | DDC 801/.92—dc23
LC record available at https://lccn.loc.gov/2016032780

Cover design by Lisa Force
Text design by Juliet Williams
Type set in Futura, Palatino, and Scala Sans
Published by The Ohio State University Press

∞ The paper used in this publication meets the minimum requirements of the American National Standard for Information Sciences—Permanence of Paper for Printed Library Materials. ANSI Z39.48-1992.

9 8 7 6 5 4 3 2 1

Remembering objects as mundane as a bicycle basket was a not insignificant part of my vocation [as a writer]. The deal worked out for me as a novelist was that I should continuously rummage around in memory for thousands and thousands of just such things. Unlikely as it may seem, a passion for local specificity, the expansive engagement—something close to fascination—with the seemingly familiar . . . object like a lady's kid glove, or a butcher shop chicken, or a Gold Star flag, or a Hamilton wristwatch . . . is all but at the heart of the task to which every American novelist has been enjoined since Herman Melville and his whale and Mark Twain and his river. . . . Its concreteness, its unabashed focus on all the particulars, its passion for the singular and pronounced aversion to generalities is fiction's life blood. It is from a scrupulous fidelity to the blizzard of specific data that is a personal life, it is from the force of its uncompromising particularity, its physicalness, that the realistic novel . . . derives its ruthless intimacy.

—Philip Roth, Pulitzer Prize–winning author, from the symposium
"The Life and Work of Philip Roth," aired on C-SPAN March 19, 2013

CONTENTS

Foreword by Eric Schwitzgebel   ix
Acknowledgments   xi

FIRST PART: PRELIMINARIES

Messages to the reader   3

Chapter I	In which Marco asks Russ about reading, but he responds about presuppositions	11
Chapter II	Russ performs a small study that surprises Marco	24
Chapter III	Russ presumes to identify Marco's presuppositions	35
Chapter IV	Marco's questionnaire and a "boot-like" sentence	41
Chapter V	Contrasting broad experience and pristine experience, with Amsterdam as an example	54
Chapter VI	In which Marco sends Russ his paper on the experience of reading McCarthy's *The Road*; Russ hesitates but then critiques it	68

SECOND PART: PHENOMENA

Chapter VII	Phenomena and how to explore them	83
Chapter VIII	In which Marco rankles at Russ's emphasis on delusion, and they discuss the existence of experience	95
Chapter IX	*Great Expectations* and genies reveal something about knowing others' experience	100

Chapter X	Pristine experience, broad experience, presuppositions, and tendencies; Russ challenges James Joyce	110
Chapter XI	On the adulteration of pristine experience	130
Chapter XII	Phenomena, adulteration, apples, and turkey	136
Chapter XIII	Pristine experience : broad experience :: phenomena : not phenomena	147
Chapter XIV	Phenomena, mental states, judgments, and hunger	169

THIRD PART: PERSONAL

Chapter XV	Getting even more personal	183
Chapter XVI	Similarity and familiarity, scams, and the fight to the death	198
Chapter XVII	Marco wears the beeper	210
Chapter XVIII	Ultimately personal: Twenty-four moments of Marco's pristine experience	217
Chapter XIX	A very small quibble on wording	233
Chapter XX	Salient characteristics of Marco's experience as characterized by Russ	243
Chapter XXI	Two more quibbles on wording	249

FOURTH PART: CLARIFICATIONS

Chapter XXII	Where Russ transitions back to the general	263
Chapter XXIII	Feeling hooks inside one's chest; metaphor and experience	285
Chapter XXIV	Metaphor tables	294
Chapter XXV	Retrospective prospections	301
Chapter XXVI	In lieu of a conclusion	314

| Works Cited | 317 |
| Index | 323 |

FOREWORD

This book has the potential to revolutionize both the study of the experience of reading and the study of aesthetic experience generally. But you will need to be patient with it.

Currently, we know very little about what people actually experience when they read a text. Do people form visual images of scenes depicted in the text? Do people hear the voice of the narrator as though speaking in their heads? Do they immerse so deeply that they no longer visually experience the page before them? How much variation is there between people, within the same person over time, and depending on features of the text or reading context? How do differences in readers' experiences relate to their understanding and appreciation of the text? There is virtually no systematic work on these topics that adequately confronts the methodological challenges of studying readers' conscious experiences as they stream past. The academic community is similarly ignorant about aesthetic experience while encountering music, movies, photography, painting, dance, cathedrals, sunsets . . .

Russell T. Hurlburt ("Russ," in this book) is the world's leading practitioner of "experience sampling" methods in psychology—"beeping" people to discover what was in their stream of inner experience at the moment immediately before the beep. (I have been critical of Russ's methods in Hurlburt and Schwitzgebel 2007, but as I said in 2007, I know of no better method for studying consciousness.) Marco Caracciolo, a postdoctoral researcher in literary theory, contacted Russ, thinking that Russ's experience sampling could help him explore readers' experiences when confronting a text like Kafka's *Metamorphosis*.

Russ's reaction is perhaps somewhat surprising: he confronted Marco about the presuppositions that Marco was bringing to the enterprise, presuppositions Russ thought likely to ruin Marco's potential to discover the truth about readers' experiences. Thus, Russ led Marco away from the study of others' experiences to an exploration of himself. This book is a record of that encounter, as it took place in Russ's and Marco's email exchanges. It is characteristic of Russ's work that he starts with such personal encounters, collaborative but also frankly confrontational, whether between himself and a research subject or between himself and another researcher. These personal encounters, coupled with a thorough exploration of specific details before drawing general conclusions, often yield novel insights otherwise unlikely to have been obtained, insights both for the people encountering each other and for the almost-voyeuristic observer.

The format of the book will require you, as I said, to be patient. If you are like me, when you are confronted with an academic text, your first, hurried reaction will be to home in as quickly as possible on the takeaway message, to determine how much time to invest and on which parts. This book is not an expository essay that can effectively be approached in that way. It is a journey, so you'll have to buckle in for the ride at the beginning. If you are interested, scientifically or personally, in the experience of reading, you should find the journey worthwhile.

You might think that Russ and Marco could save the reader's time by editing the exchanges down to the essentials. To understand why they have not done this, you need to know another central and distinctive feature of Russ's approach: Russ believes that toxic presuppositions are often reflected, invisibly to us, in our decisions about what is worth paying attention to and what can be omitted without loss. He fights this tendency by employing random beepers that force the researcher and subject to consider in detail whatever experience happens to be present at the moment of the beep, whether that experience seems deep or mundane, typical or unusual, on-topic or off-topic. Often, what one is initially inclined to dismiss proves to be the thing one *regularly* dismisses—the very thing perpetually in one's blind spot, the very thing one needs finally to learn to see. Russ and Marco, by presenting the full text of their exchange, only lightly edited, similarly refuse to prejudge what details matter, letting it all hang out for the reader's evaluation. The result is a conversation of profound importance for both aesthetics and consciousness studies, revealing the evolving perspectives of two cutting-edge researchers in their full, unguarded humanity and authenticity.

Eric Schwitzgebel
Professor of Philosophy
University of California, Riverside

ACKNOWLEDGMENTS

This book, which is essentially a protracted epistolary duet, is part of an even larger symphony of voices and conversations that shaped, directly or indirectly, our thinking on the subjects we explore in these pages. Some of these voices read this book, or parts thereof, and helped us improve its conception and presentation. For their comments and suggestions, we are thankful to Vanessa Arreola, Chris Heavey, Jason Kelsey, Herbert Lindenberger, Marta Meana, Alan Moore, Eric Schwitzgebel, Doug Unger, and one anonymous reviewer. Other voices can be heard more in the distance, but their interest and encouragements still served as essential accompaniment to the composition of this book, and to the email exchange that preceded it.

We thank Lynn and Alex for their willingness to participate in and have us discuss the preliminary study reported here.

While working on this project, Marco held a grant from the Netherlands Organization for Scientific Research (NWO; file number 446–11–024), which he gratefully acknowledges. Marco thanks his Groningen colleagues (particularly Julian Hanich, Miklós Kiss, and Liesbeth Korthals Altes) and the colleagues and friends who have shared many of the questions explored in this book (Porter Abbott, Marco Bernini, Emily Troscianko, and Anežka Kuzmičová). Thanks also go to those who have witnessed, not without some amusement, Marco's first DES experiments in and around his Oude Boteringestraat office (Paolo Maffezioli, Virginia Pignagnoli, Thom van Duuren, Bram van Leuveren, and Nadja Zadorina).

This book wouldn't have been possible without the support of Cécile Guédon and Bobbie Hurlburt.

Eric Schwitzgebel, regarding his foreword, notes the following: "It has largely been in collaboration with my graduate student Alan T. Moore, who has been working on the topic for his dissertation, that I have come to appreciate the potential of applying experience sampling methods to aesthetic experience. See Moore and Schwitzgebel 2013 for some of our preliminary results."

FIRST PART
PRELIMINARIES

To: The reader
From: Marco Caracciolo
        Groningen, The Netherlands

We spend a significant part of our lives engaging with stories told in conversation, literary fiction, movies, theater, comics, and video games. We do so not just because stories can be entertaining, interesting, and informative, but also because these qualities have an experiential "feel" attached to them: narrative can elicit powerful emotions or evoke vivid mental imagery; it can stir up the audience's past memories and invite them to consider existential or ethical questions.

Armed with these ideas, and prompted by the recent rise of interest in the so-called "experientiality" or "consciousness factor" of narrative within my field, narrative theory, I emailed Russ Hurlburt, asking his advice on an empirical study that I was planning. I had just finished reading Russ's book-length conversation with philosopher Eric Schwitzgebel, and I had a hunch that Russ would be responsive and helpful. What I did not expect, however, was that our correspondence would end up challenging many of my assumptions regarding narrative and experience.

In my first email to Russ I wrote that I wanted to set up an empirical study of narrative experientiality on the basis of his Descriptive Experience Sampling (DES) method. We decided to run a pilot study where "Lynn" and "Alex" would read Franz Kafka's *The Metamorphosis*. The participants were two skilled DES subjects, so we could expect them to deliver high-fidelity descriptions of their experiences. We would "beep" them in the DES way a few times while they read; they would take notes on whatever was in their experience just before each beep; and then Russ would interview them about their beeped experiences.

The results of these interviews are described in the body of this book, and I don't want to spoil it for you. Here's a glimpse: Lynn's experiences while reading were approximately what I (and probably you, dear reader) anticipated. But Alex's experiences (as Russ described them) surprised me, almost alarmed me. Baldly stated, I didn't believe him. Alex's reading experiences couldn't possibly be like that; or if they were, Alex couldn't possibly be reading with comprehension. My temptation was to disregard Alex's DES report on the grounds that it was apparently irrelevant to my study.

Russ suggested that my disbelief and inclination to disregard were likely the products of my own presuppositions, which blinded me to actual experiences while reading. I parried, saying that Russ undervalued the big picture of the experience of reading: the DES method was biased in favor of experiences of a narrow temporal scope, stripping down the richness of the reading experience and leading to reports as bizarre as Alex's. There ensued an email correspondence where we hammered away at my presuppositions or Russ's narrowness regarding issues central to both consciousness science and literary studies: the methodological pitfalls involved in the investigation of experience; the difference between "pristine" experience as can be apprehended through the DES method and the "broad" experience that forms the backbone of narrative experientiality; the degree to which experience can be shared with others; the role of language and metaphor in shaping experience and experiential reports; what it means for a text to convey a character's experience; the dividing line between a humanistic and a scientific approach to experience. Eventually I, too, wore the DES beeper, in a kind of participant-observation. I don't want to spoil that part of the book for you, either, but when the time comes you'll see that my first-person encounter with DES left a mark on my views about experience.

A few months ago I was invited to present my work on narrative experientiality at a conference on psychological approaches to literature. The audience was a small but extremely competent group of literary and psychological scholars. As part of my presentation, I explained the *Metamorphosis* study and described Alex's experience. The audience laughed out loud at the obvious absurdity of such a description. Their reaction was strikingly similar to my own surprise/alarm when Russ first described Alex's experience to me. You might expect that I would have found these scholars' laughter congenial, a validation of my view of the reading experience. Indeed, a year ago I would have been one of the laughers, but now the laughter irritated me: I recognized it to be the noise of presuppositions being stirred up in the audience, the same presuppositions that I had been trying hard to work through over the course of my dialogue with Russ. My reaction to the laughter made it clear that Russ's and my interchanges had been transformative for me.

It was then that I understood that others might value a vicarious participation in the Russ/Marco interchanges, and that technology would make it possible. I have never met Russ, so our dialogue has been entirely electronic, and as a result, whatever had been transformative for me continued to exist in its original email-exchange form. We should make that accessible.

This book presents a mostly verbatim account of Russ's and my interchanges. We have edited out a few places to make your reading easier, but those alterations are minor and, I think, do not appreciably alter the flow, content, or energy—they continue to display the tension that results when two people try to be honest with each other about important matters that might involve personal blindnesses on one side or both. Much of the conversation is about my own presuppositions, and, dear reader, you have every right not to care much about that—they are, after all, only one person's small or large delusions. Yet, as the laughter of my colleagues evidenced, I think some of my presuppositions about experience may be broadly shared. I don't want to be dogmatic about that, however, so I invite you into the fray. You may come to believe, as Russ suggested, that my initial views were presupposition-ridden, that your own views were similar to mine, and that you have profited from our skirmishes. Or you may come to believe that Russ has duped me into accepting his overly narrow way of looking at experience. But either way, I think you will appreciate the genuine struggle that is conveyed in these pages.

In the course of my conversations with Russ I have often been struck by the poetic quality of his DES descriptions. Virginia Woolf suggested that art isolates one instant from the stream of time and turns it into a single, clear-cut "moment of being." To me, this process bears a striking resemblance to the rigor and determination with which Russ pursues a randomly chosen instant of his participants' existence. To use Woolf's favorite metaphor, Russ's experience sampling can be said to "crystallize" human time. Here artistic and scientific methods seem to converge. As Russ himself put it when I drew his attention to the poetry of DES: "when you get down deep enough into genuineness, [every human endeavor] looks pretty much the same." Such genuineness and painstaking attention to detail surround all of our exchanges, giving them the personal tone and resonance which—I hope—will make the puzzles of experience concrete and relevant to you.

Marco

To: The reader
From: Russ Hurlburt
        Las Vegas, Nevada, USA

When Marco Caracciolo asked for some advice in applying my Descriptive Experience Sampling (DES) method to study the phenomena of the experience of reading, I replied that I thought his study underappreciated the sensitivities required to study phenomena, that if he really wanted to take inner experience seriously, he needed to start over. I expected that to be the end of it.

Instead, it was the beginning of an email correspondence where we confronted each other about many of the crucial issues involving experiential science and humanism. I am a grizzled scientist who, across five decades, has pioneered the exploration of inner experience (thoughts, feelings, sensations, etc.). Marco is a vigorous humanist whose work deals with the "experientiality" of literary narrative—its capacity to draw on the audience's past experiences and turn them into novel imaginative experiences. Those intersecting interests but divergent histories and personalities energized the confrontations: Marco thought I was too narrow in my approach and wanted me to respect his broad view of experience. I thought Marco was unknowingly ambiguous in his thinking about experience and that his overconfidence reflected presuppositions about experience rather than facts.

This book presents our exchanges as they happened, not sanitized or bowdlerized. I think you will find those exchanges to be genuinely confrontational. Confrontation has acquired a bad connotation, implying intemperate argumentation, but genuinely to confront means to come face to face with. Genuine confrontation begins with a personal disagreement (the real Russ suggesting to the real Marco that Marco's comments may reflect presupposition rather than fact; or the real Marco suggesting to the real Russ that Russ's comments overlook important aspects) and then, face to face, exposing relevant details until the disagreement is clarified or resolved.

I've written rather a lot about presuppositions (particularly in Hurlburt, 2011a; Hurlburt and Schwitzgebel, 2007, 2011), that they are delusions that warp one's view of the world. I fancy myself as having quite a bit of practice in sniffing out presuppositions in myself and others, the result of 35 years of investigating the details of inner experience, and in helping others to grind away or set aside ("bracket") their presuppositions. From that experience I highlight three aspects: First, presuppositions (aka delusions) are blindnesses. If Marco has presuppositions, he will not, in fact cannot possibly, recognize them and must energetically deny their existence—that's the nature of delusion. Second, no one (unless they have attained perfection) has direct knowledge of the presuppositions of others. What looks to me like Marco's presupposition might actually reflect my own blindnesses or hypersensitivities. Third (really a corollary of the first two), if there is progress in the bracketing or grinding away of a presupposition, it will require repetition and more repetition, and progress will be uneven.

The conversations displayed in this book are always on the scent of Marco's or my presuppositions or blindnesses. The value of this book, if value it has, derives from the likelihood that you, dear reader, share Marco's presuppositions or my blindnesses/hypersensitivities, and that you might profit from our transformative confrontations. If what I said in the previous paragraph about the nature of presuppositions is correct, then you also will require repetition and more repetition. Trying not to spoil the conclusion for you, here is an example. Marco and I disagreed about pristine experience and broad experience: I thought they were fundamentally different whereas Marco thought they were largely the same (you'll find the details of that distinction inside this book). We battled back and forth, trying, eventually successfully, to work through our differences. We could (as would most authors) have written a book that explicates our conclusions: pristine experience is like this, broad experience is like that. Instead, we have provided a book that seeks to change your way of apprehending distinctions such as between pristine experience and broad experience. That is, this is *not* a book about *it* (types of experience); this is a book about *you* (potentially abrading away some presuppositions about experience).

So I warn you that the conversations in this book meander. Conversations that are effective in bracketing presuppositions *must* meander. I might call these conversations "braided" in the sense that there are multiple strands that wind around each other, reaching backward and forward to make a stronger structure. Each plait retreats behind the others but then emerges again at a deeper level, exposing presuppositions from a new perspective. I think the interwovenness of our confrontation is essential to the bracketing of presupposition process, and the good news is that the result of the braiding is a stronger structure than would result from exposing each plait one at a time. (By the way, the book's cover is inspired by the braided nature of our confrontation.)

This book therefore displays our interchanges, word for word, no holds barred. We have provided some landmarks to make your reading easier, edited out a few strands that led farther afield than we judged desirable here, and provided some occasional edits to correct misspellings and the like, but what remains is essentially verbatim, preserving the tension that ran through our interaction. I hope it engages your (slightly prurient) interest in genuine human exchange. There is no jargon employed, no special expertise required, and I hope you will find that our emails read more like fiction than technical scholarship, making our exploration of experience personally compelling as well as valuable to psychologists, consciousness scientists, literary scholars, and humanists of all stripes.

Last but by no means least, I salute Marco's commitment to genuine discovery, wherever that path leads, and his unflinching willingness to present this book, which reveals aspects of the private Marco (as revealed by the beeper and otherwise) at an uncommonly personal and not always flattering level. I respect greatly his willingness to open these conversations to public scrutiny and trust that you will find his commitment revelatory and motivating as well as just plain interesting.

Russ

Q: *Why should I want to participate vicariously in your argument? Why don't you two just work out your differences, figure out what you jointly believe, and tell us about that? That would be much more efficient!*

RUSS AND MARCO: *As in many things, the journey is more important than the destination. If there is value in the reading you are undertaking (and we think there is), it comes from the transformation, not merely the acquisition of a new set of facts. That kind of transformation requires taking one perspective and then another and then another on the same material, requires confrontation, requires* repetition, requires growth, requires time for stubbornness or pride to melt away.

Q: I'm new to this topic. What is Descriptive Experience Sampling?

RUSS: Here's what you need to know at the outset: Descriptive Experience Sampling (DES) is my attempt at presenting a method that produces high-fidelity descriptions of inner experience. If you are a subject in DES research, you carry a random beeper into your natural environments (work, driving, shopping, recreation, etc.). When it beeps, you are to notice your inner experience (thoughts, feelings, sensations, perceptions, etc.) and jot down its characteristics. At the end of a sampling day (after you have collected about six beeps), you participate in an "expositional" interview designed to help you provide faithful accounts of your experience.

Q: What do you mean by inner experience?

RUSS: Thoughts, feelings, sensations, tickles, seeings, hearings, etc.; anything that directly presents itself "before the footlights of consciousness" (as William James would say) at a particular moment. The details will become clear as we progress.

I

IN WHICH MARCO ASKS RUSS ABOUT READING, BUT HE RESPONDS ABOUT PRESUPPOSITIONS

January 7
Dear Dr. Hurlburt,
I am a postdoctoral researcher at the Department of Arts, Culture, and Media of the University of Groningen in the Netherlands, and my work deals with the phenomenology of reading literary narrative. In particular, I am interested in correlations between the experiential components of people's engagement with literature (mental imagery, emotions, etc.) and higher-order judgments concerning the ethical, social, or aesthetic relevance of literary texts.

I've recently come across your Descriptive Experience Sampling (DES) method, and after reading up on your work I started thinking of applying a version of your methodology to the study of the reading experience. As far as I know this hasn't been attempted before (although in several cases your subjects did get a beep while they were reading), so I would be greatly interested in any comment or suggestion you may have on the experimental design described below. My project is still in its infancy, so feel free to suggest radical revisions to the set-up.

First of all, your subjects typically carry the beeper with them throughout their day; but since I am interested in a very specific activity here I think it would be impractical to ask my participants to ignore the beeps when they are not reading, or to turn on the beeper only when they start reading. My guess is that a relatively controlled experimental situation would be more suitable to this study. For instance, I could ask each [1] participant to read a novel in my office (or in a more "natural" setting such as a coffee shop) for a couple of hours, informing them that the beeper will go off at random intervals after they have been reading for 30 minutes. I think this warm-up period is important for readers to be able to immerse themselves in the novel, letting go of the thought that they are participating in a psychological study etc.

Immediately after the beep, participants would stop reading, jot down some notes, and come to me in order to be interviewed about their experiences. This procedure would be repeated several times over three or four reading sessions, with the participant picking up at the point where he or she was interrupted by the beep. The plan is to sample the reading experiences of a group of 10 readers, who would be asked to read the same novel (I need the same novel because the purpose of the project is to gain insight not just into the reading experience per se, but also into how stylistic and narrative strategies can interact with and perhaps constrain the reading experience).

Before the first session, each participant would receive a minimal phenomenological training (mainly in order to agree on the terminology used in the interviews); I will also make clear that the purpose of the study is to gain accurate information on how participants respond to the text at an experiential level, not assessing their literary competence or interpretive skills (I imagine institutional pressures are to be taken into account here, especially if the subjects are recruited among literature students—something that I'd rather avoid).

If you have any thought or suggestion about this variation on your methodology I'd be most interested in hearing it! In any case many thanks for your fascinating work.

All the best,

Marco Caracciolo

NOTE: Before you read on, we encourage you to note your reaction to Marco's proposed study. We strongly urge you to jot down a few notes about it—we'll wait! You might think that you don't need to jot down notes—that you'll be able to recall your reactions later. That is likely not true (it's one of the themes of this book). For now, we advise you to humor us: jot down a few words about Marco's study and your reaction to it.

January 8

Hi Marco—

I agree that understanding the phenomenology while reading would probably be of great value to literary folks, to psychological scientists, and to those engaged in pedagogy.

I agree that there are (to my knowledge) no good studies of the phenomenology while reading.

I agree that applying DES to the experience while reading might be extremely fascinating as well as worthwhile from the two perspectives above, so I applaud your project.

In my opinion, the main difficulty of a study such as the one you propose is the overcoming or bracketing of presuppositions, both by yourself and by your subjects, but your description does not seem to address that. Unless you are successful in that bracketing, I think your study's results will not be very interesting. If you are successful, your study's results will likely be incredibly interesting. That is, I think that if you really want to know about the phenomenology while reading, then by far the most important part of your design will be your ability to enable yourself and your subjects to bracket presuppositions. All other design features are secondary to that.

In that light, I think there is no such thing as the "minimal phenomenological training" to which you refer.

I think that any training you might do on the terminology to be used in the interviews will reify your own presuppositions and assist the subjects in entrenching their own presuppositions, and is therefore undesirable.

I think that any attempt to make "clear that the purpose of the study is to gain accurate information on how participants respond to the text at an experiential level" will precipitate a collusion between you and the subject that will substantially undermine your ability genuinely to find what you're looking for. There is only one possible DES phenomenological task—to apprehend whatever experience happens to be ongoing at the moment of a beep. In your study, that implies that your sincere interest must be to apprehend whatever experience happens to be ongoing at the moment of the beep while the subject happens to be reading. That is, if you want to apprehend phenomenology in high fidelity, you must be equally interested in seemingly unrelated phenomena ("distractions") as in those phenomena that seem on target.

And I do mean *equally* interested. If you (think you) "know," prior to your investigation, what phenomena are interesting, then you might as well not conduct the investigation—you'll just underscore your presuppositions.

If you have developed an effective way to bracket your own and your subjects' presuppositions, then it probably doesn't matter whether they read in your office or at home.

If I were to conduct such a study, I would have each subject begin by engaging in 3–5 DES sampling days (including an interview about each day's samples before proceeding to the next sampling day) while they go about their everyday *nonreading* activities. That is, I would learn how to talk to my subjects on turf that is *not* particularly of interest to my study. During those iterative interviews, I would try (and probably be successful) to awaken an interest in them and in me to apprehend their experiences, *whatever they are*, in high fidelity. That is, I would try to foster the notion that getting their experience right (that is, in high fidelity) is more interesting than getting it in line with their (or with their perception of my) presuppositions. That is not an easy task, but it is attainable if you are sincere and skilled.

Then, and only then, I'd ask them to read, and beep them while doing so, and emphasize that I'm interested in their experience at the moment of the beep, in high fidelity and whatever it is (whether related to reading or not).

That may well be more difficult for you than for them.

You likely will have the reaction that that is a lot of work, and so it is. But bracketing presuppositions is a lot of work. If you can figure out a more streamlined way to bracket presuppositions, I'm all for it, but I'm pretty sure that any attempt at streamlining is probably motivated by some presupposition and therefore counterproductive.

I think your study is unworkably ambitious. Your question ("how stylistic and narrative strategies can interact with and perhaps constrain the reading experience") is what I would call a validation question, and to answer it you would need many stylistic and narrative strategies, many subjects, and many samples from each subject. Most behavioral scientists ask validation questions, and on that altar sacrifice phenomenological adequacy. I think that is bad science in areas where phenomena might be important.

At this point in the history of the world, I think validation studies regarding experience are premature. If you want phenomenological adequacy, I'd suggest reorganizing your study to ask a straightforwardly phenomenological question: What are some experiential phenomena that occur while reading? I'd use a variety of subjects (probably fewer than 10) reading a variety of materials, and see what emerges.

I'd take seriously the trying to figure out how to bracket presuppositions effectively, by whatever means are necessary. For example, I'd suggest co-interviewers whom you respect but who have interests different from yours.

I'd recommend that you take individual differences seriously. There is no reason to believe that people have the same experiences while reading, even if they are reading the same passage.

I'd read my 2011 book.

I suspect all that may seem daunting and/or disappointing. If psychological science had a real commitment to the phenomena it studies, then there would be an infrastructure that supports the kind of work that you'd like to do, an infrastructure that has already done some of the basic work (of the kind that I am suggesting here). However, that is not the state of the world. So I think if you are really interested in phenomena, then you need to start at the beginning.

Please let me know if you have questions or comments.
—Russ Hurlburt

MARCO: *After exchanging the hundreds of emails that are displayed in this book, I find it impossible not to notice the naïveté of my planned study. My remarks on the "relatively controlled experimental situation" and the "minimal phenomenological training" appear to express what I now see as a (largely false) confidence in my own experience-sampling skills.*

RUSS: *Show of hands, please: A few pages back, did you jot down something about Marco's naïveté or overconfident self-assurance? (If you didn't jot it, it doesn't count.) I suspect there are not many hands showing, because I think Marco in this regard is very much like most people who consider exploring experience.*

RUSS AND MARCO: *One of the themes in this book is Marco's transformation from self-assurance about his phenomenological skill to the recognition of the naïveté of that self-assurance. Such transformation is crucial, as Epictetus noted: "What is the first business of one who studies philosophy? To part with self-conceit. For it is impossible for* any one to begin to learn what he thinks that he already knows" (108 AD/1865, II, 17).

Abrading away overconfident self-assurance is accomplished not by acquiring a new set of facts or attaining a higher level of erudition/competence, but rather by cultivating the valuing of naïveté. That cultivation is a large part of the journey that is this book, a part that requires multiple perspectives and repetitions.

January 9
Dear Russ Hurlburt,

Many thanks for your extremely rich reply! I completely agree with the importance of bracketing presuppositions, for me as well as for the participants. I will certainly try my best both while illustrating the purposes of the study and in the interviews. [2]

It's a great idea to sample the participants' everyday experiences *before* examining their reading experiences. As you say, it's a lot of work and I will probably have to reduce the number of participants. But I see the point of setting the stage for the study by interviewing the participants about their nonreading experiences. Thanks a lot for the suggestions! I will have to think about all this.

One comment on the issue of validation: I agree, in principle, that it's problematic to make generalizations about the experiences provided by reading the same novel.

Even though I understand your cautiousness ("There is no reason to believe that people have the same experiences while reading, even if they are reading the same passage"), I still think that if our experiences of the world were not broadly similar, it would be impossible to *share* experiences with others, for instance in so-called "joint attention" (see Seemann, 2011). You may have a different experience from mine while you read the same passage or, say, view the same painting, but the fact that we can discuss and compare our experiences suggests that there is no unbridgeable difference between my experiences and yours. They may not be the same, but they are sufficiently similar to be discussed and negotiated in social interaction. (And the reason why they are similar, I would say, is that they are based on the same object—novel or painting; see Caracciolo, 2012, on the sharing of experiences between writers and readers.) Maybe you'll say that this is, in itself, a presupposition. But isn't this kind of presupposition built into any episode of linguistic sharing of experiences—including, of course, interviews? [3]

[4]

In any case, thanks once again for the great feedback.
All the best,
Marco

Q: *I can accept that this book will meander and repeat—I understand that that is necessary if one is to abrade away conceit. But so I don't drift away, can you give me at least a hint of the direction we will take?*

RUSS AND MARCO: As Russ points out in his introductory note, our conversation is "braided": the division into chapters is designed to help you orient yourself through our exchanges. However, bear in mind that there are no clear-cut boundaries, because the same themes keep recurring in all (or most) of the chapters.

Here's a rough list of the themes we'll address:

a) *Broad/pristine experience:* The status of experiences in the broad sense vis-à-vis pristine experience: do they fall into the same category?
b) *Shared experience:* Whether and to what extent experiences (pristine and broad) can be shared, linguistically or otherwise.
c) *Talk about experience:* The difference between pristine experience and what people say about their experiences (broad experience).
d) *Humanistic/scientific:* The difference between a humanistic and a scientific approach to experience.
e) *Presuppositions:* The role of presuppositions and delusions.
f) *Judgments:* Do judgments always involve pristine experience?
g) *Mentalism:* Skinner's notion of "mentalism" and pristine experience.
h) *Metaphor:* The role of metaphor in conveying experience.
i) *Personal:* The personal dimension of our conversation.
j) *Concepts:* The relationship between concepts and experience.

When Marco writes on January 9 (near where [3] is in the margin above) that people's experiences are broadly similar, he is opening up the discussion of theme (b). As here, we'll provide "road map" comments to signal (often very approximately) where each theme starts and where it ends.

January 10
Hi Marco—
Please see my comments below.
—Russ

RE [2] "I will certainly try my best [to bracket presuppositions]." [The "2" refers to the number in the margin of the previous email.]

Perhaps you expected that I would be pleased to hear that you will try your best to bracket presuppositions, but actually I am dismayed. I'm not surprised, because your response is typical of scientists I have encountered. I think bracketing presuppositions is a high skill (Hurlburt, 2011a; Hurlburt and Heavey, 2006; Hurlburt and Schwitzgebel, 2007, 2011), perhaps on a par with violin playing. If you were to say "I agree with the importance of virtuosic violin playing, and I will certainly try my best," we both would think that statement is absurd. "Trying my best" has only a little to do with violin playing skill (which depends far more on method, practice, repetition, instruction, feedback, instrument, etc.). Your statement implies that if you try to bracket presuppositions, you can be successful, and that is, I think, very far from the truth. Presuppositions are delusions, and their bracketing requires method, practice, repetition, instruction, feedback, instrument, and so on, applied consistently over time.

It is, of course, desirable (in violin playing and bracketing presuppositions) to try your best at each step of the way, but without method, practice, repetition, instruction, feedback, instrument, and so on, trying is useless.

So my dismay comes from the fact that you, like others, seem drastically to underestimate the required rigor of effective bracketing of presuppositions, and that can't be a good thing.

RE [3] "If our experiences of the world were not broadly similar, it would be impossible to *share* experiences with others."

When Mary (sincerely, skillfully) says "I feel a pain in my heart about Jill," she describes a stabbing sensation in her chest, so painful that she nearly doubles over. When Sally (sincerely, skillfully) says "I feel a pain in my heart about Jill," she describes a cognitive process that judges Jill's situation to be extremely important and problematic (and she feels no chest pain). Mary thinks (delusionally) that Sally feels chest pain; Sally thinks (delusionally) that Mary is judging

Jill's situation. Mary and Sally can bridge their (unnoticed) differences because both do indeed find Jill's situation problematic. However, Mary's and Sally's experience is *not* the same. Whether it is similar or not is a matter of definition of "similar." Mary and Sally will typically never notice the differences between their experiences, even though those differences are immense (Mary is nearly doubled over; Sally cognitively engaged).

I think that to overlook these differences (as I think most psychology and probably most literary criticism does, but I'm no expert there) is, as you predicted, a presupposition (aka a delusion).

RE [4] "But isn't this kind of presupposition built into any episode of linguistic sharing of experiences—including, of course, interviews?"

Yes, indeed. There are (broadly) three ways to deal with that: (1) (ostrich) I've got presuppositions about experience but so do you, so I won't do anything about mine; (2) (behaviorist) I've got presuppositions about experience and so do you, so science should ban all reports of experience; and (3) (genuinely bracket) I've got presuppositions about experience and so do you, so we should both apply our collective intelligences to develop methods that might rationally be expected to be effective in keeping presuppositions at bay.

DES tries to fit into option (3). It has developed a method that explicitly seeks to help the investigator and the subject bracket presuppositions in these ways: it discusses specific, brief moments; it randomly selects moments to discuss (avoiding the selection of "favorite" moments); it asks open-beginninged questions; it uses an iterative method; it uses co-interviewers of different persuasions; it discusses brief moments because it expects to take a long time to check and recheck the meanings of words and their intention; and perhaps 100 more ways that are discussed in Hurlburt (2011a).

You might say that even though I intend to bracket presuppositions, I am not adequately skilled in so doing. To which I would reply: fine; then either be a behaviorist and rule out all discussion of experience; or develop a procedure that allows you to do better than I do; or examine my work carefully and see if what you say is true.

ROAD MAP: Note that this (January 10) email introduces both the presuppositions theme (e) and the personal theme (i).

January 11
Dear Russ,
Many thanks for your further thoughts and comments, lots of food for thought here!

[5]   I didn't mean to be dismissive when I wrote "I will try my best," since I genuinely share your concern about presuppositions. But I'm not sure I follow you when you draw such a sharp distinction between "trying one's best" and things like "method, practice, repetition, instruction, feedback, instrument." To me, all these count—or could count at least—as trying one's best.

At any rate thanks again for the feedback, I think I have a much clearer picture of the strategies I should implement to make my study methodologically sound now. And of course I'll keep drawing inspiration from your work.
All the best,
Marco

January 12
Hi Marco—
Preliminarily, let me say that I am no mind reader: I happily accept that I didn't and don't know exactly what you meant by "try my best." (And while I'm on this topic, I also should state explicitly that I am not the judge of who is or who is not deluded—I happily accept my ignorance on that score also. In particular, I do not feel anything remotely close to "You're deluded and I'm not, ha ha!" As I tried to state explicitly and repeatedly in my 2011 book, my sense is much more "You're deluded and so am I." The question is how to keep the ramifications of our (as in my) delusions from debilitating.)

RE [5] Distinctions about "trying one's best."
I've been teaching DES interviewing for a long time. Suppose I'm working with "Jack," and I point out what seems to me (imperfectly, to be sure) to be his presupposition about some particular something that has emerged in an interview. I suggest the desirability of bracketing that presupposition. The typical "Jack" response is something like "I will try my best—I am genuinely concerned about presuppositions" with the implication that he will do better in the next interview. But I think trying his best will *not* make Jack a better interviewer in the next

interview, any more than trying his best will make him a virtuoso the next time he picks up a violin.

Over the course of years of work and practice, trying one's best will make for better interviewing (and virtuosic violining), so I am indeed in favor of trying one's best. But it's a long-haul kind of thing.

True presuppositions operate out of sight, or prior to sight. If I'm right when I point out a presupposition to Jack, he *must* think I'm wrong. If he says, "Oh! You're right!" then I'm pretty sure I'm mistaken, because presuppositions don't give up without a fight. If I'm right, then Jack *must* think I'm exaggerating, that I really don't understand what he meant, that I might be right about this detail but it's really just a trivial detail, that he's actually much more skilled than I think he is, that he's much more knowledgeable about this topic than I am (but he's a kind and polite person so he wouldn't say that, at the risk of hurting my feelings), that it's my presuppositions that are in play, not his. And of course he might be right about all that, because I am not in a position to judge my own presuppositions. Therefore I have no right to be dogmatic. On the other hand, I have been doing this a long time and have a track record of being a pretty good (not perfect) sniffer of presuppositions, so I have no right simply to cave in, either. As a result, by their fundamental nature, presuppositions bring real people into direct conflict about very personal things.

So the best I can hope for from Jack is for him to say, sincerely, "I accept that you might know something about presuppositions in general, but I think you're mistaken about this one; I'll do what you say out of regard for your track record." But he won't actually do what I say, because he doesn't and can't understand what I say. So at the next interview (continuing the scenario that my presupposition-sniff was in the ballpark) he will do the same thing that he did in the first interview (or perhaps worse). I will point it out again, he will deny it again, this time with perhaps more vehemence. In the third interview (if there is one, because Jack's valuable time might seem to him to be being wasted on my obvious incompetence) Jack will do the same thing again, and I will point it out again, but this time there will be a glimmer of comprehension about what I'm talking about and a real recognition that something needs to be done about it. In the fourth interview, he will do it again, but this time he will recognize it by himself and be mad at himself for not having been able to change his behavior. In the fifth interview, he will correct the problem on his own.

But in the sixth interview, the problem will be back, and he will be frustrated by its return; but he will recognize that he has to work at it some more. And so on, the problem coming and going, working and working, until eventually it mostly doesn't come anymore.

That's the typical presupposition bracketing scenario at its best.

If that's what you had in mind by "I will do my best," then I'm all for it.

RE [1] Your study.

[6] I could do a very brief version—like a pilot—of your study. For example, I could beep two experienced subjects in two or three passages. If that's of interest to you, please suggest a shortish work that could be read with interest by undergraduates—say, an hour of reading—and I'll figure out how to beep people in at least approximately the same place (e.g., 8 seconds after they turn page 11).
—Russ

January 13
Dear Russ,
RE [6] "Please suggest a shortish work."

I'd suggest Franz Kafka's *The Metamorphosis*. It's long enough to beep the subjects a couple of times but short enough to be read in one sitting. It lends itself to multiple readings and interpretations [see Russ's comments in RE 42] while remaining highly readable in style and captivating in its subject-matter. But *The Metamorphosis* is also a text that foregrounds and problematizes experience: Kafka is well known for his ability to evoke narrative junctures that have a tangible experiential "feel" (think only of the adjective "Kafkaesque" and how we use it to describe situations that are somehow reminiscent of Kafka's paradoxes and absurdities; see Troscianko, 2010). In *The Metamorphosis*, for instance, we are told that the protagonist turned into an insect of some sort, but he is never described directly: despite its central importance in the story we have little information about the character's new body. How do readers cope with this indeterminacy in their imaginings? It is this kind of question that makes *The Metamorphosis* a good case study for investigating the reading experience.

If you like this choice, I could send you a pdf and a list of key passages within a day or two.
Marco

NOTE: In an exchange of emails, Russ and Marco agree that Russ will run a pilot study that delivers four beeps during the reading of The Metamorphosis. *The beeps will be delivered in such a way that the participants will be reading more or less the same passages when they hear the beeps. A screen shot of the Metamorphosis text reader can be found on the Companion Website.*

COMPANION WEBSITE: Additional materials accompanying this book can be found on the book's companion website. A link can be found on this book's page on The Ohio State University Press website (or simply Google "caracciolo hurlburt companion").

II

RUSS PERFORMS A SMALL STUDY THAT SURPRISES MARCO

January 23
Hi Marco—

I have now run the *Metamorphosis* study with two participants; see the raw data in tables 1 and 2. Lynn is an undergraduate who did four days of DES training before she participated in the *Metamorphosis* study. Alex is a grad student fairly knowledgeable about DES but not yet skilled at it as an interviewer. As you will see, they have very different experiences.

As you know, Lynn and Alex each received four beeps, which occurred some fixed number of seconds (the same for Lynn and Alex but different for each page) after they advanced to the quasi-randomly determined page; table 1 shows where Lynn and Alex reported they had been reading when they heard the beeps. Then I conducted standard DES interviews within 24 hours of Lynn's and Alex's participation and immediately thereafter prepared descriptions of their beeped experiences. Those descriptions are in table 2. You have mentioned that you take it as widely understood by most in the literature business that experiences while reading are very similar. (1) Could you point me to a place or two where that is written down? (2) What do you think of that after looking at the Lynn and Alex descriptions in table 2? (3) What do you think about the timing of the beeps and the use of the *Metamorphosis* story in general?
—Russ

[7]
[8]
[9]

TABLE 1. Where Lynn and Alex heard the beeps in *The Metamorphosis*

BEEP	TEXT WITH APPROXIMATE BEEP POSITION[a] INDICATED FOR <u>LYNN</u> AND A<u>L</u>EX
1	Was it really not enough to let one of the trainees make enquiries—assuming enquiries were even necessary—<u>did the chief clerk have to come himself, and did they have to show the whole, innocent family that this was so suspicious that only the chief clerk</u> could be trusted to have the wisdom to investigate it? And more because these thoughts had made him upset than through any proper decision, he s<u>w</u>ang himself with all his force out of the bed.
2	He was e<u>specially fond of hanging from the ceiling</u>; it was quite different from lying on the floor; he could breathe more freely; his body had a light swing to it; and up there, relaxed and almost ha<u>pp</u>y, it might happen that he would surprise even himself by letting go of the ceiling and landing on the floor with a crash.
3	Gregor crawled a little further forward, keeping his head close to the ground so that he could meet her eyes if the chance came. Was he an animal if music could captivate him so? It seemed to him that he was being shown the <u>way</u> to <u>the unknown nourishment</u> he had been yearning for.
4	He could already hardly feel the decayed apple in his back or the inflamed area around it, which was entirely covered in white dust. He thought back of his family with emotion and love.[b] If it was possible, he felt that he must go away even more strongly than his sister. He remained in this state of empty and peaceful rumination until he heard the clock tower strike three in the morning. He watched as it slowly began to get light everywhere outside the window too. Then, without his willing it, his head sank down completely, and his last breath flowed weakly from his nostrils. When the cl<u>ea</u>ner came in early in the morning—they'd often asked her not to keep slamming the doors but with her strength and in her hurry she still did, so that everyone in the flat knew when she'd arrived and from then on it was impossible to sleep in peace—she made her usual brief look in on Gregor and at first found nothing special.

[a] Approximate beep positions indicated by double underline for Lynn and by wavy underline for Alex.
[b] Lynn broke off reading about here.

TABLE 2. Lynn's and Alex's experiences at four moments while reading *The Metamorphosis*

BEEP	LYNN'S EXPERIENCE	ALEX'S EXPERIENCE
1	Lynn was reading about the chief clerk going to look for Gregor. Lynn innerly sees an open brown door with a circular glass window, opening inward from the right, revealing a bright white light outside the door, as if opening into bright sunlight. This is seen from the perspective as if she had just opened the door. In the doorway is a man; the details of the man are not clear, as if the brightness behind him makes it hard to see his details. [This seeing was taken to be a still image of a moving scene, a congruent illustration of the scene she was reading about.]	Alex is reading the word "swang." His experience seems wrapped up in the word "swang," that is, there is nothing else present in his experience. He does not articulate this word or innerly see it or hear it. Alex is of course in reality seeing the word swang on the screen, but he does not attend to any of the visual details of this word as seen. The process seems to be going from word to word, and the beep happened to fall on the word swang.
2	Lynn was reading about Gregor, who is talking about liking to hang down from the ceiling. Lynn innerly sees a dimly lit room with a bat (perhaps a foot tall) hanging from the ceiling over a bed with white sheets. She doesn't see much else about the room (no furniture, etc.), but she knows there is a window off to the right that supplies the light for the room. [The bat was somewhat a misrepresentation of the scene—Gregor is really a bug—but Lynn felt no incongruence—she is simply illustrating the story she is reading.]	Alex is reading the word "happy." It's just he and the word—he's moving word by word by word. There is no speaking or hearing or imaging in any other way. This experience is the same as sample 1 except that the word is different. Other than that different word, the experience seems identical.
3	Lynn is innerly seeing an illustration of a scene she had read about on the previous slide. That is, the beep occurs on slide 92, but her inner seeing pertains to slide 91, where Gregor had been crawling toward where his sister was playing the violin. Lynn innerly sees a spider crawling on the floor, from left to right, as if coming from one room into another. The sister is seen to be sitting at a table in the kitchen; the violin may have been seen [Lynn wasn't sure]. The focus of her seeing is on the spider crawling. [Lynn was reading the new slide apparently without comprehension—her understanding was that in a parallel universe where the beep had not occurred, she would have had to go back and read that slide again. (Whether that is true is unknown.)]	Same as sample 1 and sample 2 except that the word is "way." [When asked whether there was any experienced difference in emotional tone or meaningful comprehension of the words, Alex denied that. The word could be common or rare, emotionally laden or neutral, and the experience would be the same, he thought.]

4   Lynn had broken off from reading and at the moment of the beep was occupied by noticing the pressure on the wooden arm of the chair against her left forearm. She had stopped reading, leaned to the left, putting some weight on her left forearm. She had taken her eyes off the computer screen and looked to her right, although Lynn was not seeing what her eyes were aimed at. She feels the pressure of the chair on her arm, a narrow strip that conforms to the flat wooden arm of the chair.

At the moment of the beep Alex is innerly saying "cleaner." This saying is in his own voice but at a somewhat higher pitch than his experienced actual voice. He experiences the voice as being rushed [in reality, Alex is coming up on a time deadline]. His experience seems much more a speaking than a hearing, although it is possible that the rushed aspect (but not the higher pitch aspect) is more heard than characteristic of the speaking. It seems that Alex is speaking the word and then the next word and then the next word, and the beep happens to catch "cleaner." That is, it seems more a word—word—word experience than a speaking-a-sentence experience. [Alex reported retrospectively that if this kind of speaking gets to the end of a sentence, there is no inflective drop or pause for the period—the stream of words continues word—word—word across a period with no experienced pause or any other acknowledgment of the period.]

Alex was surprised that he had three of the same kinds of experiences.

Notes: There was apparently a computer malfunction: it froze up while trying to load page 98. Furthermore, Lynn was somewhat time pressured to make the sampling meeting on time, so she came to the interview with three beeps, which we discussed.

Then we suggested that she could read the end of the story in the lab; after the fourth beep we would interview her. Thus beep 4 was delivered under somewhat different circumstances from those of beeps 1–3.

Q: *Could you please clarify how the descriptions in table 2 were produced?*

RUSS: *I wrote them as the result of separate interviews with Lynn and with Alex using the Descriptive Experience Sampling (DES) procedure. We will describe the DES procedure in some detail below (see April 26), and I have described it in much detail elsewhere (e.g., Hurlburt, 2011a). For now, it will be sufficient to understand that these are intended to be high-fidelity descriptions of moments of Lynn's and Alex's experiences produced by a method designed expressly to produce such descriptions. Whether these descriptions actually do faithfully capture Lynn's and/or Alex's experiences is a matter of debate, as is exemplified in some of what follows.*

January 24
Dear Russ,
Thanks a lot. The data provided by both participants is extremely interesting. Lynn's and Alex's experiences are about as different as they could be! Lynn reports mental imagery at her beeps, while Alex reports this word—word—word thing.

[10] I'm a little puzzled by Alex's report. Should I really understand him to be experiencing merely one word after the other, each word with no experienced meaning? That doesn't seem possible. Perhaps it would be useful to ask participants to complete a text comprehension questionnaire after the interview, just to check whether they understood the story they were reading. I don't know what you think about this, but Alex seems to be concentrating on the task itself (the words that appear on the screen)

[11] rather than on the story. His reading seems to be an extreme case of nonimmersive reading, in which the linguistic medium becomes so opaque that he doesn't have any mental access to the storyworld *beyond* the text. Perhaps it is the artificiality of the lab setting that distracted him. Do you know if he's used to reading books on a screen (computer, e-book reader, etc.)?

[12] It is difficult to imagine how someone could understand the meaning of a narrative text without forming a mental representation (however vague and sketchy) of the described situation. Discourse psychologists such as Rolf Zwaan (see, e.g., Zwaan and Radvansky, 1998) have argued that "situation models" play a key role in narrative comprehension, and

that they have an experiential component. It's hard to believe that these mental operations take place in a *completely* unconscious way for Alex. Which doesn't mean that it's impossible, of course, but first of all I would need evidence that he's actually understood the text he was reading. There are some other inconsistencies that make me wonder about the reliability of his reports. For instance, Alex seems to be an extremely fast reader at times: on screen 102, he read up to line 9 in 14 seconds, whereas I predicted that participants would be reading line 3 or 4 at the time of the beep. But on screen 92 he seems to have read just one line in 8 seconds (I predicted lines 2–3). I don't know how to explain this discrepancy—perhaps the beginning of screen 92 was linguistically or syntactically more difficult—but at any rate it reinforces my suspicion about Alex's nonimmersive reading.

Lynn's reports are much more in line with my expectations and with previous studies of the psychology of reading narrative.

I have a question about Lynn's first sample. Was Lynn imagining standing on Gregor's side of the door (i.e., in his room) or on the clerk's side (i.e., in the corridor)? I have the sense that she imagined being in the room, but maybe you can clarify this point on the basis of the interview. Interestingly, at this point in the story the door to Gregor's room has not yet been opened, which means that Lynn made up that detail (with respect to the story, not with respect to her own experience—although we have to remember that this is the first beep, so we shouldn't be too confident about the report). A possible way to interpret this finding is that Lynn was aware of the emotional salience of the door for Gregor, and that she imaginatively opened the door on his behalf. (As you can see from both of these remarks I'm suggesting that Lynn might be adopting Gregor's spatio-temporal and perhaps emotional perspective—through a form of identification—at this point in the story.) [13]

Another clarification question concerns Lynn's second sample. Do I understand correctly that Lynn was visualizing Gregor as a bat even though she knew that he was actually a bug? This hesitation reflects the text's indeterminacy as to the exact nature of Gregor's body after the metamorphosis. Lynn seems to visualize different bodies depending on the type of posture or movement described: hanging down from the ceiling is probably more typical of a bat than of a bug, and consequently she imagines Gregor as a bat. By contrast, crawling is more strongly associated with bugs than with bats, and therefore Gregor becomes a bug. Many critics have seen him as a cockroach-like insect, while Vladimir

Nabokov—who had a second career as an entomologist—suggests that Gregor is a "brown, convex, dog-sized beetle" (1980, 259).

Now to your questions.

RE [7] "Could you point me to a place or two where [it is claimed that experiences while reading are very similar]?"

I don't think any literary scholar would actually make the argument that all readers experience literary texts in exactly the same or even in similar ways. If questioned about this, most literary scholars would probably acknowledge the diversity of readers' responses. You can have a look at the preface and at the introduction of James Phelan's *Experiencing Fiction* (2007), for example, for a clear statement of this. The problem, rather, is that most literary criticism and theory has, so far, tended to downplay that diversity, either because of a disregard for experience itself or because of normative assumptions (along the lines of "it doesn't really matter if readers tend to read in substantially different ways; they *should* read in the way that I am advocating here!").

[14]

There are, of course, studies that do focus on readers' experiences. Some of them are empirical, such as those conducted by Marisa Bortolussi and Peter Dixon (2002), David Miall (2006), and others. But even these studies focus on experiential patterns that involve much bigger "slices" of readers' engagement with stories than can be studied through the DES method. The question of the temporal structure of readers' experiences is perhaps worth exploring in more detail. It could be argued that DES cannot provide useful data for the literary scholar precisely because it "freezes" too small a chunk of readers' engagement to enable us to study larger experiential patterns and dynamics.

[15]

Q: *Could you say a bit more on why experience would be important for literary studies?*

MARCO: *Literary studies has traditionally concerned itself either with questions of literary history or with offering interpretive readings of literary texts—readings that seek to connect the themes, style, and structure of a particular text with broader frames and cultural interests (for instance, feminist or postcolonial theory). A partial exception to this historical or textual emphasis was the work of reader-response theorists such as Norman Holland (1975), Wolfgang Iser (1978), and Umberto Eco (1979), who stressed the importance of audiences' role in making sense of literature.*

Over the last twenty years some literary scholars have taken this reader-response approach in a more decidedly psychological direction, giving rise to the field of so-called "cognitive" approaches to literature (see Hogan, 2003; Richardson, 2004). Monika Fludernik (1996) was the first scholar to theorize about the "experientiality" of literary narrative, or the ways in which it taps into experiential predispositions and interests. In a parallel development, several researchers have started employing empirical methods to investigate aspects of literary texts and their reception (see van Peer, Hakemulder, and Zyngier, 2007). However, even in these fields the reading experience remains relatively marginal: with a few exceptions (e.g., Kuiken, Miall, and Sikora, 2004), the phenomenological framework is entrenched less in literary studies than in neighboring disciplines like film studies. More recent work (including my own) seeks to further explore this dimension of literary texts (see Caracciolo, 2014b; Kuzmičová, 2014; Troscianko, 2014).

RE [8] "What do you think of [the widespread literary understanding that experiences while reading are very similar] after looking at the Lynn and Alex descriptions in table 2?"

It's clear enough that Alex and Lynn experienced the text in radically different ways. As I pointed out above, however, I'm not convinced that Alex was actually experiencing the story (as opposed to just skimming through the text). I think it would be interesting to repeat the study with a larger number of participants.

RE [9] "What do you think about the timing of the beeps and the use of the *Metamorphosis* story in general?"

I think the *Metamorphosis* story was probably a bit too long for a two-hour time slot. Both readers got the feeling of being pressed for time, and this seems to have had a significant impact on their experiences. Ideally, it would be good to give readers as much time as they want to finish the reading task. As for the timing of the beeps, I think the idea of placing them shortly after the page turns worked well, because they were sufficiently close for both readers. But of course the fact that Alex's and Lynn's reports were so dramatically different makes it difficult to compare or contrast their experiences in any meaningful way.

All best wishes,

Marco

[16]

January 25
Hi Marco—
I'm traveling so can give only a limited reply.

RE [10] "Ask participants to complete a text comprehension questionnaire after the interview."
    I agree that in a real study that would be a good idea.

RE [11] "[Alex's] reading seems to be an extreme case of nonimmersive reading."
[17]   I think it is highly likely that Alex understood the text he was reading. I suspect it is entirely untrue that "the linguistic medium becomes so opaque that he doesn't have any mental access to the storyworld *beyond* the text."

RE [12] "It is difficult to imagine how someone could understand the meaning of a narrative text without forming a mental representation."
    I suspect that "difficult to imagine" is a characteristic of your imagination, not Alex's reading. I think yours is a widely held and quite likely untrue presupposition. I told you at the outset that people's experience is (I think) widely different, despite the fact that most people think it is mostly the same. Those people are vastly mistaken, I think.

RE [13] "Was Lynn imagining standing on Gregor's side of the door?"
    Yes. This was Lynn's first beep *today* but her 25th beep overall. I have very little doubt that her account of the door being open in her experience is correct about her experience, even though it is incorrect with respect to the text. People who visualize as they read make up details all the time; many of those details subsequently turn out to be incorrect. Most people then update their inner seeing without realizing that they have done so.

RE [14] "Most literary criticism and theory has, so far, tended to downplay that diversity."
    Most people (wrongly) assume that everyone's experience is like their own. That probably applies to literary critics.

RE [16] "Of course the fact that Alex's and Lynn's reports were so dramatically different makes it difficult to compare or contrast their experiences in any meaningful way."

I think the fact that they were so dramatically different makes it *imperative* to compare or contrast, although what is then to be examined is the literary presupposition that (incorrectly, I think) assumes that they should be more similar.

RE [15] "[DES] 'freezes' too small a chunk of readers' engagement."
Please see Hurlburt (2011b).
More later.
—Russ

January 26
Dear Russ,
Thanks a lot for the clarifications as well as for referring me to Hurlburt (2011b).

RE [17] "I think it is highly likely that Alex understood the text he was reading."
I'm ready to concede this. Perhaps it was misleading on my part to focus exclusively on the issue of linguistic comprehension. The question, rather, is whether Alex was having any conscious experience of the *meaning* of the words he was reading. [18]

If he was, then the results must reflect Alex's concern for providing a "molecular" rather than a "referential" description (in the terms of Hurlburt 2011b) of the moment before the beep: in other words, he confines himself "entirely to those bits of material that exist within the [experiential] slice" (Hurlburt 2011b, 280)—a molecular description—instead of providing the external reference points that would allow us to make sense of those bits of material (a referential description). Suppose that Alex gets a beep while he's engaged in conversation. Is he likely to concentrate only on the word his interlocutor was uttering before the beep, or will he give us at least some context, e.g., the topic and whereabouts of the conversation? I doubt that the description of an experience qualifies as such without *any* context at all. And sketching the context, in this [19]

[20]

case, would have required engaging at least in part with the meaning of the passage Alex was reading.

[21] If, on the contrary, Alex wasn't experiencing any meaning at all (whether he understood the text or not), then I doubt that his descriptions can be considered relevant to the study of the experience of reading *narrative*. I completely agree that we should be open to differences between people's experiences, but on what grounds can Alex be said to be experiencing the story, if he only perceived its words?

Just my five cents' worth. I may be wrong; I may be presupposing too much. But I'm very interested in your thoughts about this and other issues.

All the best,

Marco

III

RUSS PRESUMES TO IDENTIFY MARCO'S PRESUPPOSITIONS

January 27
Hi Marco—
I think that the issue of bracketing presuppositions in an investigation of experience is more important (at this stage in the history of the universe) than is the result of that investigation of experience. That is, it is more important to discuss how to fish than to give you a fish. Your reactions are exactly what I would expect from a thoughtful, bright guy, so my upcoming critique applies not merely to you but would, I expect, apply to most of your peers.

[22]

Actually, I think you are somewhat out in front of your peers in the sense that you are inquiring about experience before most of them are so doing. However, to my presupposition sniffer (and I wholeheartedly re-emphasize my fallibility), you are still locked in by your presuppositions. Below is what I take to be evidence of that.
—Russ

RE [21] "The study of the experience of reading narrative."
This study is *not* "the study of the experience *of* reading narrative." It is instead "the study of the experience *while* reading narrative." The distinction between *while* and *of* is a huge difference, as huge as the difference between "horses" and "unicorns." We did in fact beep Lynn and Alex *while* they were reading narratives. We did *not* have a right to say that we beeped them while they were engaged in the experience *of* reading narratives. First, they may *not* have been experiencing the *Metamorphosis* narrative (as was probably true for Alex at all his beeps and for Lynn at her fourth beep). Second, even if they were directly experiencing something about *Metamorphosis* (as was probably true for Lynn at beeps 1, 2, and 3), they were *not* experiencing reading narrative. Lynn was innerly seeing a brown door, innerly seeing a bat

[23]

hanging, innerly seeing a spider crawling. None of those is remotely similar to the experience of reading narrative.

You may think I am quibbling with words here, but if so, I think that is your presupposition defending itself. If you are interested in a faithful account of the experience *while* reading, it would likely be a fatal error to instruct a subject to report about the experience *of* reading narrative. That that error would be made by most or all of your colleagues is evidence only of mass fatality. The instruction for investigating experience *has to be* to report whatever experience happens to be ongoing at the moment of the beep, regardless of whether that experience happens to seem to be related to the experience of read-

[24] ing a narrative. There has to be explicit room for reporting that there was no experience whatever ongoing at the moment of the beep, or that there was seemingly irrelevant-to-the-subject experience ongoing at the moment of the beep (as Lynn's arm pressure), or that there was seemingly irrelevant-to-the-investigator experience ongoing at the moment of the beep (as Alex's word—word—word).

[25] This is a very big deal. Investigating phenomena is like fishing. You throw your line into a pond where you expect reading experiences to occur, but then you reel in whatever you get, whether it is a reading experience or a rubber boot. I say again: if you think this is a small detail, your presuppositions are fighting for their lives.

RE [19] "The results *must* reflect Alex's concern for providing a 'molecular' rather than a 'referential' description. . . . Sketching the context . . . *would have required* engaging at least in part with the meaning."

Your use of certainty-implying modal verbs (*must* and *would have required*) betrays (to my sniffer) a confidence that is far from warranted. There is in the world of experience no grounds for certainty about anything, not by me and not by you, not by anyone short of omniscience. Experience does not follow the rules of physics or the rules of grammar or the rules of logic. Experience is what it *is*; it is *not* what it *must be*. So as a general rule, when you feel certainty arising in you about anything experiential, I advise you to take that as a sign that your presuppositions are in control, that they are baffling you, that they are trying to make you feel stupid if you should feel anything that aligns with anything other than their (unwarranted) certainty.

In that same passage, you use softer verbs that express uncertainty ("I *doubt* that the description of an experience," "I *doubt* that his descriptions can be considered relevant," "is he *likely*," "on what *grounds* can Alex be said"). What I am going to say here is on thinner ice. If those phrases express honest skepticism, then great. But usually, at this stage in the presupposition battle, they arise from the same kind of unwarranted certainty as does "must," but are politely disguised. I re-emphasize that I am no mind reader, so I have no reason to be confident of what I am saying here. But if it applies to you, I suggest that you consider this: there is an important way that politely hidden certainty is *worse* than bald certainty. It gives the (false) impression of generosity and virtue—that is, it uses the appearance of virtue to hide vice. Presuppositions are wily. It's harder to attack a generous-seeming virtue.

(I've written here about presuppositions as though they are entities of their own, but I actually don't know anything about the ontology of presuppositions. My aim is to paint colorfully the admittedly metaphorical battlefield on which the struggle with presuppositions (whatever they are) is pitched.)

Now with one more recognition that I have no standing which grants me the right to discover your presuppositions, and with apologies if I have missed the mark, I return to the questions that you asked.

RE [19] "The results must reflect Alex's concern for providing a 'molecular' rather than a 'referential' description."

I doubt that that is true. I think Alex is providing a referential description, but the bounds of the experience are narrow, far narrower than you(r presuppositions allow you to) suppose. I highly doubt that his description of attending to a word followed by another word, etc., is due to any mistaken view of the task. I think Alex described word—word—word because his experience was of word—word—word. That you find that hard to believe is a characteristic (I think) of you and your presuppositions, not of Alex and/or me. I accept that that is not the usual experience of most people (probably including you), but that does not make it (as it appears that your presuppositions would say) impossible. As my mother would say, "Don't judge others by yourself."

[26]

RE [20] "I doubt that the description of an experience qualifies as such without *any* context at all."

It is really quite simple, Marco. If there is an experience of context, then a description of experience should include context. It there is *not* an experience of context, then a description of experience should *not* include context. That you think there must always be at least some context is (I think) your presupposition about the way the world is.

RE [21] "I doubt that his descriptions can be considered relevant to the study of the experience *of* reading narrative . . . but on what grounds can Alex be said to be experiencing the story, if he only perceived its words?"

I dealt with this mostly above, but it is important so I will recapitulate: If you insist that Alex tell you about his experience of *reading the story,* he will make up an account of his experience of *reading the story.* Your presuppositions will be happy, but you may well have missed the most important thing of all—that you're wildly mistaken about how reading takes place.

We've only looked at two people who have played our *Metamorphosis* game, but I have seen lots of beeps while people are reading. I'm not pulling rank here, insisting that I'm right and you're wrong and by god you'd better do it my way. I'm trying to say as clearly as I can and in as many ways as I can that presuppositions die hard; and that if experience is to make its way into science, we have to figure out how to deal with presuppositions more effectively.

January 28
Dear Russ,
Thanks a lot for your further thoughts on this. See my comments below.
All the best,
Marco

RE [22] "I think that the issue of bracketing presuppositions in an investigation of experience is more important (at this stage in the history of the universe) than is the result of that investigation of experience. That is, it is more important to discuss how to fish than to give you a fish."

[27] Well, yes, but that presupposes that your audience is already interested in fish. I doubt that this is possible without giving them at least some fish.

RE [23] "Lynn was innerly seeing a brown door, innerly seeing a bat hanging, innerly seeing a spider crawling. None of those is remotely similar to the experience of reading narrative."

If I understand you correctly here, you're saying that Lynn was not experiencing the fact that she was reading a story, but only (part of) the *content* of that story, through her mental images. I would agree with this.

There is a longstanding debate within literary studies as to whether an "immersive" style of reading similar to Lynn's is compatible with being aware that one is (only) reading a series of words on a page or screen (see Nell, 1988; Ryan, 2001, on being immersed in a story). In other words, can we be simultaneously conscious of the representational content of the story—its characters and situations—*and* of its fictional, artificial nature? Alex and Lynn seem to fall on opposite ends of this scale, since Alex seems to be aware only of the language, whereas Lynn experiences only the content of the story (through her visual imagery). I wouldn't be surprised if other readers could experience both dimensions at the same time. It would be interesting to see if this varies according to the reader's expertise. For instance, I suspect that literary scholars may be capable of attending to both linguistic form and representational content at the same time—but is this really the case? DES could help us address these questions going forward.

RE [24] "There has to be explicit room for reporting that there was no experience whatever ongoing at the moment of the beep, or that there was seemingly irrelevant-to-the-subject experience ongoing at the moment of the beep (as Lynn's arm pressure), or that there was seemingly irrelevant-to-the-investigator experience ongoing at the moment of the beep (as Alex's word—word—word)."

I completely agree that there *has* to be room for reporting experiences that are unrelated to the narrative. The question, however, is what to do with those apparently irrelevant reports (see my response to your next point).

RE [25] "Investigating phenomena is like fishing. You . . . reel in whatever you get, whether it is a reading experience or a rubber boot."

That makes a lot of sense. My further thought, however, would be that you have to decide what is relevant and what is not at some point. If you're a fisher you're not likely to be interested in boots, even if you may fish a rubber boot from time to time. I'm not saying that there is the same difference between Alex's and Lynn's reports as between a fish and a boot, of course. Looking at what happens when readers do *not* experience the story might actually be very productive. Still, I don't know how to sidestep the fact that my discipline deals mainly with experiences *of,* not with experiences *while.*

RE [26] "I accept that [Alex's] is not the usual [reading] experience of most people (probably including you), but that does not make it (as it appears that your presuppositions would say) impossible."

[31] OK, I'm ready to grant that Alex may not have had any experience of the context, and that his description is as referential as Lynn's—just much more "bounded." (I think this ties in with the question of the richness of experiences, and it may well be that there is no way to address that question because interpersonal differences are too vast.) The fact remains that I, as a literary scholar more interested in experiences *of* than in experiences *while,* wouldn't know how to use Alex's reports. They just seem to be too "boot-like" to yield any insight into people's experience of narrative. But then, I may be missing an important element right now. Maybe if I saw similar reports from other readers, I would change my mind.

At any rate I'd be curious to have Alex's (and Lynn's) impressions about the *Metamorphosis* story. For instance, I could ask them to complete a simple questionnaire about their engagement with Gregor, their emotional reactions, etc. I know that this wouldn't be standard DES, but I wonder if you (and Alex and Lynn) would agree to this. Feel free to say no, of course. I think it might be interesting to contrast the results of the DES interviews with their overall responses to the story.

IV

MARCO'S QUESTIONNAIRE AND A "BOOT-LIKE" SENTENCE

NOTE: Here Marco sends Russ a modified version of a questionnaire used by Miall and Kuiken (1995) in their psychological studies of reader-response. Russ asks Lynn and Alex to fill out the questionnaire. Their responses are shown below at January 31.

January 29
Hi Marco—
Please see below.
—Russ

RE [18] "The question . . . is whether Alex was having any conscious experience of the meaning of the words he was reading."
    A few days ago I emailed the following request to Alex:

> I'd appreciate a clarification of your reading samples. We established, as I understand it (please let me know if I am mistaken), that your experience at three beeps was of word—word—word, without any or much indirect-experience of the implications of those words; that is, little or no indirect-experience of the story (even though you were comprehending the story, but that comprehension was outside of your awareness).
> What I didn't ask was whether the words themselves ("swang," "happy," and "way") were recognized as meaningful words, or were they just chunks of experience, not experientially wordy (but of course known to be words when you and I talked about it)? Maybe the way to tease this apart is to ask whether it would have made any experiential difference if the words had been in Greek or Italian, or if the "words" had been nonsense syllables. So, for example, at the first beep, you were reading ". . . proper decision, he swang himself

with . . ." Would your experience have been the same had you been reading ". . . pwipsie durasiot, ek stolt hiftral worf . . ." ? Here, as usual, I'm asking only about your experience, not about any presumed underlying process that might be derailed by such nonsense syllables.

And if your answer is No, that is, that you somehow in direct experience recognized them to be English words, can you describe how that recognition was experienced? Did you, for example, recognize the meaning of each word, and, if so, how?

Thanks very much. As usual, any light you can shed on this would be appreciated, and "I don't know" is an OK answer.

Alex's response, arriving yesterday, is this:

[32]   I feel like I would have experienced the exact same thing as if I had been reading it in another language. Nothing was in my experience besides the words. No impression of their definition or identity as English or whatever was in my experience at the moment of the beep.

January 30
Dear Russ,
That's all very helpful, many thanks for sending on your exchange with Alex. Well, that kind of report does seem to shatter a lot of presuppositions in literary studies.
All the best,
Marco

January 31
Hi Marco—

RE [32] Alex: "I feel like I would have experienced the exact same thing as if I had been reading it in another language."

I interviewed him about exactly what he meant. The clarification is that had he been reading a sentence that said "The man went to the durasiot and bought a sandwich," he would have experienced word—word—word—word—word, etc., including the nonword "durasiot," in exactly the same way as the other actual words. Eventually his outside-of-his-awareness processor would have detected that he didn't understand "durasiot," but that would not have happened in the originally experienced stream of words.

I still have more to say about your previous email, but it will have to wait a bit.

Here's a summary of Alex's and Lynn's characterizations of their usual reading habits as reported on your questionnaire: Lynn said she had read two novels in the past year for pleasure, including Young's *The Shack*. Alex said he had read four novels in the past year including Vonnegut's *Timequake*, Lovecraft's *Bloodcurdling Tales of Horror and the Macabre*, and Saki's *Beasts and Super-Beasts*. His favorite authors are Vonnegut, Lovecraft, and Conrad Aiken.

I'm also attaching the items about reading *The Metamorphosis* from your questionnaire (see table 3).

—Russ

February 1
Dear Russ,
Please tell Alex and Lynn that I really appreciate their taking the time to complete the questionnaire.

It looks like Alex is a more experienced reader than Lynn, and there can be no doubt that he understood the story. Do you know if Alex and Lynn reread the story, or if they filled out the questionnaire on the basis of their memories of the reading task?

Judging from his answers to the questionnaire it seems that Alex did have some non-word—word—word experiences while reading the *Metamorphosis* story. He reports visualizing Gregor's body (occasionally) and feeling sympathy for him (quite often). What I would still like to ask Alex—maybe in person if we can arrange a Skype call, or maybe you can relay the question to him—is whether he thinks that his word—word—word experiences just depended on the *timing* of the beep. In other words, if he had been beeped at other points in time, would he have reported a visual image of the character, or sympathy for him? Or were those experiences interpolated after reading the story, as if Alex had realized feeling all those things only in retrospection, while his online experience of the story was consistently word—word—word?

All the best,
Marco

[33]

TABLE 3. Questionnaire items about reading *The Metamorphosis*, with Lynn's and Alex's responses

QUESTIONNAIRE ITEMS[a]	LYNN'S RESPONSES	ALEX'S RESPONSES
Please choose the answer that best describes your reaction to this story, and, where indicated, briefly describe your reaction in your own words.		
1. To what extent were you absorbed in your reading of *The Metamorphosis*? a. not at all b. a little c. somewhat d. quite a lot e. very much	e. *very much*	c. *somewhat*
Explain briefly what, if anything, you found absorbing about this story:	*The rare situation Gregor was in.*	*I liked the contrast between Gregor's indifference at becoming a giant insect and his preoccupation with the mundanities of dealing with his boss. I also was absorbed in the decay in of the relationship of Gregor with his sister and his family, it seemed to mirror the tensions that I have seen in the families of those with disabilities.*
2. Did you visualize Gregor's body? a. never b. occasionally c. fairly often d. quite often e. very often	e. *very often*	b. *occasionally*
If you can, describe how you visualized Gregor:	*I visualized Gregor as a giant spider, lots of legs, crawling, grayish color, dirty, covered in a sticky, gray, liquid substance.*	*Like a giant brownish black beetle.*
3. As you were reading, did you have any awareness of your own body? a. never b. occasionally c. fairly often d. quite often e. very often	b. *occasionally*	b. *occasionally*
If you can, describe one of the bodily experiences you've had while reading *The Metamorphosis*:	*My arm felt the pressure of me leaning on it while reading.*	*The feeling of the chair on my body, the pressure and occasional uncomfortableness.*

4. Did you feel sympathy for Gregor?
   a. never
   b. occasionally
   c. fairly often
   d. quite often
   e. very often

   If you can, describe an episode in which you felt sympathy for Gregor:

e. very often	When Gregor's sister wanted to get rid of him. I felt like his family, especially his sister whom he loved the most, betrayed him.
d. quite often	At the end most of all, when he was coming out of his room listening to his sister play violin.

5. Did you feel disgust for Gregor?
   a. never
   b. occasionally
   c. fairly often
   d. quite often
   e. very often

   If you can, describe an episode in which you felt disgust for Gregor:

a. never	
a. never	

6. As you read *The Metamorphosis*, how often did you see things from Gregor's perspective?
   a. never
   b. occasionally
   c. fairly often
   d. quite often
   e. very often

   Describe an episode in which you saw things from Gregor's perspective:

e. very often	When Gregor's mother and sister wanted to move everything out of his room. He did not want the painting of the woman gone, so he was guarding it. I felt I would have done the same thing if something was that meaningful to me and I was threatened to lose it.
e. very often	The whole story was told from his perspective, it was hard to see it from a different perspective. One episode when I saw something from Gregor's perspective is when he was trying to get out of bed.

[a] Abridged. The complete questionnaire results are on the Companion Website.

ROAD MAP: *The discrepancy between Alex's word—word—word experience while sampling and his reporting mental imagery and sympathy for Gregor in the postreading questionnaire inaugurates the discussion of differences between pristine experience and what people say about their experiences, which we called theme (c) above.*

February 2
Hi Marco—
I talked with Alex.

I asked him whether he reread *The Metamorphosis* in responding to your questionnaire. He said No. He also said he had read *The Metamorphosis* when he was a junior in high school (6?? years ago), so he had some prior familiarity with the story. He said he thought that most (80%) of the answers to your questionnaire came from his reading during the study. He said his reading during the study was entirely with comprehension.

I asked him whether he knew anything about his word—word—word experience prior to this study, and he said No, that it came as a complete surprise to him. He said he would have predicted, prior to this study, that he would have frequent visual images while reading. And of course, he said, that still might be true—we have only four samples.

I asked him whether, prior to sampling, he would have thought it possible to experience a series of words while reading. He said he would have thought it possible in general, but not for him.

RE [33] "If he had been beeped at other points in time, would he have reported a visual image of the character, or sympathy for him?"

[34] He said that he believes that he did occasionally have visual imagery and feelings while reading *The Metamorphosis* during this study. But he said it with the wry smile of someone who from his own data knows that he is not to be trusted. That question is about his pristine experience while reading, and I think we (including Alex) have established pretty convincingly that he is not to be trusted when he retrospects about his pristine experience. (He is not alone in this regard.) He didn't know that he had word—word—word; why should we believe him if he says that he did have imagery?
—Russ

P.S. I forwarded this email to Alex, saying "Please correct anything that I misrepresented." He responded, "I think that captures it nicely."

February 3
Hi Marco—
I wrote Lynn:

> Marco has one additional question for you: When you filled out the questionnaire, did you do it from memory of the original participation in the study, or did you go back to *The Metamorphosis* again to refresh your recollections?

Lynn responded:

> I did it based on what I remembered from *The Metamorphosis*. I did go back and finished reading the whole story but I did not go over what I had already read.

—Russ

February 4
Hi Marco—
Below please find my responses to your January 28 email.
—Russ

RE [27] "I doubt that this is possible without giving them at least some fish."

This is an example (actually two examples) of the catch-22 I discussed in my 2011 book: It is difficult (if not impossible) to tell someone about pristine experience until they think that pristine experience is important. But it is not possible to think that pristine experience is important until you tell them about it.

The second catch-22 is: It is difficult (if not impossible) to tell them about case studies (like Lynn/Alex) until they think that case studies are important. But it is not possible to think that case studies are important until you describe case studies. You ask for a larger study, but a (generally unacknowledged) characteristic of any large study is that the details of the individual get averaged out and therefore lost.

[35] The reason that you are impacted by our interchange (assuming that you are impacted) is that you have been forced to encounter Alex as a solitary individual who challenges your deeply held presuppositions. I'm pretty sure that a study of 10 individuals would have had less impact, and a study of 1000 individuals even less.

RE [28] "You're saying that Lynn was not experiencing the fact that she was reading a story, but only (part of) the *content* of that story, through her mental images."

Actually, I am not saying that. I agree with the part that Lynn was not experiencing the fact that she was reading a story. However, [36] I think she was also *not* experiencing the content of that story, if by "experiencing" you mean what I would call "pristinely experiencing." As she read, she innerly saw things that were related, closely or distantly or not at all, to the content of the story. That is quite different from "experiencing the content of the story through her mental images." She innerly saw a door that was open when the story content was that it was closed; she innerly saw a bat when the story content was of a bug. And so on. The best you can say, I think, is that she innerly saw *along with* the content of the story. That is, Lynn is a free agent, innerly seeing things that are to some degree inspired by the story, innerly seeing other things that are incongruent with the story, innerly seeing other things that have nothing to do with the story, and experiencing things in ways other than innerly seeing (sensory awareness, innerly speaking, etc.), all sometimes sequential, sometimes separately parallel, sometimes combined in ways that have much or little to do with the story.

RE [29] "There is a longstanding debate within literary studies as to whether an 'immersive' style of reading similar to Lynn's is compatible with being aware that one is (only) reading a series of words on a page or screen. In other words, can we be simultaneously conscious of the representational content of the story—its characters and situations—*and* of its fictional, artificial nature?"

There is a similarly longstanding debate in consciousness studies, and I think both are fueled by the same confusion, which arises out of the failure to look carefully enough at the phenomena of interest. Lynn is *not* immersed in the reading, if by "immersed" one means totally engrossed to the exclusion of all else. She innerly sees things that are more or less (but not completely) driven by the read content, so even at her most engrossed she is still not entirely engrossed. She is simultaneously processing at an intelligent (if not pristinely experienced) level hundreds or thousands of other things in the welter of her environment, inner and outer, past, present, and future. She no doubt does not have to stop her inner seeings to click the *Next page* button on the *Metamorphosis* reader, because that part of her that is keeping track of the computer and the mouse is doing so simultaneously with the inner seeing of the bed and the bat. And at the same time she is interacting in an intelligent (if not pristinely experienced) way with the pressure on the arm of her chair, the temperature in the room, the argument she had with her boyfriend last Tuesday, the dinner plans she has with her parents next Friday, and thousands or millions of other things that are reverberating around in her neurons at one level or another. Every fiber of her being knows at some level (with no cognition implied here) that she is merely reading a story—she doesn't cover her hair when she sees the bat like she would if a real bat were hanging there.

The confusion arises because pristine experience is not carefully examined. When it is, it becomes obvious (I think) that much processing is going on that is not pristinely experienced. Any other explanation of Alex's understanding of the story seems farfetched by comparison to that simple explanation.

So I think your "Alex and Lynn seem to fall on opposite ends of this scale, since Alex seems to be aware only of the language, whereas Lynn experiences only the content of the story (through her visual imagery)" is on the wrong track. Alex is *not* aware of the language; his word—word—word experience is more elemental than is usually meant by "language." "Pwipsie durasiot" does not belong to language. And Lynn is not experiencing only the content of the story—she (pristinely) experiences some combination of some things related to the content of the story and some things not. Alex and Lynn are at the same end of the scale in the sense that both have multiple (probably counted in the hundreds, millions, or more) simultaneous ways of processing the neural impulses that originate in the retina when the eyeballs are aimed at the page (and all the other neural impulses that are arising simultaneously). Both make it abundantly clear that there is intelligent processing going on outside of pristine experience. [37]

RE [30] "Still, I don't know how to sidestep the fact that my discipline deals mainly with experiences *of,* not with experiences *while.*"

[38]   No, your discipline does *not* deal with experiences *of*; it only mistakenly thinks it deals with experiences *of*. That may be worse, as far as sidestepping is concerned.

RE [31] "The fact remains that I, as a literary scholar more interested in experiences *of* than in experiences *while*, wouldn't know how to use Alex's reports. They just seem to be too 'boot-like' to yield any insight into people's experience of narrative."

[39]   FYI, I showed our entire conversation to Alex, and this "boot-like" sentence is the one to which he had the strongest reaction, something like: *I am a reader. I read with comprehension. I understand and react to the story and its characters. You can't dismiss me merely because my experience doesn't align with your presuppositions.*

I agree with Alex. But it is a typical strategy that presuppositions use in their battle against annihilation: When a fact that threatens the presupposition presents itself, the presupposition says, "It's irrelevant," or "I'd need to see more reports like that." (Here again, I'm giving presuppositions a life of their own; I mean that as a literary device, not an ontological claim.) Whatever their ontological status, presuppositions don't give up without a fight to the death.
—Russ

February 5
Dear Russ,
Thanks a lot for your comments. See my responses below.
All the best,
Marco

RE [34] "I think we (including Alex) have established pretty convincingly that he is not to be trusted when he retrospects about his pristine experience. (He is not alone in this regard.) He didn't know that he had word—word—word; why should we believe him if he says that he did have imagery?"

Actually, I think this highlights the differences between the aims of a "literary" study of the reading experience and your own work. The fact is that most literary scholars, including me, are only slightly worried about the problem of the fidelity of people's reports. Perhaps you will say that we should be *more* worried—and I can see the point of that reply. But keep in mind that the standards of fidelity are likely to be very different for a psychologist interested in pristine experience and for a literary scholar who deals with larger experiential dynamics such as empathy for characters or the emotions elicited by reading fiction. Exploring these topics *only* through the DES method seems unfeasible to me, because of the divide between the relatively small slices of experience that can be sampled through DES and the broad experiential patterns literary scholars tend to focus on. (This doesn't mean that DES cannot be used to complement other methods of literary investigation, of course.) I wouldn't know how to study these larger phenomena without retrospection. And this also explains why the standards of literary theorists and scholars when it comes to assessing the reliability of readers' reports are less rigorous than yours. We *have* to trust people's descriptions of their experiences; otherwise the study of reader response would never get off the ground.

[40]

[41]

Surely, from your perspective this must sound like a messy business. But really, it all depends on the aims of your project. You have a professional interest in getting the details of people's experiences right, but I'm sure that when a friend of yours tells you "I felt so happy yesterday," you don't cast into doubt his words (other things being equal) only because they are based on retrospection. Studies of reader response are probably closer to this more casual way of dealing with others' experiences—they don't need completely reliable data, only reasonably reliable data.

Further, another thing to take into account is that for the average literary scholar, what people do with stories *after* they've finished reading them matters more than what happens *while* they read them. Discussing, analyzing, interpreting stories—all are of key importance to the literary scholar. Take, for instance, Alex's judgment that the "decay in the relationship of Gregor with his sister and his family ... seemed to mirror the tensions that I have seen in the families of those with disabilities." This is an extremely interesting interpretation of *The Metamorphosis* in my view, one that—to my knowledge—hasn't been offered before. But it's hard to think that Alex formed this judgment while he was reading Kafka's story (although we can't rule out this possibility, of course); it's much more likely that Alex arrived at this idea while reflecting on the story *after* reading it. Still, Alex's judgment is a way of thinking about— and therefore, in some sense of the word, experiencing—*The Metamorphosis*. It deserves attention in its own right, regardless of whether it was formed during or after reading the novella. This is not to say that pristine experience doesn't matter. It does matter, at least to me. But it's important to remember that literary scholars (including me) are likely to

[42]

be also interested in dimensions of people's engagement with literature that can be captured *only* through retrospection and post-hoc reflection on stories.

RE [39] "I showed our entire conversation to Alex, and this 'boot-like' sentence is the one to which he had the strongest reaction."

Alex's reaction to my comment is quite understandable. I obviously shouldn't have said this—at least, not in that way. Of course he comprehends the story and reacts to its characters, but since all of that seems to happen in an unconscious way (at least judging from the four beeps we have), there is no reason to include it in an investigation of the *experience* of reading literature. As for the experiences that he did have, again the problem is that there is no way to distinguish those experiences from experiences he could have had while reading an essay, a newspaper, or even a street sign. It's not they are completely irrelevant to literary studies—but they don't seem to be specific or distinctive enough to tell us something about the way in which the phenomenology of reading literary texts differs from the phenomenology of reading in general.

RE [35] "The reason that you are impacted by our interchange (assuming that you are impacted) is that you have been forced to encounter Alex as a solitary individual who challenges your deeply held presuppositions."

Literary theorist Norman Holland provided a detailed (and mostly idiographic) description of the reading experiences of five readers in *5 Readers Reading* (1975). The method is very different from DES, but Holland can still serve as a precedent for this kind of study.

RE [36] "I think [Lynn] was also *not* experiencing the content of that story, if by 'experiencing' you mean what I would call 'pristinely experiencing.' As she read, she innerly saw things that were related, closely or distantly or not at all, to the content of the story. That is quite different from 'experiencing the content of the story through her mental images.'"

I see what you mean here, but I think the divergence between us is merely terminological. There is no way to experience the content of a story *as such* because that content is always filtered through the reader's mind. It has no independent existence (unless as a series of words on a page/screen perhaps, but that's not the "content of a story" in my view—it is just a series of words on a page/screen). Therefore, when I say that Lynn is "experiencing the content of the story through her mental images," I am actually saying something along the lines of your "seeing things that are related, closely or distantly or not at all, to the content of the story."

RE [37] "Alex and Lynn are at the same end of the scale in the sense that both have multiple (probably counted in the hundreds, millions, or more) simultaneous ways of processing the neural impulses that originate in the retina when the eyeballs are aimed at the page (and all the other neural impulses that are arising simultaneously). Both make it abundantly clear that there is intelligent processing going on outside of pristine experience."

I agree that Lynn and Alex are both unconsciously processing (and comprehending) the story. But I can still see a difference between them: Lynn is experiencing "some combination of some things related to the content of the story," while Alex is not. Whether what he is experiencing is language or something "more elemental than language itself" is an interesting question (and I think you may be right), but either way the difference between Lynn and Alex still seems highly significant to me. [45]

RE [38] "No, your discipline does *not* deal with experiences *of*; it only mistakenly thinks it deals with experiences *of*."

As I pointed out at RE 25, I think my discipline does deal with experiences of. Except that those experiences are not at all "pristine," in your term: on the contrary, they are heavily influenced by post-hoc reflections, interpretations, judgments, presuppositions. They are still in an important sense experiences of (they are intentionally directed at the story), but they do not comply with your standards of fidelity and absence of presuppositions. [46]

V

CONTRASTING BROAD EXPERIENCE AND PRISTINE EXPERIENCE, WITH AMSTERDAM AS AN EXAMPLE

February 6
Hi Marco—
I still think these issues are at the center of both of our disciplines.
    Please see below.
—Russ

RE [41] "We *have* to trust people's descriptions of their experiences; otherwise the study of reader response would never get off the ground."

[47]   The word "experience," as you know, is tricky because it means different things in different contexts. In particular, sometimes it means what I call pristine experience—something actually directly before the footlights of consciousness at some moment. I think that meaning of "experience" is pretty definite—there is some gray at the edges about what is and what is not pristine experience, but for the most part the distinction between pristine experience and all else can be made with (good but not perfect) reliability. But at other times the meaning of "experience" is far less specified, as when you write "Alex's judgment is a way of thinking about—and therefore, in some sense of the word, experiencing—*The Metamorphosis*." So it makes reasonable sense, in the less-specified kind of way, for a tourist to say to her companion, "I really enjoyed the experience of Amsterdam," or for a literary theorist to say to his colleague, "The experience of reading *Anna Karenina* is different from the experience of reading *The Metamorphosis* or of reading *The Adventures of Tom Sawyer*." I accept that there can be a bit of truth to such statements.

However, the less-specific use of "experience"—let's call it "broad experience"—has at least two important perils. The first is that it fails to distinguish between the pristine and the less-specified uses of the term "experience" and thence to presume that the tourist's use of (the less-specific) unspecified "experience" implies something about pristine experiences while in Amsterdam. I think our *Metamorphosis* ministudy (and the rest of my work) demonstrates that that is simply not true, even though it is widely presumed to be true or thoughtlessly acted upon as if it were true.

The second peril is to presume that (the less-specific) term "experience" refers to something that is well and uniformly grasped. I think that is usually far from true. When the typical tourist says, "I really enjoyed the experience of Amsterdam," and her companion says "I did too," they usually uncritically believe that they are talking about the same experience. But it is usually not true. The tourist refers primarily to the freedom to smoke dope in public without fear; the companion refers primarily to the number of museums. Much everyday conversation is based on the mistaken presumption that I know what you mean and you know what I mean.

I think both perils apply to our reading situation.

ROAD MAP: *Our discussion of the status of experiences in the broad sense vis-à-vis pristine experience (theme a) starts with Russ's remarks here.*

RE [46] "My discipline does deal with experiences of. Except that those experiences are not at all 'pristine,' in your term: on the contrary, they are heavily influenced by post-hoc reflections, interpretations, judgments, presuppositions. They are still in an important sense experiences of (they are intentionally directed at the story), but they do not comply with your standards of fidelity and absence of presuppositions."

I think you risk the second peril. I said above that I preferred "experience while" to "experience of," and now I will expand that logic to say that regardless of whether it is contrasted with "while," I think "experience of" is a dangerous term. As a general principle I don't really care much about what terms one uses as long as one keeps importantly different things distinct, but "experience" is sufficiently problematic that I think some terminological consideration is required. To say "the experience of Amsterdam" connotes misleadingly that there is something like an essence of Amsterdam that gets transmitted to the tourist, whereas I think that Amsterdam is a collection of a large number of mostly diverse things (coffee shops, canals, red-light district, architecture, the Dutch people, the distinction between the northern and the southern people, etc.). The Amsterdam of one visitor can be dramatically different from the Amsterdam of another. Furthermore, "experience of" connotes that this experiencing is a one-way affair, originating with Amsterdam and received by the experiencer. I don't think that is true. The tourist's interactions with Amsterdam are substantially reflective of the tourist, as well as reflective of Amsterdam. It is very difficult to use "experience of" and reflect this two-way-ness: perhaps one must say "I had the experience of that very small slice of Amsterdam that my proclivities and desires and fears led me to procure for myself, and not of the remainder of Amsterdam that others might experience," or something like that.

[48] So I might suggest that your phrase "engagement with" (as in "literary scholars (including me) are likely to be also interested in dimensions of people's engagement with literature that can be captured *only* through retrospection and post-hoc reflection on stories") is less problematic than "experience of." "Engagement with" is desirable because it does not connote an essence—I can be engaged with something that I know very little about, and I can be engaged with some perhaps minor aspect of something. And it hints at the bi-directionality of the process: "with" suggests an interaction between; "of" suggests a unidirectional introjection.

Thus to say "the engagement with Amsterdam" connotes informatively that the tourist herself had some impact on her tourist/Amsterdam interaction—one tourist (on the basis of her proclivities) visits the coffee shops, another focuses on the canals, another on the red-light district, another on the architecture, another on the people, etc.

So it seems preferable to me for a literary theorist to say to his colleague, "My engagement with *Anna Karenina* is different from my engagement with *The Metamorphosis* or with *The Adventures of Tom Sawyer*."

RE [44] "I think the divergence between us is merely terminological. There is no way to experience the content of a story *as such* because that content is always filtered through the reader's mind. It has no independent existence (unless as a series of words on a page/screen perhaps, but that's not the 'content of a story' in my view—it is just a series of words on a page/screen)."

I agree; that's part of the logic behind my suggestion of "engagement with." The literary community may well have already argued this and agreed on a terminology; as I say, I don't really care what terminology we use as long as we don't fall into the traps that "experience of" sets for us.

RE [40] "Exploring these topics *only* through the DES method seems unfeasible to me."

I agree. DES is a tool, and like all tools, is useful only in its range of convenience. I do think it likely that DES would be a useful tool in understanding the ways in which readers engage with texts.

RE [42] "Discussing, analyzing, interpreting stories—all are of key importance to the literary scholar. . . . Literary scholars (including me) are likely to be also interested in dimensions of people's engagement with literature that can be captured *only* through retrospection and post-hoc reflection on stories."

I have no objection to discussing, analyzing, or interpreting. I suspect that the best stories are those that can be discussed, analyzed, and interpreted in many different ways (further evidence for "engagement with" rather than "experience of").

RE [43] "There is no way to distinguish those experiences from experiences he could have had while reading an essay, a newspaper, or even a street sign . . . they don't seem to be specific or distinctive enough to tell us something about the way in which the phenomenology of reading literary texts differs from the phenomenology of reading in general."

The word "phenomenology," like "experience," is fraught with peril because of its usual less-specific nature and the shared but often incorrect view that what you mean by phenomenology is the same as what your reader means. For example: Are Lynn's four beeps examples of the phenomenology of reading literary texts? Are Alex's? In what way is the phenomenology of reading different from the experience of reading? Is discussing, analyzing, and interpreting stories part of the phenomenology of reading literary texts? Is the examining of the literary texts in preparation for the discussing, analyzing,

[49]

58 • CHAPTER V

and interpreting stories part of the phenomenology of reading literary texts? And so on. I suspect there is not universal agreement about the answers to those questions among literary scholars.

RE [45] "Either way the difference between Lynn and Alex still seems highly significant to me."

I agree, but for me it is too soon to tell what that significance is. Much more research with many more subjects (and investigators!) is necessary. Perhaps it will be discovered that the pristine experience while reading is of no significance—it is epiphenomenal. Perhaps it will be discovered that Alex and Lynn are examples of the range of differences in the mechanics of reading across people, and if so, then that might lead to the recognition of differences in the development of the reading skill, and if so, then there may be differences in the ways people might be helped to learn to read. That might not be of particular interest to a literary scholar, but reading is a highly important skill and if we happened upon something that led to the improvement of its acquisition, that would be a big deal. Perhaps it will be discovered that exploring the pristine experiences while reading can shed some light on the way literary texts are apprehended (and the individual differences thereabouts). I don't know. All are worth knowing.

February 7
Dear Russ,
See my comments below.
Marco

RE [47] "The word 'experience,' as you know, is tricky because it means different things in different contexts. In particular, sometimes it means what I call pristine experience—something actually directly before the footlights of consciousness at some moment. . . . But at other times the meaning of 'experience' is far less specified."

[50] I completely agree that the term "experience" in the broad sense is more problematic than experience in the sense of pristine experience. I am aware of both of the dangers that you highlight above, and one of the reasons why I admire your work is that it insightfully exposes the limitations and pitfalls of the commonsensical understanding of "experience." However, I also think that when people refer to reading *The Metamorphosis* or visiting Amsterdam as an experience, they are not wrong

or misguided. There is something irreducibly experiential about these activities, something that cannot be broken down into a series of distinct moments, something that makes sense as a whole because it is intertwined with people's reflections and emotions and memories in a specific—and perhaps unique—way.

I think these processes are well worth investigating. But again the key lies, in my view, in not essentializing the experience of a Kafka story (or of Amsterdam). The tourists may believe that they're talking about the same thing for the first three minutes of their conversation, but as soon as they start discussing the reasons for their enjoying Amsterdam, they're likely to realize that they've had quite different experiences. The same applies to the experience of reading *The Metamorphosis*. As soon as we ask readers to talk about their experience, the differences between them become evident. Thus, the second peril can be solved by going beyond appearances and inviting people to describe their experiences. As for the first, I agree that it's important to distinguish between pristine experience and experiences in the broad sense, but I also think that we should try to do justice to both of them. In order to do so, we should develop tools for exploring the diversity—as well as the structural similarities (more on this soon)—of people's experiences in the broad sense.

RE [48] "So I might suggest that your phrase 'engagement with' (as in 'literary scholars (including me) are likely to be also interested in dimensions of people's engagement with literature that can be captured *only* through retrospection and post-hoc reflection on stories') is less problematic than 'experience of.'"

I think you're right about the versatility of the phrase "engagement with," and yet I wouldn't draw such a sharp distinction between "engagement with" and "experience of." In my view the problem has to do with a certain generalizing *use* of these phrases rather than with the phrases themselves. If I say "the reader's engagement with Kafka's story," I may be collapsing differences between readers in the same way as "the experience of Kafka's story" does. The issue is not so much with terminology as with the speaker's awareness that experience is a bi-directional process that involves both "reality" and the experiencer's predispositions and interests.

[51]

[52]

RE [49] "Is discussing, analyzing, and interpreting stories part of the phenomenology of reading literary texts? Is the examining of the literary texts in preparation for the discussing, analyzing, and interpreting stories part of the phenomenology of reading literary texts?. . . . I suspect there is not universal agreement about the answers to those questions among literary scholars."

My take on this is that phenomenology is an investigation into the structures of experience more than a description of its contents. Talk about "the phenomenology of reading (narrative)" is therefore both more abstract and more general than the description of particular experiences that can be had while reading (narrative). People's experiences are widely diverse in terms of contents, but they share some underlying structures. Intentionality in the philosophical sense of "being directed toward an object" is one of these. Further examples of experiential structures are what Kevin O'Regan and Alva Noë (see O'Regan and Noë, 2001; O'Regan, Myin, and Noë, 2005) call "corporality" and "alerting capacity" in their enactivist theory of perception.

I believe these structures or patterns are extremely important in readers' interaction with literature, too. Both Lynn and Alex, for example, seem to engage in some sort of perspective-taking—they adopt Gregor's point of view on the world. But this structural resemblance surfaces in the questionnaire, not in the DES reports, because it involves a large experiential dynamic rather than a small slice (however referentially described) of readers' engagement with the text. Of course, it may be possible to identify recurring structures through DES, too. Yet I have the sense that setting DES reports in a broader context (possibly in the context of an experience in the broad sense) may help us with this.

February 8
Hi Marco—

RE [50] "However, I also think that when people refer to reading *The Metamorphosis* or visiting Amsterdam as an experience, they are not wrong or misguided. There is something irreducibly experiential about these activities."

I agree. However, the question is not whether there is experience, but whether it makes sense to say that the experience is *of Amsterdam* (or *of* The Metamorphosis).

RE [52] "The issue is not so much with terminology as with the speaker's awareness that experience is a bi-directional process."

I agree—that's what I meant when I said "As a general principle I don't really care much about what terms one uses as long as one keeps importantly different things distinct."

RE [52] "Experience is a bi-directional process that involves both 'reality' and the experiencer's predispositions and interests."

This is what I understand you to be saying here: that the Kafka story (or Amsterdam) is the "reality," about which one reader (or tourist), because of her predispositions and interests, has one experience and another reader, because of different predispositions and interests, has a different experience. Is that what you mean? If so, then I think that essentializes the Kafka story (or Amsterdam) and implies that there is an essential reality of the Kafka story (Amsterdam) that is separate from the reader (tourist). I think that there is not such an essential reality. It seems to me that supposing the existence of such an essentiality is the enemy of experience, whether pristine or otherwise. It is perhaps easier to see with Amsterdam. The two tourists do *not* each bi-directionally interact with Amsterdam per se. One sees the inside of coffeehouses, the other the inside of museums. They do not interact with the same reality (Amsterdam) but with different predispositions. Each tourist has experiences, to be sure; those experiences physically take place within the Amsterdam city limits; those experiences reflect some characteristic that is found more in Amsterdam than in most elsewheres; those experiences are usually uncritically called "experiences of Amsterdam"; the tourists who spend more than three minutes talking with each other will discover that they've had quite different experiences of quite different things, but they are likely to continue to call those two different things "Amsterdam" and to believe that they are referring to the same essence-of-Amsterdam. But I don't think that bears careful scrutiny. I think that the more carefully one looks, the more confident one becomes that there is no essential Amsterdam of which one tourist has one experience and another tourist has a different experience. Instead, there are lots of essentially different things/experiences to which the grunt "Amsterdam" can be applied.

I think the same applies (although somewhat hiddenly) to *The Metamorphosis*. This does not in any way diminish the importance of discussion of literary themes or reactions or significances. It suggests that assuming that there is an essential reality of *The Metamorphosis* is likely to be a distraction.

[53]

RE [51] "I wouldn't draw such a sharp distinction between 'engagement with' and 'experience of.' In my view the problem has to do with a certain generalizing *use* of these phrases rather than with the phrases themselves."

I agree there is no sharp distinction, and I didn't intend one. What I was trying to say was that I think "experience of" leans toward essentializing in a way that "engagement with" does not. For example, saying "the experience of Amsterdam" tends to lead one to presume that there is an essential Amsterdam (or the "Amsterdam of reality"), whereas saying "engagement with Amsterdam" has less of that tendency. I think that avoiding the essentializing tendency is in general a good thing, and because the essentializing tendency is ubiquitous, insidious, invisible, and taken for granted, anything that aids that avoidance is a good thing.
—Russ

February 9
Dear Russ,
See my response to one of your comments below.
All the best,
Marco

RE [53] "I think the same applies (although somewhat hiddenly) to *The Metamorphosis*. This does not in any way diminish the importance of discussion of literary themes or reactions or significances. It suggests that assuming that there is an essential reality of *The Metamorphosis* is likely to be a distraction."

Part of the problem with "the experience of Amsterdam" may lie in "Amsterdam," which is actually a collection of relatively heterogeneous things, places, situations—and therefore experiences to be had. If you replace "Amsterdam" with something more spatio-temporally bounded (like "*The Metamorphosis*"), then the phrase starts making sense. You're still likely to find a diversity of responses (and therefore of experiences), but I believe that these experiences will have more in common than people's "experiences of Amsterdam." Why is that? Because *The Metamorphosis* is a semiotic artifact that has been constructed by a person in order to tell a story about a traveling salesman who suddenly turns into an insect, etc. In other words, readers' engagement with *The Metamorphosis* will be much more guided than will be their engagement with the countless things, places, and situations that make up Amsterdam. Kafka did write some things and not others, talking about one character and not another, doing so in specific ways and not others, etc. We can discuss all of these things, and reach an agreement on some of them. Saying that there is an "essence" to Kafka's story is going too far, of course, and I agree with you that this kind of talk is misleading and even dangerous. But I do think that our engagement with *The Metamorphosis* is related or intentionally directed to something "out there," which has a certain structure and properties—which in turn influence our engagement in important ways (see again Caracciolo, 2012).

February 10
Hi Marco—
I think we are approaching a core issue; if we can get straight about it, we will have accomplished something.

I accept that Amsterdam is more heterogeneous than is *The Metamorphosis*. So I think it is possible, even likely, that the experiences of two randomly selected people while reading *The Metamorphosis* will be more homogeneous than will be the experiences of two randomly selected people who are visiting Amsterdam. I further accept that because Kafka did write some things and not others, it is more likely that a reader of *The Metamorphosis* will be experiencing an insect or a violin than a raft on the Mississippi River or women's role in 19th-century Saint Petersburg.

However, I also think it possible, even likely, that *The Metamorphosis* as an experiential occasion is more heterogeneous than you give credit. That is, I think it possible, even likely, that the literary scholar's way of proceeding (discussion, analysis, comparison, etc.) gives an impression of more homogeneity than actually exists. [55]

RE [54] "*The Metamorphosis* is a semiotic artifact that has been constructed by a person in order to tell a story about a traveling salesman who suddenly turns into an insect, etc."

I accept that *The Metamorphosis is* a story about a traveling salesman who suddenly turns into an insect. But whether it *was constructed to tell* that story is not at all obvious. Perhaps it was constructed to shed light on the stresses of families with disabilities (and the salesman-ness and insect-ness of the story are incidental details). Perhaps it was constructed to <option C>. Perhaps it was constructed to <option D>. I [56] presume that a literary scholar could advance coherent arguments for any of these constructive options, citing relevant passages of the text, noting the occurrence of certain words and the absence of certain other words, and so on. Those arguments will all be bound to *the text*, that is, to something out there, and they will point to some structural properties of the text that are understood to advance the argument. All the while they radically turn away from whatever real experiences actually take place while reading the text or while discussing the text or while analyzing the structural properties of the text. That is, they radically turn away from experience, even though they claim to be interested in experience.

[57]

I accept that it is possible, perhaps even likely, that the DES way of proceeding (exposing pristine experience) gives an impression of *less* homogeneity than actually exists. The DES virtue is that it is aimed directly at actual experience as it is undergone by real people at real times. So one might say it radically turns toward experience and away from the text itself.

My prediction: If we examined a variety of readers in the DES way, you would come to a more heterogeneous view of passages that you now accept as homogenous. An essential part of the DES art is to be genuinely open to that possibility: to the extent that you are convinced that a particular passage has only one (or a few) legitimate understanding/experience, you will be deaf to any alternative.

[58]

Can a literary scholar discover something important about *The Metamorphosis* in the DES way? I don't know. That's what we're trying to find out, and that will require substantially more people reading and faithfully describing their experiences while doing so. Were I a betting man, I would bet yes.

—Russ

February 11
Dear Russ,
These are key issues indeed. See my responses to your comments.
All the best,
Marco

RE [55] "I think it possible, even likely, that the literary scholar's way of proceeding (discussion, analysis, comparison, etc.) gives an impression of more homogeneity than actually exists."

I agree with you that this is possible, even likely, and it's part of the reason why I became interested in DES in the first place.

RE [56] "I accept that *The Metamorphosis is* a story about a traveling salesman who suddenly turns into an insect. But whether it *was constructed to tell* that story is not at all obvious."

Note that whether readers and scholars can attribute intentions to authors is a very old question in literary studies. Already in the 1940s the so-called New Critics condemned this "intentional fallacy" (as they dubbed it), arguing that it is neither legitimate nor desirable to judge literary texts on the basis of their authors' intentions. The debate goes on, and the intentionalist position has gained some ground recently (see Herman, 2008; Abbott, 2011). I'm largely sympathetic with this revival of intentionalism.

Suffice it to say here that it is one thing to attribute complex intentions, which reflect a particular interpretation of the story ("*The Metamorphosis* was constructed to shed light on the stresses of families with disabilities"). It is another thing to argue that Kafka's novella was written to tell a story about a traveling salesman. The latter attribution of intention is much more elementary but also, I believe, much more widely shared among readers. We don't treat stories as if they were "found," natural objects. We treat them as if they were intentionally constructed by a human being in order to call our attention to some characters, action sequences, and so on. Call this a primary intention, because it is cognitively much more basic and bound up with the action itself of telling a story. There might be secondary authorial intentions (say, about the effects of a story or the meanings it is supposed to generate), but I agree with you that it can be difficult to reach a consensus about these. And even if it is possible to discover the author's original intentions (in the secondary sense), it might just be more productive to disregard them and strike out in other directions through our own interpretations.

RE [57] "[Literary scholars] radically turn away from whatever real experiences actually take place while reading the text or while discussing the text or while analyzing the structural properties of the text. That is, they radically turn away from experience, even though they claim to be interested in experience."

I think you're right that these arguments turn away from pristine experience, or from "whatever real experiences actually take place while reading the text." But I'm not sure that these interpretations turn away

[59]

[60]

from the experiences that take place "while discussing the text or while analyzing the structural properties of the text." This offline engagement with literary stories is still, in my view, experiential in an important sense. Further, pristine experience and offline discussions might be connected. In my view, it is possible, even likely, that some kinds of reading experiences result in or otherwise affect people's discussions of and arguments about literature. I am specifically interested in correlations between these two dimensions, and I think DES is invaluable because it helps us zoom in on reading experiences in unprecedented ways.

RE [58] "Can a literary scholar discover something important about *The Metamorphosis* in the DES way? I don't know; . . . [but were] I a betting man, I would bet yes."

And so would I.

February 12
Hi Marco—

RE [59] "Whether readers and scholars can attribute intentions to authors is a very old question in literary studies."

I didn't intend to enter that debate. I would observe (1) that Alex was hugely mistaken in his prior-to-sampling grasp of his own (reading) experience; our DES work leads me to conclude that Alex's mistakenness is by no means the exception. So I think it prudent to begin with the premise that people don't or at least may not know their own experience, and if they don't or may not know their own experience, they may well not know their own intentions. I have no reason to believe that novelists are exempt. Whether readers and scholars can attribute intentions to authors seems like a more difficult question than whether *authors* can attribute intentions to *themselves*.

And (2) I can see no way of determining the truth of a claim about an author's intention, whether that claim is made by the author or a reader.

Life is short; I for one cannot see the utility in worrying about a question to which perhaps no one can know the answer, and even if they did, we can't be confident about it. That is exactly the logic that led me to focus on pristine experience, which I think is pretty darn knowable by the subject and ascertainable by the investigator.

RE [60] "But I'm not sure that these interpretations turn away from the experiences that take place 'while discussing the text or while analyzing the structural properties of the text.' This offline engagement with literary stories is still, in my view, experiential in an important sense."

I think we may make headway on this question only by examining some concrete examples of discussion/analysis. If you would like to send me an example or two of offline engagement that is experiential, I'd be happy to look at it. (By the way, you may recognize the interest in concrete examples as being another example of a congruence between our conversation and DES.)

—Russ

VI

IN WHICH MARCO SENDS RUSS HIS PAPER ON THE EXPERIENCE OF READING McCARTHY'S *THE ROAD*; RUSS HESITATES BUT THEN CRITIQUES IT

February 13
Dear Russ,
I think you're perfectly right that it is impossible to verify the reader's attributions of intentions to an author, or even an author's attributions of intentions to him- or herself. But this is not one of the commitments of the intentionalist view of narrative. Rather, this should be seen as a descriptive claim: people tend to make attributions of intentions when they discuss a text (as in "Kafka wanted to do x") regardless of whether their attributions can be proven right or wrong.

I think that the best thing is to send you a manuscript of mine ("Narrative Space and Readers' Responses to Stories: A Phenomenological Account"[1]) where I discuss readers' responses to the representation of space and landscape in Cormac McCarthy's novel *The Road* (see the accompanying box). I do so by analyzing a corpus of online reviews of this novel. Writing reviews is an example of readers' offline engagement with literature. Yet I argue that even this mode of engagement is experiential, because it brings into play issues that are emotionally and evaluatively salient for the reviewers. See section 4, in particular the subsection titled "Thematic Evaluations," and section 5. I have the sense that you may disagree with this use of the term "experiential"—or consider it too broad to be productive—but I'd be very interested in your feedback.
All the best,
Marco

---

1. Later revised and published as Caracciolo, 2013a.

EXCERPTS FROM MARCO'S THE ROAD PAPER
1. INTRODUCTION
My article explores how the mental imagery evoked by spatial descriptions can become bound up with emotional responses and with judgments about the thematic (ethical, social, aesthetic) relevance of a text. I choose narrative space as the lens through which to study readers' engagement with literature for two reasons. First, since spatial references in narrative have a strong perceptual component, they are likely to produce visual—or more generally sensory—imagery, which makes it easier for the analyst to explore the interrelation between mental images and other responses to stories. Second, narrative space remains relatively under-theorized in narrative theory and related disciplines, and I would like to advance our understanding of this domain of storytelling by developing a phenomenological account centered on the concepts—derived from human geography—of "meaning-making" and "sense of place." Indeed, as a philosophical framework, phenomenology is in a unique position to capture the complexity of the interactions between different aspects of the reading experience. I will argue for the continuity between two aspects of readers' engagement with narrative literature that are often construed as distinct and mutually impervious: their experiential responses (mental imagery, sense of physical immersion, emotional reactions) and higher-order meaning formations such as thematic interpretations.

. . .

4. ZOOMING IN ON THE CORPUS

. . .

VISUAL IMAGERY
The landscape of The Road seems to have such a stark visual quality that it becomes difficult for some readers not to visualize it. One reviewer writes: "From the moment I picked it up, I couldn't put it down and even when I did, the bleak landscape that McCarthy paints for us so eloquently would not leave my mind" (Angry Warrior, 2008). Many readers attempt to capture the visual "feel" of the setting through the metaphor of the novelist as painter: in the corpus, the words "painting," "paint," and "picture" are used in this sense 215 times. For instance, a reader states

that McCarthy's "use of the language paints detailed pictures, albeit gray bleak ones" (Akhenatonio, 2009). This parallel between literary description and painting has a long pedigree, dating back to Horace's "ut pictura poesis," and has been extensively discussed in 20th-century literary theory (see Mitchell, 1994, chap. 3). But what is it that gives this pictorial quality to the storyworld? Partly, this is due to the repetitive nature of McCarthy's spatial descriptions: since the landscapes seen by the man and the boy in their peregrinations are all monotonously alike, it becomes increasingly easy for readers to visualize them as they read further in the text.

The uniform grayness and colorlessness of the landscape also seem to be responsible for its visual impact. These features are explicitly thematized by the novel from the very first page, where the motif of the discoloration of the storyworld is introduced: "Nights dark beyond darkness and the days more gray each one than what has gone before. Like the onset of some cold glaucoma dimming away the world" (McCarthy, 2006, 1). Many readers remark on the pervasiveness of the adjective "gray." "I think the word 'gray' is mentioned hundreds of times, because that is the one word that can now describe the entire world," one reader (Craig, 2006) writes. Responding to complaints about the excessive use of this adjective, another reviewer remarks: "I didn't necessarily mind it. It actually aided in reminding you of the dread and gloom that consumed the world, things like snow were presently gray and the ocean black" (Black Brain, 2011). As this statement shows, the visual "feel" of the storyworld is closely bound up with its emotional connotations—a point that I will develop in the next section. Another interesting finding is that the colorlessness of the storyworld reflects itself in the mental imagery of some readers, who report imagining the novel in black and white: "The book is written in language almost like watching black and white TV which adds to the setting" (Lutz, 2007).

We can take the word "vivid" as a rough indicator of the pictorial quality of McCarthy's novel. 71 readers use this adjective in their reviews. Its occurrences fall into three groups: in group a (32 occurrences), "vivid" refers to the spatial dimension of the storyworld; in group b (32 occurrences), it describes either the story as a whole, or its characters, scenes, and themes; finally, in group c (7 occurrences) it is used to characterize McCarthy's style. Out of the 71 readers that use the word "vivid," 24 explicitly mention the visual imagery they experienced while or after reading the novel. Most of these references to visual imagery fall into group a (19 occurrences), whereas 5 belong to group b.

The correlation between vivid visual imagery and the spatial dimension of the novel is hardly surprising, of course, since spatial descriptions are the most visually rich passages in a narrative text (see Esrock, 2005). As one reader colorfully puts it, "McCarthy's representation of the setting is so vivid that the images are burned into your brain right off the bat" (maya j, 2007).

February 14
Hi Marco—
Thanks for sending me "Narrative Space and Readers' Responses to Stories." I don't really have too much to say about this other than it highlights why I am not a literary scholar—I personally feel the need for purer data, data whose provenance I understand. I'm not sure that is possible in literary scholarship.

I suppose that "it highlights why I am not a literary scholar" might sound glib, but I do not mean it that way. It also highlights why I am not an orthodox psychologist, and that has been a long daily struggle of one kind or another.
—Russ

February 15
Dear Russ,
I completely understand. There is a large gap between your work on experience and the way in which literary scholars (myself included) talk about reading experiences, and I can see why the latter project may seem messy and ungrounded to you.

Actually, I agree with you about these shortcomings—it's just that I don't have any other way to talk about the kinds of phenomena I want to talk about. Realizing this may be part of the reason why interdisciplinary dialogue is important. On a more pragmatic level, DES may help us overcome at least some of the problems with theorizations of experience in literary studies.
All the best,
Marco

February 18
Hi Marco—

RE [61] "It's just that I don't have any other way to talk about the kinds of phenomena I want to talk about."

DES itself grew out of the same kind of problematic, except within psychology rather than literary scholarship. I wanted to talk about what I thought was important (experience) at a time (the 1970s) when psychology was either behavioral (in which case one could not talk about experience at all) or humanistic (which loved to talk about experience but did so in a way I found messy and ungrounded). DES was my solution. There may be other, better solutions. DES may not be an adequate solution (the jury is still out) either for psychology or for literary scholarship.

I spent last night continuing to try to work through whether I have been too cavalier/reticent in my (lack of) response to your *The Road* paper. I still have not really explicitly said what I thought of your paper, other than my almost-glib response. I could rationalize that failure-to-mention as an act of kindness—Russ, magnanimous person that he is, doesn't wish to make Marco's life difficult. But I could also see my almost-glib response as avoidance—Russ, insecure person that he is, doesn't wish to expose his view to attack; or condescension—Russ, strong person that he is, wishes to protect the much weaker Marco from the force of his opinion.

So I will be more forthcoming, and you can feel free to take or leave what I say.

This is the opening sentence of your paper:

> My article explores how the mental imagery evoked by spatial descriptions can become bound up with emotional responses and with judgments about the thematic (ethical, social, aesthetic) relevance of a text.

I think, rightly or wrongly, your article does nothing of the sort. I think it does not explore mental imagery. I think that the mental imagery that is evoked by (for example) *The Road* is not (or at least not necessarily or not completely) particularly evoked by the spatial descriptions. I think your article does not explore how mental imagery is bound up with emotional responses. I think your article does not explore how mental imagery is bound up with judgments about the thematic relevance of a text.

In your defense, I have similar reactions to reading the opening lines of many, probably most, papers that seek to explore experience. I think, rightly or wrongly (from here on, I will, out of a prosaic sensibility, omit the repetitive expression "rightly or wrongly," which, I hope you will understand, should be felt as a pedal tone of every phrase), that opening lines are often more aspirational than introductory. That is, I think your opening lines would be more accurate if they said:

> I wish my article were exploring how the mental imagery evoked by spatial descriptions can become bound up with emotional responses and with judgments about the thematic (ethical, social, aesthetic) relevance of a text. I can't do that, but I hope that you (and I, for that matter) will not notice and will pretend that I actually conducted such an exploration.

Your paper states that it is going to use the 2500 Amazon reviews of *The Road* as the vehicle to this exploring, and you get to the heart of your paper in section 4. "Zooming in on the Corpus." This is where it would seem that you would examine the data—the Amazon reviews. But I don't think you do examine the data, or if you do, you don't do it in a way that is convincing to me. I will examine in detail the section on visual imagery, which is the first and presumably most important data-analysis section.

Here is the opening sentence of that section: "The landscape of *The Road* seems to have such a stark visual quality that it becomes difficult for some readers not to visualize it." That statement implies causality: stark visual quality leads to visualization. But where does that imputed causality come from? Your method would seem to imply that you have examined the corpus, and out of the corpus arises the stated causality. That may well be true, but if it is, the method of that arising is not made clear and the data of that arising are not made transparent. That leads me to suspect that the imputed causality arises more from your presuppositions than from the corpus; then you try to buttress your own conviction with the corpus data. But even that buttressing is not convincing to me. Angry Warrior (2008) is the only reviewer you cite in this regard, but the Angry Warrior quotation you provide does not support your causality. Angry Warrior says the imagery won't leave him (her?) alone, and says that the landscape is bleak; but Angry Warrior does *not* say that the cause of this stubborn imagery is the bleakness. And even if he did, he is talking about the bleakness of the landscape that would cause the imagery, not (or at least not necessarily) the *visual* bleakness of the landscape. The landscape is bleak in a lot of ways other than visually. To the extent that Angry Warrior implies causation, it is McCarthy's eloquence that is given credit; and if that is true, then Angry Warrior would be seen as implying that any eloquent prose (not just stark visual prose) would elicit imagery.

In this I am taking no position on whether your imputed causation is or is not correct. My point is that I can't see a warrant for claiming that the causation arises from the corpus rather than from your own (perhaps correct) point of view.

You write:

> Another interesting finding is that the colorlessness of the storyworld reflects itself in the mental imagery of some readers, who report imagining the novel in black and white: "The book is written in language almost like watching black and white TV which adds to the setting" (Lutz, 2007).

I think that you mischaracterize Lutz. Lutz did *not* say that his (her?) imagery was in black and white. Lutz is not (or at least may not be) talking about his imagery at all: Lutz talks about McCarthy's language, not Lutz's imagery.

You write:

> We can take the word "vivid" as a rough indicator of the pictorial quality of McCarthy's novel. 71 readers use this adjective in their reviews. Its occurrences fall into three groups: in group a (32 occurrences), "vivid" refers to the spatial dimension of the storyworld.

But as far as I can tell, you provide no examples whatsoever of group a. It is not obvious to me what you mean by "vivid" referring to a spatial dimension; not obvious to me how you would determine whether a use does or does not count as such; not obvious to me how you keep your own suppositions in check when making such determinations.

The bottom line: I think it possible or even likely that your conclusions come from your suppositions, not from the corpus, and that the corpus is used (not very convincingly from my point of view) in an attempt to buttress those conclusions. I accept that I may have missed something; or that you may not have presented something that demonstrates how tightly the conclusions are bound to the corpus, but

I have not seen any methodological or procedural evidence that shows that you have a way of keeping your suppositions under control.

From my point of view, performing a convincing analysis of qualitative data is quite difficult, particularly when the data are as unconstrained as are the Amazon reviews. For it to be convincing to me, there must be some demonstration of rational attempt(s) to keep presuppositions at bay. Otherwise my default assumption is that there were no potentially adequate ways to keep presuppositions under control.

I accept that your paper might strike a literary scholar much differently than it strikes me—that's what I originally meant when I said that your paper "highlights why I am not a literary scholar." Literature itself clearly does not have any obligation to keep presuppositions under control, and perhaps that is true of literary scholarship as well. That is difficult for me.

—Russ

February 19
Dear Russ,
Many thanks for your comments on my paper. I think you're right on many counts, particularly when you call attention to the shortcomings of my qualitative analysis.

Also, it's true that I could have done a better job of quoting reviews that support my claim in the section about visualization. But I don't think that this is a substantial problem with my methodology—there are so many reviewers who talk about the relationship between McCarthy's style and mental imagery in the corpus that it shouldn't be hard to convince my reader that there *is* a relationship (at least from those reviewers' perspective). Take these statements, for instance: "McCarthy's writing is very visual and reading the book created a very vivid picture of the world he had created" (Peter G., 2007); "Great story and so descriptive you can vividly imagine the scenery" (5TooRMTR00PER, 2011); "the writing was good in that it is memorable and creates a vivid (though grey) world very different from ours" (Roxane, 2009); "[McCarthy] paints vivid pictures that almost make it seem like the reader should be sitting in a red, fold-up, theatre chair, rather than in the comforts of their own home" (Zachary Breakstone, 2008). It's entirely my fault that I didn't quote these—and many other—reviews, of course, but this is more a matter of rhetorical effectiveness than a problem with my claim about the relationship between language and mental imagery. Therefore, I think the issue can be more or less easily solved, and I really appreciate your pointing it out.

With regard to the question of causation: note that I'm not saying that the readers are objectively right in suggesting that McCarthy's style caused their rich visual imagery. I don't have the tools to evaluate this claim. All I am saying is that some of the reviewers subjectively saw a causal connection between these two phenomena, and this is an interesting fact in itself (whether it is objectively true or not).

[62] I agree that I didn't make any effort to limit or keep presuppositions in check in this particular paper. I believe this is a more substantial problem than the ones I've discussed above. In my defense I can say two things: (1) When I wrote this particular paper I didn't know anything about DES and I hadn't thought much about the role of presuppositions in empirical research (in fact, I sent you this paper just to show you what I meant by saying that thematic evaluations can be experiential). (2) Literary studies have been a speculative enterprise for a long time, and speculation cannot do without presuppositions. Maybe what disturbs you about my paper is that I'm disguising speculative claims as empirical research. I understand this objection, but I don't think

[63] that is completely true. What I'm trying to do, rather, is build a synergy between some (speculative) hypotheses and the discussion of empirical data. Whether this is convincing or not I don't know. Yet I have serious doubts that the project I'm embarking on in this paper (i.e., showing how readers can experience narrative space) could be accomplished in a completely presupposition-free way. Maybe this makes the project seem uninteresting or flawed to you, but I assure you that regardless of my own execution, which may be problematic, this project *is* worthwhile for a literary scholar.

All the best,
Marco

February 20
Hi Marco—

RE [62] "[Keeping] presuppositions in check."

I do not think that keeping suppositions in check is an ultimate good. On the contrary, there are many human situations where it is desirable or necessary to act on one's suppositions. DES emphasizes the bracketing of presuppositions because if one's interest is in faithfully apprehending the experiences of another, then bracketing presuppositions seems to me to be a necessary step. [64]

RE [63] "What I'm trying to do, rather, is build a synergy between some (speculative) hypotheses and the discussion of empirical data."

That seems to me to be a fair statement about literature in general, including literature creation and literary scholarship, and literary folks have every right to try to build such synergies. It "disturbs me" when that synergy-building involves (I think) unwarranted statements about experience. My reaction to your particular paper is not unusual for me—I am frequently disturbed in this way. I fully accept that literature has the right to disturb me; but I also have the right to think that it might be to literature's advantage to know the difference between statements about experience that are (I think) warranted and those that aren't. [65]
—Russ

February 21
Dear Russ,
See my responses to your comments below.
All the best,
Marco

RE [64] "DES emphasizes the bracketing of presuppositions because if one's interest is in faithfully apprehending the experiences of another, then bracketing presuppositions seems to me to be a necessary step."

I agree with this, but a lot turns on the adverb "faithfully." If I understand correctly, you're defining faithfulness in terms of a description's adherence to an original ("pristine") experience. To some extent I share this concern with you. But in other cases the criterion of faithfulness is less important for me, because I'm interested in what people say about their experiences regardless of whether it accurately captures a pristine experience (if there is one) or not. This is where my work comes closer to the approach of Pollio, Henley, and Thompson (1997), who in *The Phenomenology of Everyday Life* interview participants about broad experiences such as their stance toward their body, their perception of time, etc. I don't think these projects are mutually exclusive: sometimes [66] it makes sense to zoom in on a small "slice" of people's experiential stream, as DES can be said to do (let's call this a "high-resolution" approach). In other cases, however, it might be interesting to examine larger experiential patterns and structures by asking people to generalize about their experiences: this is what happens in "low-resolution" methods such as those of Pollio et al. Both high-resolution and low-resolution methods have limitations: the first lack temporal "depth," since they are tied to extremely small-scale experiences; the second can reveal larger experiential dynamics but cannot say much about pristine experience because of the reflective stance they encourage in participants. Further, there is a trade-off between the temporal resolution of the research method and its fidelity to the original pristine experience: the larger the scope of the experience to be described, the more presuppositions are likely to make their way into the participants' reports, so that these reports should be taken not as accurate descriptions of pristine experience but rather as the result of retrospective elaboration. Thus, in the case of the phenomenology of literary reading, my suggestion is that only a combination of high-resolution and low-resolution methods can paint a comprehensive picture of people's engagement with literature, since it can offer insight into the ways in which pristine experience and retrospective generalizations are related.

RE [65] "I also have the right to think that it might be to literature's advantage to know the difference between statements about experience that are (I think) warranted and those that aren't."

But again the distinction between "warranted" and "unwarranted" depends on a criterion of faithfulness to pristine experience. I think it's legitimate to look at the reviews in themselves, as statements that are more or less closely related to the reviewers' past experiences (in the broad sense), including their reading experiences. Of course, this kind of work is messy and unspecific, and does not meet DES standards because it is anything but presupposition-free. But here I would distinguish between presuppositions on the participants' side and presuppositions on the researcher's side. I agree that it is crucial to minimize researchers' presuppositions (and it is possible that I'm not doing enough to minimize them in my own work); but I don't think that it is always crucial to minimize participants' presuppositions—if only because, as you say, presuppositions are in the world, and it might be interesting to see them at work.

February 23
Hi Marco —

RE [66] "High-resolution" vs. "low-resolution methods."

I think it makes sense to talk, for example, of Google Maps as having high-resolution and low-resolution modes (actually, a continuum thereof), because at all times, from all "altitudes," Google Maps is aimed at the same thing — the earth in a particular locale. But I don't think that your "high-resolution" and "low-resolution" explorations of experience are aimed at the same thing, and therefore I find it misleading to speak of high- and low-resolution methods. What you call high-resolution (DES) methods aim at pristine experience, which I think is a directly apprehendable phenomenon. (It is private, to be sure; and people can be mistaken about it, to be sure; and one can never apprehend another's pristine experience in its entirety or with perfect fidelity. But at any given moment, for any given person, there is, within some limitations, only one answer to the question "What is in your experience at this moment?") By contrast, what you call low-resolution explorations aim at constructs such as "the reading experience," which is not the same thing as pristine experience, and in fact (I fear) is not any distinct phenomenon at all. (I certainly accept that there is something experiential about reading, and that there is something experiential about discussing reading. But the fact that we use the same word "experience" does not imply that we always mean the same thing by experience, or that we know what we mean when we use that term, or that we recognize that our meaning of experience shifts on successive uses of the term, or that two people engaged in conversation about reading understand the same thing by experience. That is, I see no reason to believe that we generally do, or perhaps ever can, really understand each other when we talk about the reading experience as your paper on *The Road* talks about it.)

So I think that DES and what you discuss about the reading experience are not high- or low-resolution explorations of anything. I think DES is (or at least can be) a fairly high-resolution investigation of pristine experience, but I don't think your investigation is a low-resolution investigation of the reading experience, because I don't think the reading experience exists.

The problem is not merely that "experience" is polysemous — that would be a far easier problem to solve. The problem is that, except in the sense of *pristine* experience, the term experience is always (to my ear) slippery: people proceed as if that term had a shared meaning even if it doesn't; if they discover that it has different meanings, then they can try to nail the meaning down; and they may reach agreement that they have nailed it down, but that agreement is likely to be illusory.

I don't know whether there is a proper term for the kinds of terms I am calling "slippery." Similar terms are "momentum" as applied to sports and "self" as used by psychologists. Sports people use "momentum" as if it were meaningful and well understood ("The Lakers have the momentum heading into overtime"), but I think there is little or no evidence for the existence of momentum in sports (as locutions such as "The momentum has shifted" should indicate to a careful observer). There are many psychologists who with conviction hold that the self exists and is amenable to scientific investigation, but as far as I can see, that has always been a scientific dead end. I think "experience" as you use it is in that category.

In summary: The only use of "experience" that I think does not have this slipperiness is pristine experience. Therefore I think that the exploration of pristine experience may have scientific merit that is substantially different from other scientific investigations of experience. Pristine experience does not differ from the reading experience only in the degree of resolution. The difference is much deeper than that.

I'm not trying to be dogmatic about this—I fully accept that I might be mistaken. And I fully accept that literary scholars may have different constraints and points of view.

—Russ

SECOND PART
PHENOMENA

VII

PHENOMENA AND HOW TO EXPLORE THEM

February 25
Dear Russ,

    I can see why distinguishing between pristine experience and loose experiential talk (as in "the reading experience") makes sense from your perspective. But the claim that "the reading experience" in the broad sense doesn't exist seems to me exaggerated. You write: "the fact that we use the same word 'experience' does not imply that we always mean the same thing by experience, or that we know what we mean when we use that term." I think you're right. But I don't see why it should follow from this that experience in the loose sense doesn't exist, or that people are necessarily wrong when they refer to "the reading experience." [67]

    You go on: "I see no reason to believe that we generally do, or perhaps ever can, really understand each other when we talk about the reading experience." This seems to condemn human beings to a tragicomedy of errors in which they generally misunderstand what other people think and feel. I think this view of intersubjectivity is fundamentally misguided. We can understand and even share other people's experiences because we share a lot in terms of perceptual and cognitive systems, bodily structures, and even cultural assumptions and values. The fact that DES shows that the fine details of people's pristine experiences vary significantly does not imply—as far as I can see—that we misunderstand one another all the time. It probably just implies that in most situations those fine details do not matter, and we can get on with our lives and practice intersubjectivity without paying too much attention to DES-level differences. To put this point otherwise: when you argue that people do not "really" understand one another because the experiences they refer to are not sufficiently similar, I think your standards of similarity are unreasonably high. If it is true that my "high-resolution and low-resolution explorations of experience are [not] aimed at the same thing," then you cannot draw any conclusion about experience in the broad sense on the basis of DES findings. Certainly, you can't say that people [68] [69] [70] [71] [72]

[73] do not "really" understand others' experiences. But then I disagree with the premise that "high-resolution and low-resolution explorations of experience are [not] aimed at the same thing." Experience is a phenomenon, not a thing, and if people—lots of people—use the same word to refer to activities such as reading a book or becoming ill, their usage cannot be discarded only because it does not meet your strict DES criteria. If these "things" seem experiences to them, they *are* experiences.

[74] Further, I think you're overlooking the fact that DES descriptions and reports rely heavily on language. Yet language is inherently experiential in the broad sense. When Lynn says "I innerly saw a bat," she says so because she learned to recognize a certain kind of experiential events (mental imagery) and call them in this way. Her reference to the mental image in her pristine experience is bound up with previous mental images—and thus with a background of experience in the broad sense.

[75] Again, I don't think it's desirable to drive a wedge between pristine and nonpristine experience, even if I grant that they are distinct phenomena and that they may be susceptible to different research methods.

All the best,
Marco

February 26
Hi Marco—

Thanks for your thoughtful comments. I still think this discussion is at the heart of many important issues, and trying to advance the straight talk about them is worth the effort.

RE [67] "I don't see why it should follow from this that experience in the loose sense doesn't exist."

Let's start by examining the parallel statement that schizophrenia doesn't (or at least may not) exist. Certainly there are severe behaviors and phenomena that are called schizophrenia—I do not deny that or discount their importance or the severe problematics that are involved for the individuals and their families. But to believe or to say that schizophrenia exists goes beyond that, and goes beyond, I think, the science. There may well be many different kinds of physical or neurological or behavioral patterns that are called by the same word "schizophrenia."

"Schizophrenia" in one manner of speaking is a useful term: it points to a severity of disturbance, and certainly it has a different meaning from "depression," or "influenza," or "Cadillac." But many people who use the term "schizophrenia" imply (intentionally or not) that they are referring to a homogeneous existing disease entity "schizophrenia," and that may have substantial undesirable ramifications for understanding, treatment, and research. For example, as I read the literature, there are far too few investigations of the (perhaps very disparate) phenomena that are called schizophrenia. The problem is that most who use the term "schizophrenia" would deny that they are referring to a homogeneous entity, and yet their locutions (such as "What is the treatment for schizophrenia?") betray them.

In sum: Were I to say that schizophrenia doesn't exist, I would *not* want to be understood as saying that hallucinations don't exist, or that sudden shifts in affect don't exist. I would want to be understood as saying that there is probably not a homogeneous existing disease entity "schizophrenia," and perhaps not even a discrete number of separable entities. [76]

It seems to me that your use of the term "experience" is far looser than the term "schizophrenia"—that is, the range of situations in which one invokes "experience" is greater than the range of situations in which one invokes "schizophrenia." You acknowledge that yourself, giving examples ranging from traveling through India to reading a text like *The Metamorphosis*. It seems to follow that there is nothing that remotely resembles a homogeneous "experience" phenomenon. So when I say "experience" doesn't exist, I do *not* wish to be understood as saying that pain (an experience) doesn't exist; I do *not* mean that reading *The Metamorphosis* doesn't occur; I do *not* mean to deny that it makes sense to say that I had a different experience traveling through India than I did traveling through Paris. What I intend to say is that the term "experience" is used in many different ways (which you acknowledge), that people in conversation often don't realize that they use the term in different ways (which I think you acknowledge), that with the possible exception of pristine experience it is very difficult and perhaps impossible to nail down agreement about the referent of "experience" in any given use (which you might not acknowledge), because there is nothing that remotely resembles a homogeneous experience phenomenon, and any approach thereto is slippery.

RE [67] "Or that people are necessarily wrong when they refer to 'the reading experience.'"

I don't think I said it is wrong to refer to "the reading experience." I said that when they so refer, they often (perhaps usually or maybe always) don't know exactly what they refer to, that people who in conversation make such references often (perhaps usually or maybe always) don't understand each other, and they often (perhaps usually) don't realize that they don't understand each other, and they often (perhaps usually) don't realize that there is no homogenous reading experience phenomenon.

RE [68] "This seems to condemn human beings to a tragicomedy of errors in which they generally misunderstand what other people think and feel."

That seems like pretty much the same question I answered in my 2011 book:

> *We often don't know what we think or feel or experience.* We know to some extent but are deluded to some extent about our own experience. . . . We as individuals often (probably usually) don't take the trouble to distinguish between what we actually think, feel, experience and what we are told we should think, feel, and experience.
>
> *Are we a bunch of fools?* I'd prefer to say we are a bunch of human beings, which, in my view, means that we are a bunch of complex beings that are partly logical, partly delusional. Some of us are doubtless more delusional than others; I know of no one who is free of delusion (although I accept that freedom from delusion may be possible). Many of us pretend, including to ourselves, that we are free of delusion, and that is foolish, because to the extent that we believe our own pretendings we dig ourselves deeper into whatever delusions we may have—confidence in your own nondelusion is probably evidence of delusion. Delusions are tenacious because they seem so unquestionably true, so incontrovertible, so completely acceptable, so downright virtuous. (Hurlburt, 2011a, 412–13)

RE [69] "We can understand and even share other people's experiences because we share a lot in terms of perceptual and cognitive systems, bodily structures, and even cultural assumptions and values."

I agree, but at the same time, and largely unexamined, and often to a large extent, we overbelieve and, if asked, overstate the degree of that understanding/sharing. And the science of experience does not do much or any better with its questionnaires or structured interviews.

When you say "we share a lot in terms of perceptual and cognitive systems," I remind you of Alex and Lynn. If you claim that similarity of perceptual and cognitive systems leads to similarity of experiences, it would seem that the highest degree of similarity ought to be in pristine experience, because pristine experience is the least affected by outside (e.g., interpersonal, cultural) influences. However, Alex's and Lynn's experiences while reading are *much* different. Therefore I think it is particularly unwise to presume that similar perceptual and cognitive systems lead to similar experience. If there are similarities in experience, they must come *after* (or "higher," if you prefer) than perceptual and cognitive systems.

RE [70] "The fact that DES shows that the fine details of people's pristine experiences vary significantly does not imply—as far as I can see—that we misunderstand one another all the time."

I didn't say, nor do I think, that we misunderstand one another all the time. I said we *often* misunderstand one another, and we don't generally know when or whether we are misunderstanding one another. *Time 1*: We interact, assuming we understand one another, and (as an omniscient being might observe) we do in fact understand one another. *Time 2*: We interact, again assuming we understand one another, and (as an omniscient being might observe) we do in fact understand one another again. *Time 3*: We interact again, again assuming we understand one another, but (as an omniscient being might observe) this time we do *not* in fact understand one another, and furthermore fail to recognize this lack of understanding. Suddenly, for no apparent reason, you're angry at me, or I think you're stupid, or whatever. The omniscient being knows the reason—we didn't understand each other and we didn't know that we didn't understand each other, and that made you angry at me or you to look stupid to me. I think that is, at least in part, why husbands and wives get in trouble, and Republicans and Democrats, and Israelis and Palestinians.

The human condition, as it seems to me, is that we often misunderstand each other without realizing it. The misunderstanding itself is not too problematic; the not realizing it gets us into trouble.

RE [71] "We can get on with our lives and practice intersubjectivity without paying too much attention to DES-level differences."

I think we can get on with our lives just fine, practicing not realizing that we don't understand our differences, until one day your wife leaves you "out of the blue," or the economy collapses "without warning," or whatever, at which time you will say, "Man, nobody really understood the risks of the subprime mortgages!" Why not? Because people were motivated (by money, time, convenience, or whatever) to assume that the fine details are not important, to assume that because we share results (we're all getting rich together), we all must understand each other and the structure of the market. We go blissfully along, assuming we understand enough until forced to realize it wasn't true.

You may think my market-collapse metaphor is too extreme, and perhaps it is. So here it is without metaphor: It requires hard work to understand details. The understanding of the details is often (perhaps usually) not rewarded by society, because it is easy to presume that understanding the details is unnecessary (because it requires hard work to recognize the value of the details). In fact, in what Freud might have called a defensive maneuver, it is easy to presume that understanding the details is (not only unnecessary but) positively the wrong thing to do (it wastes valuable time while the market is surging). But I think that sooner or later, that lack of understanding and, worse, that lack of recognition that such understanding is important, may bite you.

I happily accept that DES-level differences might not be important—I certainly am in no position to state positively the conditions under which they are or are not important. I can say that I think it is worthwhile to try to find out if and when they are important and for what and to what extent. That's what science does, and it seems to me to be undesirable to presume without investigation the answers to those questions.

RE [72] "If it is true that my 'high-resolution and low-resolution explorations of experience are [not] aimed at the same thing,' then you cannot draw any conclusion about experience in the broad sense on the basis of DES findings."

I agree. I think I have no warrant to draw conclusions about experience in the broad sense. But I have warrant to worry about it. On the basis of DES, I can, I think, confidently say that people are often mistaken about their pristine experience. Alex, for example, prior to his DES sampling, would have confidently said that his pristine experience while reading involved frequent imagery; I think (as does he, now) that he was wrong about that. So people can be majorly mistaken about their (at least pristine) experience. Does that apply only to pristine experience, or to experience in your broad sense? I don't know. It certainly seems that many people, including perhaps you, do seem to be confident that they know the answer to that question. I think that confidence is misplaced.

I think the DES findings are enough to warrant a substantial skepticism about the fidelity of people's claims about their experiences. Skepticism as I use the term does not imply disbelief; it means the suspension of belief. But the source of my skepticism about experience in the broad sense is not primarily an extrapolation from pristine experience; it is that you and others don't really know what you mean by experience.

RE [73] "Experience is a phenomenon, not a thing."

The word "phenomenon" is very tricky. Webster would say that a phenomenon (for our purposes) is "an observable fact or event" or "an object or aspect known through the senses rather than by thought or intuition." By those definitions, pristine experience is a phenomenon; the experience of traveling through India is *not* a phenomenon. You have never observed *traveling through India* through your senses. You observed the Taj Mahal with your senses; you observed the sitar performance with your senses; you observed the curry with your senses; and out of all those Webster-happy phenomena you said something about the experience of traveling through India. But that saying of "experience" does *not* refer to any phenomenon; it refers to some (mental or cognitive or affective) processing (of some things that may have originated in phenomena), processing that is closer to the "thought or intuition" that Webster expressly says are *not* phenomena than to phenomena itself.

A primary reason why I explore pristine experience is that pristine experiences are indeed phenomena that present themselves directly to the person—that is, they are phenomena in Webster's sense. One gloss of the origin of DES: I was interested (more or less as you are) in experience (more or less broadly defined), and I wished to cleave to phenomena. One by one, everything that I might have called "experience" fell away except what I now call pristine experience. That is, I certainly did *not* begin with an interest in pristine experience; I am interested in pristine experience because I am interested in experience and I value knowing what I'm talking about.

RE [73] "Experience is a phenomenon, not a thing, and if people—lots of people—use the same word to refer to activities such as reading a book or becoming ill, their usage cannot be discarded only because it does not meet your strict DES criteria."

[80] It has nothing to do with DES criteria. People use the phrase "experience of reading *The Road*" in many different ways: during the reading, just after the reading, while talking about it with their friends, while watching Oprah talk about it, while reading the reviews online; and each of those can be broken down: while reading reviews they like, while reading reviews they don't like, while reading reviewers who they can't understand, while reading reviews while they are angry at their spouse/partner/whomever, while reading reviews. . . . You don't have to invoke DES to note that those are very disparate meanings of "experience." People slide from one use to the other without noticing, and without noticing that the slide might be important. So I don't recommend discarding their usage, but I do recommend being skeptical that you or they know exactly (or even approximately) what they are talking about.

RE [74] "Further, I think you're overlooking the fact that DES descriptions and reports rely heavily on language."

I get such criticisms a lot, and I don't think they are fair. The most common such criticism, which I think is related but somewhat plainer, is that when I criticize retrospective reports such as questionnaires or memoirs, people say, "I think you're overlooking the fact that DES descriptions and reports are retrospective, too." And so they are. But the size of the retrospection is, I think, important: DES retrospections are measured in seconds or fractions thereof, while short-term memory still exists, while the situation which engendered the retrospection is still active, where the developmental stage of the reporter is exactly the same as that of the experiencer, where the bodily state (fatigue, arousal, etc.) of the reporter is exactly the same as that of the experiencer. By contrast, many other retrospections are measured in days or years. Yes, both are retrospective, and I grant the possibility that the act of retrospection itself, regardless of the distance of the retrospection, may instantaneously transform everything so that millisecond-later retrospections are no better than years-later retrospections. But I think the evidence shows that the size of the retrospection *does* matter. Furthermore, the DES retrospections are prospectively prepared by the iterative nature of the DES process: a main reason we require that DES observations be iterative is so that subjects learn to be better prepared to apprehend experience when it occurs. Note I am not saying that DES overcomes the problem of retrospection; I am saying that DES takes the problem of retrospection extremely seriously and engages in systematic, thoughtful attempts to limit the ramifications of the problem. Asking an adult "What was it like for you to learn to ride a bike?" and asking that same adult, "What was your experience a second ago when the beep sounded?" are both retrospections, but one is long distance with no practice, and the other is minimal distance with substantial prospective preparation. They are not the same.

Now to "DES descriptions and reports rely heavily on language." Yes they do. But the DES art is to expose, often word by word, in high fidelity what is meant. The DES art is to presume that the subject's language does *not* match my own, to question and clarify; to be alert to discrepancies and consonances that provide *evidence* of meaning or intention; to drill down, by as many different means as possible, into the idiosyncrasies and emotionalities to get as close to bedrock as we can. Are we perfect at it? By no means. Do we spend a hundred times as much effort in so doing than does the typical interview? Probably more. Does one get better at it with practice? Probably so.

A DES subject does not typically say "I innerly saw a bat." She more likely says, "I saw an image of a bat." That triggers a series of questions about what she means by "saw"—ten questions later we are confident that she really means to be reporting a seeing—she's not merely *thinking about* a bat in the cognitive sense, nor is she remembering a bat that she has previously seen, nor is she. . . . We have nailed down that her use of "saw" is meant literally. Then we examine what she meant by a "bat": a particular bat? How big? From what perspective? What color? In motion or still? Seen clearly? etc. We have nailed down that she is indeed seeing a six-inch-long bat, gray and brown, clearly seen, etc. Then we ask what she meant by seeing "an image"? Like a picture? Borders? Frames? Edges? Movement of the image as distinct from movement of the bat? The answer to those were all No, so it emerges that she was *not* seeing an *image of* a bat, but was seeing a bat, two very different things. It has taken us several minutes to determine with fidelity the meaning of "I saw an image of a bat." Part of that sentence was true (saw, bat); part of it was not true (image). At the conclusion we write something like "Lynn innerly saw a bat." We use innerly to indicate that there was no real bat; we could as well have written "Lynn imaginarily saw a bat."

Further, the iterative essential nature of DES is designed to refine the use of language over time. As you may recall, we did not have

[81]

a naive Lynn engage in the reading task; we had already spent an hour on each of four separate occasions engaging Lynn in the repetitive, gradual-improvement-over-time effort in building our linguistic understanding of each other, refining exactly those terms that emerged as useful in understanding Lynn's individualized and perhaps idiosyncratic use of language.

Nearly all observers say that my interviews are excruciatingly slow, agonizingly repetitive in their incessant clarifications. But subjects themselves *never* say that. Why not? Maybe because I browbeat them, but far more likely because they know their words are imperfect and genuinely appreciate the struggle to get the meaning of their words exactly right.

You might say that we did not make much progress with Lynn: "I innerly saw a bat" is pretty much the same as "I saw an image of a bat." Two replies: First, there are many cases where "I saw an image of a bat" does *not* refer to anything visual at all—it might mean that she was thinking in a cognitive but not a visual sense about bats. The only way to proceed in high fidelity is to accept the proposition that *every* locution needs exposition. Second, "seeing a bat" and "seeing an image of a bat" are experientially two very different things, as different as seeing President Obama is from seeing a photograph of President Obama.

So in answer to your question: Yes, DES uses language. No, DES does not cavalierly presume that it knows what that language means, as do most interviews and conversations. Do we get a perfect understanding of Lynn's meanings? No. Do we get a higher-fidelity understanding than would most others? I think Yes. So I say the same thing about language that I said about retrospection: Note I am not saying that DES overcomes the problem of language; I am saying that DES takes the problem of language extremely seriously and engages in systematic, thoughtful attempts to limit the ramifications of the problem.

RE [75] "I don't think it's desirable to drive a wedge between pristine and nonpristine experience, even if I grant that they are distinct phenomena and that they may be susceptible to different research methods."

First let me observe that it is not I who am driving the wedge between pristine and nonpristine experience—that wedge is driven by experience itself. As I said above, when I started these investigations in the 1970s, I was interested in experience more broadly defined, much as you are. In the effort to be clear about experience, I was forced by the subject matter into noticing the wedge between pristine and non-pristine experience. I wanted to be pretty darn confident that I knew what I was talking about, and pretty darn confident that the words I used to describe experience rested pretty darn faithfully on the phenomena being described. It was forced upon me to notice (that is, the wedge was driven into me) that it is possible to be confident about what I came to call pristine experience in a way that is not possible about experience in general.

Here's one more concrete example, among the almost daily examples in the media, that occurred as I drove home thinking about what to write to you. Dave Davies, the interviewer on the National Public Radio show *Fresh Air*, asked film director Robert Zemeckis: "*Forrest Gump* was such an amazing project for you—you won the Academy Award for Best Director, right? And it sort of became a huge American cultural influence. What was it like to experience that?" Zemeckis replied that

> it's a very heady experience. In a strange way it's um quite a bit nerve wracking because y'know you end up having to be in that situation where you're thinking Oh my! You start to get insecure about thinking if you can ever top any of this, y'know, what are you gonna do next? Is everything gonna just be . . . um . . . y'know . . . uh . . . a letdown after you have a success as tremendous as we had with *Forrest Gump*? (Zemeckis, originally aired on November 29, 2012)

Do we have a warrant to believe that the insecurity that Zemeckis mentions is really a major part of the success-of-*Forrest-Gump* experience? I think the answer is No. Now, I know nothing personal about Zemeckis, and I happily accept that the possibility that insecurity *was in fact* the central part of the success-of-*Forrest-Gump* experience. So what I am saying is not at all about Zemeckis personally. That is, I would also answer No to the opposite question: Do we have a warrant to believe that the insecurity that Zemeckis mentions is really *not* a major part of the *Forrest Gump* experience? The point is that there are lots of potential ways to understand Zemeckis's reply, for example:

- I really did become insecure because of winning the Academy Award.
- I am always insecure, and was therefore insecure after winning the Academy Award but not *because* I won the award.

- I am not usually insecure, but I am insecure now and therefore likely to "recall" insecurity even about situations where insecurity was not an issue.
- My *Forrest Gump* experiences were mainly of the I-told-you-so variety, but I prefer not to mention that on public radio, so I'll mention insecurity instead.
- I'd like any actors that might be listening to see me as sensitive.
- I'd like my lover who is probably listening to see me as sensitive.

and many others. I don't know which if any of these is on target for his experience: maybe none, maybe some. Maybe others are more important.

[82]   The important part of this example is the "I don't know" part—that's what drives the wedge to which you refer. We don't know the important factor or factors that lead Zemeckis to say what he does about experience. And I think that is a *large* I don't know, not merely a quibble about details.

In my view: If one is interested in experience, and one wants really to rise above "I don't know," one is forced to acknowledge the wedge driven between pristine experience and other uses of "experience."
—Russ

VIII

IN WHICH MARCO RANKLES AT RUSS'S EMPHASIS ON DELUSION, AND THEY DISCUSS THE EXISTENCE OF EXPERIENCE

March 2
Dear Russ,
Many thanks for your insightful reply. Please find my responses to your comments below.

RE [76] "There is probably not a homogeneous existing disease entity 'schizophrenia.'"
   I agree that the term "experience" is broader than the term "schizophrenia," because it applies to a larger number of situations. But I don't think that this disqualifies talk about experience in the broad sense. Likewise, consider a simpler example, the term "car." Does it make sense to say that whenever people use the term "car" they don't know what they are talking about, because there is no quintessential car but only a large number of motor vehicles of different colors, sizes, brands, etc.? I don't think so. Thus, when I use the term "car" in "my car" I refer to my Peugeot. When you use the term "car" in "my car," you refer to your Ford. But this doesn't mean that the term is useless, or that we are "deluded" because we use the term differently. Language always slices up the world in arbitrary ways. The point is that using the term "experience," like using most other concepts, involves recognizing a situation as possessing a number of features. It doesn't necessarily involve referring to the same entity, because experience is not an object-like entity, but rather a pattern of interactions (see also the arguments advanced by "enactivist" philosophers of mind like Daniel Hutto [2000] and Alva Noë [2004]). [83]
   For "car," the defining features would be: (1) has a motor; (2) has four wheels; etc. Identifying these features for "experience" may be more difficult, and they may seem looser, but it's not completely impossible. Whenever we use the term "experience," we are referring to (1) an embodied subject; (2) who engages with an object, be it internal (a thought, a mental image) or external (a thing, another person,

or a situation); (3) the subject's engagement has a specific quality or feel, which (3a) changes over time, giving rise to a dynamic flow; (3b) depends on the subject's physical makeup but also on her memories of past interactions with the world (including her exposure to sociocultural practices); (3c) may also change the subject in significant ways. I do think this is specific enough for some purposes, and I do think all these features are implicated in people's use of the term "experience."

RE [77] "We as individuals often (probably usually) don't take the trouble to distinguish between what we actually think, feel, experience and what we are told we should think, feel, and experience."

[84]   This may be true, but I am a bit alarmed by the normativity of your discussion. Who (or what) gets to decide what counts as a delusion and
[85]   what doesn't? In every one of your statements I can detect the presence of DES, setting the standard for delusions and nondelusions, defending "pristine experience" against the onslaught of cultural presuppositions and loose terminology. Isn't your attachment to DES—a way of living more than a research method—a delusion? Or am I deluded about this? The only answer that I can give is "I don't know."

The fact is that, to me, thinking about the human condition in terms of delusion or nondelusion does not sound particularly subtle, or productive, or illuminating. It seems to go against the grain of that attention to detail that you, rightly I think, consider one of the achievements of your method. Sure, we are wrong about a lot of things. Sure, we can be (and often are) wrong about ourselves. But I can't imagine what it would mean to live without "pressures [that] distort what we think, feel, experience." I think those pressures are called "culture," to a large extent—except that I wouldn't use the word "distort" but much more neutral terms like "shape" or "inform."

RE [78] "If you claim that similarity of perceptual and cognitive systems lead to similarity of experiences, it would seem that the highest degree of similarity ought to be in pristine experience, because pristine experience is the least affected by outside (e.g., interpersonal, cultural) influences."

Fair enough, but I'm not saying that having similar perceptual and cognitive systems implies experiencing the world in the same way *at the same time*. This would be absurd, if only because our bodies occupy different spatial positions, and because our experience of the world—i.e., the way we engage with and respond to it—depends on a background of past interactions.

The point I'm making is different: because of similarities in our [86] perceptual and cognitive systems, we are at least *capable* of experiencing the world in broadly similar ways, and this capability explains why experiences can be shared. It is true that Alex and Lynn experienced the Kafka passages in significantly different ways. But my sense is that if Alex explained to Lynn his word—word—word experiences, Lynn would be surprised, perhaps, at the difference, but she would also be able to understand Alex's experience on the basis of her own past experiences. "Understanding" here does not have a purely cognitive meaning. It implies imaginatively reenacting (an approximation of) Alex's experience. Language and concepts make this possible, so in a sense I think you're right to say that "If there are similarities in experience, they must come *after* (or 'higher,' if you prefer) than perceptual and cognitive systems." Except that in my view language and concepts allow us to point out similarities *also* in preconceptual experiences (where similarity, again, is conceived in the capable-of sense).

RE [79] "The human condition, as it seems to me, is that we often misunderstand each other without realizing it. The misunderstanding itself is not too problematic; the not realizing it gets us into trouble."

As far as I can see, the only possible solution to this is talking it [87] over. To me, this means that misunderstanding is not part and parcel of human interaction, but only the side effect of incomplete, faulty, or biased interaction.

RE [80] "It has nothing to do with DES criteria. People use the phrase 'experience of reading *The Road*' in many different ways: during the reading, just after the reading, while talking about it with their friends, while watching Oprah talk about it, while reading the reviews online; and each of those can be broken down. . . . So I don't recommend discarding their usage, but I do recommend being skeptical that you or they know exactly (or even approximately) what they are talking about."

I believe you're making too much of the phrase "the experience of reading *The Road*." Few people actually use this phrase in the real world. The point is that what they say *about* McCarthy's novel can be taken as an indication of their experience of reading *The Road* (where "experience" refers to features (1)–(3) listed in RE 76).

I also have the sense that you're conflating two different projects, or rather judging the second by the criteria of the first. One thing is the scientific study of experience, in which terminological precision and the

98 • CHAPTER VIII

bracketing of presuppositions ("skepticism") are essential. Maybe pristine experience is the only aspect or dimension of experience that can be studied scientifically. Maybe DES is as good as it gets. But I would still insist that is there *another*, nonscientific way of studying experience that is based not on skepticism but on a relationship of trust between researcher and participant. You're free to think that this—humanistic?—approach to experience is messy and naive. But I am free to think—I think—that what people say about their experiences (whether they use the phrase "the experience of x" or not) is valuable, and deserves being studied as such. Now, as I understand this conversation, part of the question we're trying to deal with is the following: is there any common ground between the scientific and the humanistic project? The term "experience" seems the most likely candidate for this bridge-building. But of course if you deny the continuity between pristine experience and experience in the broad sense, then it becomes difficult or impossible to find a common ground.

[88]

ROAD MAP: *Marco's distinction between the study of the reading experience within literary theory and the psychological (and scientific) perspective of DES serves as a prelude to our discussion of humanistic vs. scientific approaches to experience (which we called theme d in chapter I).*

RE [81] "DES is designed to refine the use of language over time."

You are understandably concerned about the way language is used. I am too, in a different way, or I wouldn't be a literary scholar. But when I wrote [near marginal 73] "If these 'things' seem experiences to [people], they *are* experiences," I didn't have in mind a situation in which some particular person (let's call her Georgia) declares: "these 'things' seem experiences to me." Even if Georgia never uses the word "experience," these things would still seem experiences to her. Perhaps I should have written something like "these 'things' are experiential for Georgia." To be experiential means, quite simply, to have a relation to or to be influenced by one's background of past experiences. A circular definition, to be sure, but I don't think there's a way out of this circle, because experience *is* (it seems to me) circular—it is a two-way, and temporally unfolding, relation between present affordances (what you call "pristine experience") and a repertoire of past sensations, emotions, reflections. You're likely to

[89]

[90]

consider this account of experience too loose, metaphorical, and a matter of interpretation and presupposition rather than of science. To this I reply: sure, but I find it valuable all the same. To put it bluntly (and perhaps simplistically), this view strikes me as a more insightful way of looking at the human condition than the dichotomy between delusion and nondelusion.

RE [82] "The important part of this example is the 'I don't know' part—that's what drives the wedge to which you refer. We don't know the important factor or factors that lead Zemeckis to say what he does about experience. And I think that is a *large* I don't know, not merely a quibble about details. In my view: If one is interested in experience, and one wants really to rise above 'I don't know,' one is forced to acknowledge the wedge driven between pristine experience and other uses of 'experience.'"

As I understand the interview, Zemeckis does seem to say that he became insecure because of winning the Academy Award—we may dispute whether this is really true or not, but I don't think there can be doubts as to what he wanted to say. In any case, I don't see why the "I don't know" would be constitutive here. We could ask Zemeckis to explain what he really meant, if he had felt insecure before or afterwards, etc. We could do so in a situation in which Zemeckis does not have much to lose or win (in terms of social recognition, etc.). Surely, even in that situation there would be no way to prove that Zemeckis is not making up things or—more precisely—constructing a public identity. Perhaps that is what you mean by "I don't know." In that sense, yes, I would agree that the constructedness is more or less constitutive: people construct themselves in social interaction all the time. Still, I would say that there is something to learn from studying the ways in which people construct themselves in the same situation, when talking about similar experiences in the broad sense. For example, we could ask a group of famous people what it meant for them to deal with unexpected success. This is a different project from studying pristine experience (I agree with you that there *is* a wedge in this respect), but I would not go as far as to say (1) that these projects have nothing in common; and (2) that the only legitimate way of investigating experience is investigating pristine experience. If you replace "legitimate" with "scientific," then you may be right. But I don't think the equation is warranted.

[91]

IX

GREAT EXPECTATIONS AND GENIES REVEAL SOMETHING ABOUT KNOWING OTHERS' EXPERIENCE

March 7
Hi Marco—
I do think all these are important issues.

RE [84] "I am a bit alarmed by the normativity of your discussion. Who (or what) gets to decide what counts as a delusion and what doesn't?"

I don't know who gets to decide; certainly not me. I have tried to make clear throughout my discussion with you and in Hurlburt (2011a) that my position is *not* "you're delusional and I'm not, ha ha!" but rather, "I'm delusional and so, probably, are you." If there are places where I might have (incorrectly) implied that I get to decide who is delusional, I'd like to know about them.

I think whether something is a delusion does not depend on who gets to decide. Even if one's delusional status might be known only to an omniscient being, one's delusional status remains the same, doesn't it?

By delusion I mean believing (being convinced that) something is true when it is not true. I think it is difficult if not impossible to explain how delusion arises in the world or in any individual unless one starts with the position that we all are deluded, and that working to diminish one's delusion is a worthwhile goal (perhaps attainable, but rarely).

RE [83] "Car" vs. "experience."

I understand that all terms and concepts have ranges of convenience that are less than perfect—there is ambiguity about whether this gasoline-powered golf cart deserves to be called "car." But there is an important difference, I think, between the concept "car" and the concept "experience." There is generally no question about the existence of the thing that maybe should or should not be called a car—we will agree that the golf cart exists even though we might disagree about the concepts that should be applied to it. That is, the thingness of the golf cart for the most part stubbornly exists, independent of any definitional concept such as having a motor or wheels.

I don't think that is so easily true with "experience." I don't think there is anything (whether a thing, a phenomenon, or whatever) that is the experience of traveling through India—that's what I mean when I say "the experience of traveling through India doesn't exist." When I tell my musician friend about my experience of traveling through India, the sitar is prominent and I mention the sitar; when I tell my gourmet friend about my experience of traveling through India, the curry is prominent and I mention the curry. That does *not* imply that there is an experience of traveling through India that I can highlight from different perspectives (even though it may seem like that to me). Instead, when my musician friend asks me about my experience of traveling through India, I create a more or less coherent story that involves my musician friend's proclivities (or my take thereon) as well as some (more or less veridical) retrospections on my historical India trip. And when my gourmet friend asks me, I create a different story that involves my gourmet friend's proclivities as well as some (more or less veridical) retrospections on my historical India trip. It likely seems to me that I am consulting the thing that is my experience of traveling through India, but I don't think that is the case.

It *seems* that this is parallel to being asked about your car: when asked by a fellow Peugeot enthusiast about your car, you highlight one aspect (or set thereof) about your car, whereas when asked by a mass-transit activist about your car, you highlight another. But I think these situations are not parallel. Your Peugeot exists, and you can highlight different aspects of it, and whether you highlight or not doesn't alter the Peugeot itself, which stubbornly continues on regardless. By contrast, there is no experience-of-India that can be highlighted but which continues stubbornly on regardless. There are different manners of speaking about my India trip that seem to suggest that my experience-of-India stubbornly exists, but I think that experience-of-India-existence is a mirage.

RE [85] "In every one of your statements I can detect the presence of DES, setting the standard for delusions and nondelusions, defending 'pristine experience' against the onslaught of cultural presuppositions and loose terminology. Isn't your attachment to DES—a way of living more than a research method—a delusion?"

Doubtless Yes, and I would be the last person on earth who could be expected to have a dispassionate view of my delusions (that is the nature of delusion).

RE [87] "The only possible solution to this is talking it over."

I agree, which I suppose is my (and probably your) motivation for the present discussion (and my Schwitzgebel collaborations, etc.). So, with happy and full acknowledgment of the likelihood of my being deluded, I say that on the best self-evaluation I can muster I am not attached to DES. I think experience is important, and I value knowing what I'm talking about, and that leads me to DES. But if someone came along with a better way to investigate experience, I'd abandon DES in a heartbeat.

RE [86] "Because of similarities in our perceptual and cognitive systems, we are at least *capable* of experiencing the world in broadly similar ways, and this capability explains why experiences can be shared."

Much, of course, depends on what you mean by "we" and what you mean by "broadly similar"—Mars is in some respects broadly similar to Earth. But setting aside that quibble, I think the sentiment you state is broadly held and quite likely counterproductive for the advancement of science (and probably literature, also). I think the following sentiment is also true: regardless of some similarities in our perceptual and cognitive systems, people may have very *different* capabilities for experiencing the world, resulting in, broadly speaking, very different worldviews. (Mars is in some respects broadly different from Earth.) Experiences seem to be shared because (a) the experiences themselves are private and therefore not easily differentiated; (b) the language used to speak about experiences is shared, even if the referents are not; and (c) often, speaking does not adequately distinguish between the world and experience, so if the world situation is similar, experience is presumed to be similar. The broadly similar and the broadly different sentiments are both doubtless true in some manners of speaking and some situations. It is or should be the aim of science to tease apart those manners and situations.

So: does "we" include those in psychotic episodes—that is, do you and a psychotic individual have broadly the same capability of experiencing the world? I suspect that the answer is No. If you agree, what then is the dividing line between broadly similar and not? Does "we" include children: do you and a two-year-old have broadly the same capability of experiencing the world? I suspect that the answer is No. And if that is correct, at what age does that turn to Yes?

Note that I am not in the slightest saying that your broadly similar sentiment is not, in some important manner of speaking, true. I am saying that I think it is not always true, and in many cases it is probably less true than is the broadly different sentiment. Therefore, when you say "we are at least *capable* of experiencing the world in broadly similar ways, and this capability explains why experiences can be shared," my presupposition-detection antennae jangle by the universalizing "at least" and the categorical affirmation of "explains." I think we need to accept the possibility of incapability of similar experiencing.

Perhaps a concrete example from literature might be useful. I happen to be reading *Great Expectations*; this story is told from Pip's point of view, and often includes descriptions of Pip's (what in a real person I would call) pristine experience. For example, in the first chapter Pip describes how the church turns upside down and then back right-side up again (in reality the convict has lifted Pip up by his heels and then set him back down). I take that church-turning-over to be Dickens's attempt to describe a detail of the pristine experience of a 6-year-old (maybe he was 7; it doesn't matter), and that attempt might be faithful to a 6-year-old's experience. But most of what Dickens wrote about Pip's pristine experience is not, I think, likely or possible for a 6-year-old. I accept that my view of 6-year-old pristine experience diverges from that of most people, including most psychologists, as my writings about the Flavells might indicate (Hurlburt, in Hurlburt and Schwitzgebel, 2007, 45–47, 271–74). I happily accept that I might be mistaken. But I see no reason for anyone to be confident about the actual details of the pristine experience of 6-year-olds unless they have performed adequate investigations thereof, which I don't think anyone has done.

It seems to me that Dickens portrays Pip experientially, for the most part, as a little adult with a few experiential anomalies and not much historical knowledge. That is, in my view, a low-fidelity portrayal of a 6-year-old's experience. And that is too bad from a literary point of view. I think 6-year-olds have experience that is substantially different from that of adults, and Dickens's account of a child coming of age (as this story is generally understood) would likely have been more interesting from a literary perspective if he had actually captured the experiential differences between kids, teenagers, and young adults. Why did Dickens portray kid-Pip and teen-Pip experientially mostly like an adult with an as-yet-impoverished history? And why haven't a century of readers said, *Wait a minute! That isn't how kids are!* Of course I don't know with authority but it seems like there are two alternatives: Dickens and his readers believe, incorrectly, that we (including Pip) experience the world in broadly similar ways (with an occasional exception like churches turning upside down); or Russ is mistaken and Dickens and his readers are right so to do. If I'm right, *Great Expectations* is only half as interesting as it might otherwise be, and I mean that from a literary or humanistic or historical perspective.

I speculate about the development of experience in chapter 9 of Hurlburt (2011a).

RE [88] "Now, as I understand this conversation, part of the question we're trying to deal with is the following: is there any common ground between the scientific and the humanistic project?"

First, I rankle a bit about excluding the scientific from the humanistic because I think science is an entirely human endeavor, embodying the highest values of humanism. (That does not imply that science *alone* embodies those highest values—I think there are lots of ways in which the highest values of humanism can be embodied: art, literature, politics, etc.) So how about if we refer to it as "historical" rather than "humanistic," to emphasize that we are referring to events that take place in particular epochs and that do not admit of thorough scientific investigation. So, for example, whether I should go to India is a historical event: I have to decide more or less now, on the basis of something decidedly less than a thorough scientific study of the pros and cons thereof. Does that use of "historical" work?

Let me reiterate that I *do* think historical (humanistic) interactions are important. If I am considering a trip to India, I will ask you about your experience in traveling in India, and I will value your response, and I will make important decisions (whether to travel there and if so where and how) at least in part based on your response. I will ask you what your experience of *The Road* is and base my decision on whether to buy it on your response. So I fully and completely agree with "what people say about their experiences (whether they use the phrase 'the experience of x' or not) is valuable." If I'm an intelligent humanist, I will understand that what you say is a messy agglomeration of what you think, what you think I want to hear, what you don't want to tell me, and so on; and what I hear is a similarly messy agglomeration of what you say, what I want you to say, what I'm afraid you won't say, and so on. That understanding does not in the slightest diminish the value of what you say; it does not in the slightest diminish the relationship of trust between you and me; it merely acknowledges the human nature of communication. And regardless of the messiness of the agglomerations, I will decide, based in part on what I understand you to have said, whether to go to India or read *The Road*.

RE [89] "Experience *is* . . . a two-way, and temporally unfolding, relation between present affordances (what you call 'pristine experience') and a repertoire of past sensations, emotions, reflections."

I think that implies the thingness of the past sensations, emotions, and reflections, as if those sensations, emotions, and reflections existed on a mental shelf somewhere and now can be dusted off and put into relation with current affordances. I think that is not true. I think there is not a past sensation; there may be a current sensation that is understood as retrospectively sensed. (And the same for emotions and reflections.)

RE [90] "You're likely to consider this account of experience too loose, metaphorical, and a matter of interpretation and presupposition rather than of science. To this I reply: sure, but I find it valuable all the same. To put it bluntly (and perhaps simplistically), this view strikes me as a more insightful way of looking at the human condition than the dichotomy between delusion and nondelusion."

I did not intend a dichotomy between delusion and nondelusion. I intended to advocate an acceptance of the ubiquity of delusion. [92]

By "this view" I understand you to be referring to "To be experiential means, quite simply, to have a relation to or to be influenced by one's background of past experiences." I happily accept that as an importantly insightful way of looking at the human condition. I don't see that as being in the slightest opposed to a recognition of the ubiquity of delusion. On the contrary, if one wants an insightful way of looking at the human condition, one should both want to have a relation to one's background of past experiences *and*, as an ongoing part of that background, want to adopt a series of practices that seek to reduce the grip of delusion.

RE [91] "Still, I would say that there is something to learn from studying the ways in which people construct themselves in the same situation, when talking about similar experiences in the broad sense."

I agree. What is tricky is to keep clear the distinction between (a) whether Zemeckis became insecure because of winning the Academy Award; (b) how Zemeckis constructs his public identity; and (c) what Zemeckis says. Those are very different things, and the good humanist (including the good scientist) would keep them separate. So I worry when you write:

> I would still insist that is there *another*, nonscientific way of <u>studying experience</u> that is based not on skepticism but on a relationship of trust between researcher and participant. You're free to think that this—humanistic?—approach to experience is messy and naive. But I am free to think—I think—that <u>what people say about their experiences</u> (whether they use the phrase 'the experience of x' or not) <u>is valuable, and deserves being studied as such.</u>

because that starts out about (a) experience and imperceptibly slides into (c) what people say.

[93] Here's a thought experiment for you: At the water's edge you find a lamp, rub it, and the genie says: "I can enlighten you about experience (including whether or to what extent experience is broadly similar or broadly different across people), or I can enlighten you about what people *say* about their experience (including whether or to what extent what people say about their experience is broadly similar or broadly different across people), but not both. You may request me to provide one of those enlightenments. However, I can read your heart and I know which you genuinely prefer, and I do not provide enlightenment to someone who asks in bad faith. You may make only one request. Which enlightenment do you prefer?" (Answer the genie before going further. Take your time—I'll wait.)

RE [91] "I would say that there is something to learn from studying the ways in which people construct themselves in the same situation, when talking about similar experiences in the broad sense. For example, we could ask a group of famous people what it meant for them to deal with unexpected success."

I agree entirely. If someone actually performed such a study and wrote about it, I myself would value consulting that study were I to encounter unexpected success. I would read it for the hints it might provide as I prepare myself for unanticipated events. As an intelligent humanist, I would, as I read that study, be processing at some level what I could glean (perhaps between the lines, etc.) about the distinctions between the actual experience and the constructed-self-presentation. That would in no way diminish the value of the study.

RE [88] "Now, as I understand this conversation, part of the question we're trying to deal with is the following: is there any common ground between the scientific and the [historical] humanistic project? The term 'experience' seems the most likely candidate for this bridge-building. But of course if you deny the continuity between pristine experience and experience in the broad sense, then it becomes difficult or impossible to find a common ground."

I do think the relationship between the scientific and the historical (humanistic) may be the center of gravity of our discussion.

First, I think whether or not to "deny the continuity between pristine experience and experience in the broad sense" depends on the intention and situation. In some senses I do *not* deny that continuity: Pristine experience fits, as does experience of India, into your (1)–(3c) definition of experience (I might quibble about some of those aspects, but my point here is in broad strokes). The potential discontinuity between pristine experience and broad-sense experience is more or less like the "discontinuity" between the rim and the floor of the Grand Canyon of Arizona: it's not *really* a discontinuity (there are trails back and forth), but it's a pretty darn big distinction, and failing to recognize the distinction might be fatal.

However, in other senses I do deny that continuity: Pristine experience is, or at least is approximately, a phenomenon that presents itself directly to the person. Broad-sense experience does not (I think) have any such direct presentation.

However, regardless of whether one thinks of continuity or discontinuity, I think that pristine experience is far more directly apprehendable than is broad-sense experience.

I think it is possible, and as I have said probably desirable, for reasonable people to be interested in both pristine experience and broad-sense experience. I do not think it is desirable to confuse the two, or to mistake the properties of the one for the properties of the other.

I think it is likely that pristine experience can be explored at a higher level of reliability and fidelity than can broad-sense experience. But so far, science (and humanism broadly defined) has not expressed much willingness to do so. My crystal ball says that is to the detriment of science and humanism broadly defined, but I happily accept that were an adequate science of pristine experience mounted, it might discover that the study of pristine experience is a dead end; therefore, those who resist the study of pristine experience might be prescient.

I observe a burgeoning interest in inner experience, in science and elsewhere, and also observe that that interest is instantiated mostly by studies of broad-sense experience that do not seem to contemplate the worries that I have described above. Sooner or later, if science is to advance, that has to be recognized as a problem (I think).

So I advocate, advocate, and advocate again (some might say harp on) the investigation of pristine experience not because it is the only or the best thing to investigate, but because nearly everyone (literary, scientific, etc.) overlooks it, overlooks it, overlooks it, says it is not important, says it doesn't exist, says it is impossible to investigate. I try not to overstate the potential importance of pristine experience, try not to shout, but it is difficult to be heard against the din of ignorance (in the etymological sense).

I think a mature science of experience would explore broad-sense experience if it wished, eyes wide open to its problematics, and in parallel would explore pristine experience, eyes wide open there, too. It may discover that neither route, nor both together, is productive. It may discover that one of the routes, but not the other, is productive. Most likely, it may discover that broad-sense investigations are most effective when they are anchored, informed, or otherwise enhanced by pristine experience investigations.

We are a long way from such a mature science.

What I say here about science applies equally, I think, to literature. The literary portraits of people would be, I think, more compelling, interesting, authentic, enlightening, etc., if they portrayed experience in high fidelity.

So the question that is at the center of our discussion seems to me to be: To what extent, or in what situations, or for which people, are our experiences similar? That is not a scientific question alone, or a literary question alone, but rather a humanistic (including both science and literature) question. I think, say, shout, harp, polemicize, that we humanists should take seriously the potential for substantial differences of experience (and of course I mean the manner of experience, not merely the content). I think that there are relatively huge unacknowledged differences, recognition of which might be of substantial benefit. I happily accept the possibility that I'm mistaken, but I think the evidence is on my side. I'm not by nature a shouter, and would be happy to abandon that behavior if given the opportunity.

RE [93] The genie.

Did you take that thought experiment seriously? My own answer is that I would far rather be enlightened about experience than about what people say about experience. What people say about experience is a mush of experience, whom they say it to, what they have previously said, what situational pressures there are, etc. Therefore the mush that people say about experience is broadly similar from one person to the next. I don't see any way to rise above that mush. By contrast, experience, at least pristine experience, is a far purer deal: I experience what I experience in the privacy of my own apprehension created by solely me for solely me without regard for what you think or might say and without regard for situation, etc. Pristine experience is not a mush, and therefore might differ substantially from one person to the next. I'd love to have the genie enlighten me about the differences between experiences, or to instruct me that I am mistaken.

X

PRISTINE EXPERIENCE, BROAD EXPERIENCE, PRESUPPOSITIONS, AND TENDENCIES; RUSS CHALLENGES JAMES JOYCE

March 15
Dear Russ,

In general terms, I agree that the investigation of pristine experience is important and valuable for the advancement of science, and that it has been largely overlooked—in literary studies as well as in other disciplines. My propositions are that (1) such project should be complemented by another project concerned with experience in the broad sense, and that (2) we should look for a synthesis between the two projects going forward. I take it that you agree with at least the first of these propositions when you write that "a mature science of experience would explore broad-sense experience if it wished, eyes wide open to its problematics, and in parallel explore pristine experience, eyes wide open there, too." I also take it that you go in the direction of my second proposition when you write that "Most likely, it may discover that broad-sense investigations are most effective when they are anchored, informed, or otherwise enhanced by pristine experience investigations." I think we have a genuine common ground here.

[94]

Let me summarize (what I regard as) the five main questions addressed by our recent discussion:

a) The status of experiences in the broad sense vis-à-vis pristine experience: do they fall into the same category?
b) Whether and to what extent experiences (pristine and broad) can be shared, linguistically or otherwise.
c) The difference between pristine experience and what people say about their experiences (broad experience).

d) The difference between a humanistic (or "historical" in the sense in which you used this term in chapter IX) and a scientific approach to experience.
e) The role of presuppositions and delusions.

ROAD MAP: *Russ agrees that these are the main "questions" discussed so far; they correspond to the first five of the ten themes listed after Marco's January 9 email in chapter I.*

Here are a few further thoughts on these issues:

1) Both pristine and nonpristine experiences are—for me—patterns of interaction or engagement between a subject and a worldly affordance rather than things that can be captured in what Daniel Hutto (2000) would call an "object-based schema."

In my view, the difference between pristine and nonpristine experience lies in the nature and scope of the worldly affordance, which is actual (i.e., present to the senses) and limited in the case of pristine experience, nonactual and apprehended through memory, reflection, etc., in the case of experiences in the broad sense. Cultural and personal presuppositions have a major role in constituting nonpristine experience, but I don't think they can be completely eliminated from (descriptions of) pristine experience—more on this in a moment. [95]

[96]

2) I think you're right to say that children, or perhaps psychotic individuals, do not experience the world in the same way as I do. But this does not entail that I am *incapable* of understanding—however vaguely—what the world looks like to a child or to a psychotic individual. Take, for example, your remark that "Dickens's account of a child coming of age (as this story is generally understood) would likely have been more interesting from a literary perspective if he had actually captured the experiential differences between kids, teenagers, and young adults." I completely agree with this characterization, and with the idea that literature is centrally concerned with the problem of conveying experiential differences. But doesn't this imply that the gap between one's own pristine experience and another's can be bridged—that there is a way for me to grasp the experience of a child—even if this is by no means automatic or straightforward? [97]

[98]

Further, I am not sure that the divide between children and adults, or psychotic and nonpsychotic individuals, can be adequately captured in terms of pristine experience *only*. I think experience in the broad sense—how they talk about the world and themselves or remember past events—would be equally important to describe the engagement with the world of these individuals. Indeed, a literary representation of childhood or psychosis cannot stay at the level of pristine experience but has to involve language and larger experiential dynamics.

[99] Take, for example, the beginning of Joyce's *A Portrait of the Artist as a Young Man* (1916/2000), which conveys the world as experienced by young Stephen Dedalus. I consider this an effective representation of a child's experience, and yet it seems to focus not on an experiential instant but on recurring sensations, linguistic idiosyncrasies, and memory traces (stories listened to, lullabies):

> Once upon a time and a very good time it was there was a moocow coming down along the road and this moocow that was coming down along the road met a nicens little boy named baby tuckoo . . .
> His father told him that story: his father looked at him through a glass: he had a hairy face.
> He was baby tuckoo. The moocow came down the road where Betty Byrne lived: she sold lemon platt.
>
> *O, the wild rose blossoms*
> *On the little green place.*
>
> He sang that song. That was his song.
>
> *O, the green wothe botheth.*
>
> When you wet the bed first it is warm then it gets cold. His mother put on the oilsheet. That had the queer smell.
> His mother had a nicer smell than his father. She played on the piano the sailor's hornpipe for him to dance. He danced:
>
> *Tralala lala,*
> *Tralala tralaladdy,*
> *Tralala lala,*
> *Tralala lala.*

Uncle Charles and Dante clapped. They were older than his father and mother but uncle Charles was older than Dante. (2000, 3)

The result is, as you would say, a mush—but it is precisely because of its "mushiness" that it seems to reflect the flow of the character's experience in an effective way.

Note that the question of the literary representation of characters' experiences is an important area of investigation in narrative and literary theory (Cohn, 1978; Herman, 2011). While this line of inquiry would benefit from a deeper understanding of the distinction between pristine and nonpristine experience, it is clear that literature itself tends to integrate—or perhaps conflate—these two aspects of experience, so it won't do to limit the investigation to one of them.

[100]

3) Regarding the difference between pristine experience and what people say about their experience, it seems to me that the reason why we differ in this connection is the following: for me, what people say or think about their experiences is not necessarily a source of noise and distortion. On the contrary, it can inform experience—even pristine experience, I believe—in ways that deserve being studied. Your quest for pristine experience looks like a quest for the holy grail of unadulterated (and "pretty darn knowable") experience, while I argue that such a quest is delusional, because pristine experience is always already influenced by presuppositions. I agree that it is important to curb presuppositions—in the sense of understanding their role and heightening people's awareness of their presence—but I don't think there is such a thing as experience *without* presuppositions.

[101]

Take nonhuman animals, for example. Since animals do not possess language and culture, it could be argued that they live only in pristine experience. Heidegger (2001, 242) meant something along these lines, I think, when he wrote that animals are "poor in world." But animals too have presuppositions of a nonlinguistic kind: the instinct to survive, to find food, to burrow, etc., are all predispositions that color animals' pristine experience. In my view, this implies that pristine experience is always caught in a relationship with one's "neuro-muscular-psychological being" and cannot be severed from an organism's experiential background. For me, such background *includes* people's presuppositions about experience—their socio-cultural representations of the world.

[102]

[103] This is not to say—as a social constructionist could say—that experience is *just* a cultural construction. On the contrary, it seems to me that experience (pristine and broad) emerges from the interaction between people's biological, neurological, psychological, etc., makeup and the socio-cultural practices that guide their interaction with the world.

[104] 4) I think you're right to argue that the scientific and humanistic perspectives are closer than is sometimes thought. Yet I think the difference between the scientific and the humanistic worldview is in some sense constitutive. I can see a trace of the former in your view that cultural presuppositions are a layer superimposed on pristine experience. At the cost of oversimplifying your position, I have the sense that culture and language are, for you, means for investigating pristine experience (at best) or things that get in the way of that investigation (at worst). For me, and I believe for all humanists, culture and language are neither means nor obstacles, but objects of investigation in their own right. Likewise, methodologically, scientists tend toward clarity and simplicity in order to reduce the factors involved in a study (as is evident from your focus on pristine experience and from your wanting to do away with presuppositions), while humanists embrace the "mess" that you associate with experience in the broad sense. For a humanist, such messiness is an intrinsic part of the human condition, and can be examined by exploring—rather than short shrifting—the presuppositions that give rise to cultural experience. I don't agree that there is no way "to rise above [the] mush [of what people say about experience]." As far as I can tell, good qualitative research in the social sciences seems to do just that. Which is to say: what people say about experience may be a mush, but there is method in this mush, and there are differences—some of them cultural, others personal—that deserve being illuminated and categorized.

5) RE [92] "I intended to advocate an acceptance of the ubiquity of delusion."

We've already discussed at length the issue of presuppositions. Here let me add a few remarks on delusion. I completely agree with you that it might be desirable to accept the ubiquity of delusion as an "antidote for arrogance and self-importance." If that is a way of saying that we should learn to distance ourselves from and question our own views, that idea is at least as old as Socratic irony, and (I think) a very good maxim for negotiating the world and avoiding conflict. I share that view on existential-ethical grounds. My worry has more to do with its implications for the study (both scientific and humanistic) of experience. We are all deluded, but there is no omniscient being who can decide in what respects each of us is deluded. And so what? Where do we go from there? I don't know.

Finally, regarding the genie: that is a very good—and witty—thought experiment, but I don't buy into the basic premise that we have to *choose* between pristine and nonpristine experience. I'd rather have my cake and eat it too.

March 19
Hi Marco—

I think we are making progress in exposing each other's views. I also think the effectiveness of our ability to do that depends on concrete examples, because they "prevent us from flying away into the abstract" (Hurlburt, in Hurlburt and Schwitzgebel, 2007, 257). So let's have a look at a couple of pristine experiences that I have written about, and to which we can refer below.

Here's a typical example from Melanie in my 2007 book:

Sample 4.1. Melanie's boyfriend was talking about life-threatening sports. Melanie was thinking about scuba diving, feeling an intense bodily yearning to go diving, like her body was going forward, and she was apparently also cognitively recognizing that yearning. She also experienced her body bobbing up and down as if in waves, though she was not actually moving. (Hurlburt and Schwitzgebel, 2007, 307)

Here's a typical example from Mike Kane in my 2011 book:

Sample 2.2. Mike is in the act of pouring honey mustard onto his son Ryan's plate. He's watching the flow/shape of the mustard stream— seeing the thick liquid hit the plate, watching the shape of the honey-mustard dollop as it spreads onto the plate. He's also saying aloud, "What d'ya say?!" and he's hearing his voice say that, hearing the sing-song, leading-question-to-a-juvenile characteristic of his voice. This is a hearing experience—he does not experience himself as saying these words (although obviously he is). The experience is entirely of hearing the sounds of the words. (Hurlburt and Kane, 2011, 96)

RE [94] "My propositions are that (1) such project should be complemented by another project concerned with experience in the broad sense, and that (2) we should look for a synthesis between the two projects going forward."

I agree.

RE [95] "In my view, the difference between pristine and nonpristine experience lies in the nature and scope of the worldly affordance, which is actual (i.e., present to the senses) and limited in the case of pristine experience, nonactual and apprehended through memory, reflection, etc., in the case of experiences in the broad sense."

I think "limited" mischaracterizes pristine experience. In fact, many if not most pristine experience is not limited by worldly affordances. Much pristine experience is quite removed from the current situation—pristine experience involves recollections of past events, creations of imagination that are not at all (or at least are not tightly) related to the immediate surroundings, and so on. And even to the extent that pristine experience is related to the scope of worldly affordance, attending to the pristine experiences of a variety of individuals reveals that at any given instant the worldly affordance is incredibly rich—at any given instant there are thousands or millions of substantially different potential pristine experiences that could be said to be limited to the scope of worldly affordance. I refer to that as the "welter"; out of the welter of potential experiences, the individual creates only one or a few actual pristine experiences at any given moment.

[108] For example, consider Melanie's scuba sample described above. That pristine experience is *related to* worldly affordances—the ongoing conversation is about life-threatening sports, which might be said to include scuba—but it is not at all *limited* by worldly affordances—the conversation has not been about scuba per se, nor about yearning, nor about a sense of bobbing up and down. In fact, her sense of bodily bobbing up and down is in contradiction to the worldly affordance, in which her body is still. And consider Mike's honey-mustard-dollop sample. Mike's experience is related to the environment (he sees the dollop and hears the voice) but not limited by it. Out of the welter (the plastic feel of the mustard bottle, the color of the honey mustard, the seeing/hearing of Ryan, the recollection of what his colleague had said in the meeting he had just left, the planning for Ryan's upcoming birthday party, the thousands or millions of other things that he might

directly experience at that moment), Mike created a particular pristine experience of dollop shape and voice sound.

The point is that a pristine experience is in absolutely no way the result of a passive perceiver being acted upon by environmental stimuli. Pristine experience, even when lying relatively tightly in the scope of worldly affordance, is an act of creation of the person. Mike hears the sound of his voice, does *not* attend to the meaning of the words his voice is articulating, does *not* experience himself as creating those words, and so on. Mike creates his experience out of the welter of potential experiences. [109]

RE [96] "Cultural and personal presuppositions . . . can[not] be completely eliminated from (descriptions of) pristine experience."

I agree, and would go further, as will be seen below, although I think your use of the word "presuppositions" here is problematic and likely to lead to confusions. Let's use the following example to see why. [110]

There are some people (many, actually) whose pristine experience is (I think) predominately characterized by sensory awareness (see my paper on that topic, which is reprinted as chapter 16 of my 2011 book). Sensory awareness is the paying of specific attention to some sensory aspect of the external or internal world, not for its utilitarian but for its sensory sake. For example, when walking I reach for the door handle to open the door. The handle falls on my retina, but that is *not* sensory awareness as I define the term. But if when walking as I reach for the door handle I notice the particular glint of the goldness as it reflects the sunlight, that *is* sensory awareness. The light hitting the retina may be identical in the two instances, but out of that worldly affordance on one occasion I pass into the house without thematically noticing anything of the door knob, whereas on another occasion I create a sensory awareness of the glint.

As I have said, I am convinced that some people's pristine experience is occupied by sensory awareness much or nearly all the time. (Mike Kane, of the honey-mustard-dollop sample and chapter 6 of my 2011 book, is one such person.) There are two simultaneous sensory awarenesses in the honey-mustard-dollop sample: the visual shape of the honey-mustard dollop, and the sing-song sound of his voice. Most of Mike's samples had some kind (or, as here, kinds) of sensory awareness of the external world.

Other people (me, for one) are not so preoccupied with sensory awareness. Many people, perhaps most, have very few sensory awarenesses as DES defines that term.

Now let's return to "Cultural and personal presuppositions . . . can[not] be completely eliminated from pristine experience," where I remove the parenthetical "(descriptions of)" for the moment. I think it is misleading to say that Mike's *presuppositions* lead him to sensory awareness, whereas my presuppositions lead me to some other form of inner experience. I think "predilections," "penchants," or "tendencies" is more straightforward. I happily agree that "Cultural and personal tendencies [or predilections or penchants] . . . can[not] be completely eliminated from pristine experience." Certainly Mike's personal tendencies when it comes to pristine experience are different from mine.

Therefore I think it is not desirable and probably not possible to remove the cultural and personal tendencies that lead to pristine experience. Furthermore, I do not think it is desirable to *try* to remove the cultural and personal tendencies. Those cultural and personal tendencies are what make Mike Mike and me me.

Now let's replace the deleted parenthetical (I italicize where I remove the parentheses): "Cultural and personal presuppositions . . . can[not] be completely eliminated from *descriptions of* pristine experience." Mike believed prior to sampling that he frequently engaged in inner speech. In fact, *none* of his random samples of experience included inner speech. To be certain we would have to sample much more thoroughly, but it seems safe to say that Mike was substantially mistaken about the role of inner speech in his own experience. (Mike is a well-known cognitive psychologist, so there can be no doubt that he knows what terms such as "inner speech" mean.) The term "presupposition" seems to fit this state of affairs quite straightforwardly: it makes sense to call Mike's false belief about his inner speech a presupposition.

Therefore it seems to me that your use of "presuppositions" confounds two very different things, so I have divided that term into two: presuppositions and personal tendencies. Presuppositions are what stand in the way of making faithful apprehensions of one's own pristine experience. Personal tendencies are what lead one to create particular kinds of pristine experience in the first place. (If you don't like those two terms, I'd be happy to hear alternatives. The point is that, whatever they are called, the two processes are very different.)

The distinction is (or at least may be) important because while it does make sense to say that Mike's *personal tendencies* are what make Mike Mike, it does *not* seem nearly as sensible to say that Mike's *presuppositions* are what make Mike Mike. Now I am not entirely dismissing the constitutive importance of Mike's presuppositions—certainly Mike would be a somewhat different Mike if he had no such presuppositions. My point is relative: I think Mike would be a *very* different person if his personal tendencies were different (that is, if he often created inner speakings but never created sensory awarenesses), whereas Mike would be only a *somewhat* different person if he had a higher-fidelity view of his experience (if he accurately recognized his low frequency of inner speech and high frequency of external-world sensory awareness). I happily accept that I might be mistaken, and that I don't have a scale for measuring "very" and "somewhat," nor do I know on what the size of "very" and "somewhat" depends (age? gender? personality? etc.). A mature science of experience would have to figure those things out. All I can say, on the basis of my sampling with some hundreds of people, is that "very" and "somewhat" seem to convey the strongly different sizes of the effects that I have observed.

RE [97] "But this does not entail that I am *incapable* of understanding—however vaguely—what the world looks like to a child or to a psychotic individual."

I agree entirely. If I have ever implied that, then I have misspoken. I have not tried to say that you are *incapable* of understanding, only that you probably don't have the necessary facts at your disposal. Not understanding and incapable of understanding are two entirely different things. I don't understand nuclear physics, but I am probably capable of such understanding.

[111]

RE [99] "Take, for example, the beginning of Joyce's *A Portrait of the Artist as a Young Man*, which conveys the world as experienced by young Stephen Dedalus. I consider this an effective representation of a child's experience, and yet it seems to focus not on an experiential instant but on recurring sensations, linguistic idiosyncrasies, and memory traces (stories listened to, lullabies)."

I suspect this is close to the heart of the matter: On what warrant do you consider Joyce's words to be an effective representation of a child's experience? I'm no Joyce scholar, and I'm not even a scholar of

[112] the development of human experience. But I think it likely that Joyce's words do not effectively represent a 2-year-old's (or whatever age Stephen is taken to be) experience. I've seen enough experiences to think, for example, that "When you wet the bed first it is warm then it gets cold" is an adult's kind of thinking, not a 2-year-old's. A 2-year-old might feel warm, and then sometime later (by adult's reckoning) feel cold. So a 2-year-old's representation might be *Warm . . . cold,* or maybe *warmwet . . . coldwet,* or maybe just *coldwet* (because the discrimination of *warmwet* from *warm* hasn't yet been acquired) or maybe *coldwetMommyNo*. But that is not the experience of a sequence ("first it . . . and then it"). And a 2-year-old is not capable of thinking in the universal "you" (as in "When *you* wet the bed"); if there is any experience of sequence, it is when *I* wet the bed. Thus an adult, but not a 2-year-old, would notice: "When you wet the bed first it is warm then it gets cold."

I could make similar arguments about nearly every sentence or clause in the passage you cite. For example: I think there is no "road where Betty Byrne lives" in a 2-year-old's experience. An adult has a concept of a road to a place (an adult understands that the road is the same road whether walked or driven or bicycled), but I am not at all sure that is true of 2-year-olds. What an adult thinks of as taking the road to Betty Byrne's, a 2-year-old might experience while walking *nice blue thing . . . light feeling . . . wanna goNONO . . . wanna NO . . . Sam . . . barky Barky BARKY! walk walk walk walk Barky! Walk . . . light feeling Betty Betty!* but while being driven (down what the adult would know as the same road) something more like *Mommy pinch me . . . Vroom . . . big tree . . . big tree . . . Betty! . . . lemmeout . . . lemmeout . . . Betty!*

Similarly, I suspect there is no "his song" in a 2-year-old's experience: sometimes he sings, sometimes he sings (what an adult would know as the same song), sometimes he sings (what an adult would know as the same song), sometimes he sings (what an adult would now call *his* song). I doubt that a 2-year-old makes the causal connection between piano playing and horn piping. In short, I suspect that Joyce's *Portrait* opening should *not* be considered an effective representation of a child's experience.

I happily accept that I might be mistaken. I don't know much about children's experience. I do know quite a bit (I think) about what it would take to find out about children's experience, and as far as I know that has not been adequately done. Maybe Joyce has channeled a 2-year-old in a way more effective than I can imagine, but I know of no warrant for believing that—perhaps you can enlighten me.

I (wildly) speculate that the situation is more like this: Joyce more or less carefully observes 2-year-old's speech patterns and behavior and then writes an evocation of 2-year-old's experience that corresponds in a plausible way to Joyce's observations. Marco buys into that plausibility because it more or less corresponds to what Marco has more or less carefully observed about children's speech patterns and behavior. That is, Joyce has awakened a shared plausibility of adult-views-of-children's experience, not constrained on either side by actual children's experience.

In 2011, on a similar topic, I wrote:

> Q: I'm still struggling to understand what you mean by bracketing of presuppositions, and would like to know what you think of this: Samuel Taylor Coleridge, the novelist and poet best known for *The Rime of the Ancient Mariner* and *Kubla Khan*, talked about "suspension of disbelief" as a process that a good novelist evokes from readers. It basically consists of instilling a narrative with enough realistic or human elements for the reader to accept all sorts of fantastical elements in a story. The reader suspends his disbelief to be able to follow and become engaged in a fantastical story. So, I can enjoy the movie *Spiderman* because I have suspended my disbelief for a couple of hours and am choosing to believe that there is this guy who can propel himself across New York skyscrapers through the webs that flow from his fingers. It seems to me that you are asking your reader to do the opposite: Suspend *belief*. Put your beliefs aside, some of which may indeed be fantastical, so that you can follow and become engaged in the only real story. So Coleridge had the suspension of disbelief and you have the suspension of belief. Is that what you mean?
>
> A: Exactly! Coleridge adds enough truthiness to make a story compelling. I want to subtract enough truthiness to make an account faithful. (Hurlburt, 2011a, 181)

Similarly, I think Joyce invites you to suspend disbelief and enter into the imagined space of the child's experience. But that no more implies that the experience is veridical than that Spiderman's finger webs are veridical.

I have no objection to Joyce's "focus[ing] not on an experiential instant but on recurring sensations, linguistic idiosyncrasies, and memory traces (stories listened to, lullabies)." In fact, I have no objection to Joyce at all. Joyce did *not* claim (and he is under absolutely no obligation so to claim) that he was giving a veridical account of 2-year-old-Stephen's experience, and therefore he should not be held to account on that score. I suspect that Joyce wanted to get Marco to suspend his adult concerns (with bills and salaries and auto repairs and illnesses), and to do so, Joyce instilled his narrative with enough realistic or human 2-year-old elements (bedwetting and walking to friends' houses) to induce Marco to suspend disbelief and enliven the impression that he is entering the experiential world of a 2-year-old. Apparently Joyce was successful, and that is a testament to his skill as a novelist. So I'm not in the least critical of Joyce; my noticing the probably unfaithful nature of his account of 2-year-old Stephen's experience in no way diminishes the importance or impact of *A Portrait of the Artist as a Young Man*. (It does suggest that some other novelist might with some effect paint a 2-year-old's experience picture of higher fidelity. But that is not a criticism of Joyce any more than the use of the electron microscope is a criticism of van Leeuwenhoek.)

My criticism is that you seem to have transcended your Joyce-induced suspension of disbelief about a 2-year-old's experience into the belief that you have encountered, in Joyce, "an effective representation of a child's experience." Not disbelieving is not the same thing as believing. I don't disbelieve that Einstein's cosmological constant exists, but that doesn't imply that I believe in its existence. I'm simply ignorant.

I reiterate: I may be mistaken in my criticism: you may have a warrant for believing that Joyce provided "an effective representation of a child's experience." I would be pleased to hear the grounds for that warrant.

RE [98] "[Is] there . . . a way for me to grasp the experience of a child . . . ?"

Largely, Yes. If someone were to present to you in high fidelity a series of pristine experiences of a child, in a way that was faithful to the child's experience and yet understandable to adults, then I think you could grasp (probably not perfectly but with pretty high fidelity) that experience. Our difference seems to be that you think that Joyce has done that for you, whereas I doubt that he has. I think it possible to present children's experiences in an understandable way—I myself have tried to do that with older children. (There may well be an age where this ability breaks down; I don't know what that age is.) I think that presenting in high fidelity the inner experience of children is extraordinarily difficult for many reasons (not the least of which is the I-think-mistaken belief that it has already been done by Joyce and others, and therefore there is no need to trouble oneself to do better). One could say that my principal aim is to motivate people to try to present experiences (including children's) in high fidelity, to try to lay out why this is difficult and what must be done to overcome those difficulties, so that I, you, and others can then "grasp the experience of a child" as a child experiences it (as best that can be done).

RE [100] "So it won't do to limit the investigation to one of them [pristine experience and broad experience]."

I agree. I would be happy to stop saying "pristine experience, pristine experience! pristine experience!! PRISTINE EXPERIENCE!!!" if there were some general recognition that the pristine-experience fork in the road exists and that it might be desirable to take both forks in the road.

RE [101] "Your quest for pristine experience looks like a quest for the holy grail of unadulterated (and 'pretty darn knowable') experience, while I argue that such quest is delusional, because pristine experience is always already influenced by presuppositions. I agree that it is important to curb presuppositions—in the sense of understanding their role and heightening people's awareness of their presence—but I don't think there is such a thing as experience *without* presuppositions."

That you would think that I engage in such a quest may reflect a misunderstanding of pristine experience, so let's examine the examples from Melanie and Mike as introduced above.

As I said above, I fully accept that pristine experience is always already influenced by personal tendencies (to use "presuppositions" here, as I said above, is misleading). Melanie's scuba bobbing experience is copiously shaped by her genetic structure (she has to be capable of imagining body movement when none is present), her culture (she has to recognize scuba as life threatening), her language skill (she has to understand the life-threatening reference), her personal history (she has to have been scuba diving).

Similarly, Mike's honey-mustard-dollop pristine experience is copiously shaped by his genetic structure (e.g., he must have eyes to see the stream), his culture (which, e.g., suggests the desirability of children's saying "thank you"), his language skill (that he would say to his child "d'ya" instead of "do you"), his personal history (e.g., he apparently has said this many times), and so on.

Therefore I entirely agree that there is no such a thing as experience *without* personal tendencies and personal histories. I agree that a quest for such a thing would be delusional. However, I do not think that I engage in such a quest. I try to describe pristine experience in the full glory of its adulteration, if by that you mean as shaped by the person's genetic, cultural, language, personal, and so on, history.

RE [102] "The instinct to survive, to find food, to burrow, etc., are all predispositions that color animals' pristine experience."

If (a) by "predispositions" you mean what I have called "tendencies" above (I considered using "predispositions" instead of "tendencies," but "predispositions" has a too-cognitive connotation for my tastes—that is, it is too close to "presupposition," which is the contrast I was trying to highlight); and if (b) we now accept that neither of us knows anything about animals' pristine experience, then this sentence might be recast: "the instinct to survive, to find food, to burrow, etc., are all *personal tendencies* (or perhaps just *tendencies*) that color animals' *behavior*." If that is what you mean, I totally agree.

RE [101] "[Pristine experience is] the holy grail of . . . 'pretty darn knowable' . . . experience."

Your section (3) suggests to me that I have not communicated adequately the distinction between pristine experience and experience in the broad sense. The distinction does *not* arise from the fact that I think pristine experience is pure, or is unadulterated, or is the holy grail; I think none of those things.

I do think that pristine experience bears pretty darn close examination. The more careful the method, the higher the fidelity of the apprehension of pristine experience. (I accept that that is true only up to a point, which is why I use the "pretty darn" modifier. There is no possibility of perfection.)

By contrast, broad experience does not bear pretty darn close examination. The more careful the method, the *less* confident one will become about the apprehension of broad experience. There is no method that I know of that can improve the fidelity of the apprehension of broad experience without dramatically altering the notion of broad experience.

RE [101] "Pristine experience is . . . unadulterated."

First, as I have said above, I happily accept that pristine experience is adulterated in the sense that it reflects the cultural and personal tendencies that we have discussed. Pristine experience is *essentially adulterated*, based on cultural and personal tendencies, not just around the edges, but centrally.

But pristine experience is unadulterated in the sense that your pristine experience is created by you, of you, for you, and only by, of, and for you. It is private, created outside of the view of mothers, wives, coworkers, friends, enemies, priests, judges, lawyers, competitors, collaborators, etc., that is, out of the reach of anyone for whom you might want to create an impression. Pristine experience is unadulterated by anyone other than you.

[113]

Pristine experience is largely independent of others—Mike Kane, for example, was likely to have sensory awarenesses when with his daughter, and when with his coworker, and when by himself. Why? Because he has thousands of hours of practice creating pristine experiences, and as a result has developed (based on his physiology, history, and who knows what else) the particular skill of sensory awareness. Do the math: 30 years × 365 days × 16 hours × 60 minutes × 20 experiences (give or take); that's 200,000,000 pristine experiences, all created by the same person using the same materials (neurons, bones, etc.) for the same person. Mike is *good at* sensory awarenessing.

By contrast, broad experience is nearly always adulterated by some other(s). The notion of the experience of India arises typically in conversation with some person, and likely arises somewhat differently in conversation with a friend than with an enemy, or with a priest, or with a collaborator, etc.

So the term "adulterated" is problematic: it is fair to say that pristine experience is adulterated and that it is not adulterated. Our task is to keep the two meanings far apart.

I say that pristine experience is an easier study than broad experience because pristine experience is, in the second sense just described, unadulterated: it is always of, by, and for the same person. That does not imply that studying pristine experience is more useful than studying broad experience; being confident about that would require a mature science of experience.

RE [103] "It seems to me that experience (pristine and broad) emerges from the interaction between people's biological, neurological, psychological, etc., makeup and the socio-cultural practices that guide their interaction with the world."

I worry about a sentence like this, which has the same structure as: "it seems to me that apples (McIntosh and Granny Smith) both make good pie." That is, your sentence structure implies that pristine and broad are two subsets of the same class "experience," implies that there are far more similarities than differences between the two classes "pristine experience" and "broad experience." I think it is true that pristine experience emerges from the interaction between people's biological, neurological, psychological, etc., makeup and the socio-cultural practices that guide their interaction with the world. Also, I think it is true that broad experience emerges from the interaction between people's biological, neurological, psychological, etc., makeup and the socio-cultural practices that guide their interaction with the world. But that doesn't imply that pristine experience and broad experience are similar, any more than the two sentences "apples make good pie" and "chocolate makes good pie" implies that apples are similar to chocolate.

Therefore your sentence structure implies small differences between pristine and broad experience, when I think the differences are large. Thus we have returned (or never strayed far from) your question "(a) The status of experiences in the broad sense vis-à-vis pristine experience: Do they fall into the same category?" Table 4 provides a review.

Each of those Yeses and Nos should be understood to be only approximations—that is, I think we could probably quibble (and have quibbled) about the details of any of those. So "Yes" should be understood to mean "substantially more Yes than No" and vice versa. And perhaps you have other considerations that could be added to the table.

Of those, the central distinction seems to me to be between a directly apprehended phenomenon and an inference or construction. For example, Mike understood himself (prior to sampling) to engage frequently in inner speaking and not frequently in visual sensory awareness of the external world. It seems to me that we would

TABLE 4. Comparing pristine experience and broad experience

CONSIDERATION	PRISTINE EXPERIENCE	EXPERIENCE IN THE BROAD SENSE
Important (worthy of consideration)?	Yes	Yes
A phenomenon (present to the senses)?	Yes	No
Must be inferred or constructed?	No	Yes
Shaped by personal tendencies?	Yes	Yes
Shaped by presuppositions?	No	Yes
Exists relatively independent of the interlocutor?	Yes	No
Can training/method substantially improve the fidelity of apprehension?	Yes	No

call *I-talk-to-myself-frequently* Mike's experience-in-the-broad-sense of himself. (And those are not merely inconsequential details—Mike is a cognitive psychologist for whom thinking is an important subject matter.) Sampling revealed (to a high probability, one that could be made higher with additional investigation) that that experience-in-the-broad-sense was not a faithful account of his pristine experience.

I think it is important to try to understand both the pristine experience and the experience-in-the-broad-sense in this situation. In Mike's case, the investigation of pristine experience is what reveals that the experience-in-the-broad-sense is not faithful, and that is (or should be) an important aspect of the experience-in-the-broad-sense investigation. The experience-in-the-broad-sense investigation would reveal that many (probably most, including probably most cognitive psychologists) people believe their pristine experience to be verbal, and would try to understand where, why, and how that shared (but largely incorrect) notion arose.

RE [104] "I have the sense that culture and language are, for you, means for investigating pristine experience (at best) or things that get in the way of that investigation (at worst)."

For me (as I think for you), culture and language are sometimes means, sometimes objects of investigation. I would, for example, greatly value cross-cultural investigations of pristine experience. Nothing like that has been done (high on my list of personal failings). Do you suppose that native Chinese speakers' pristine experiences are similar to native English speakers? I don't know either. How about tribes in the Oro region of Ethiopia? An investigation of pristine experience in all those places (which I would love to do) would be simultaneously an investigation of experience, of language, and of culture. There are lots of studies that discuss the language and cultural differences among the English speakers, the Chinese speakers, and the Oro tribes. I suspect that much would be added by including an investigation of the pristine-experience differences (if they exist).

RE [105] "We are all deluded, but there is no omniscient being who can decide in what respects each of us is deluded. And so what? Where do we go from there? I don't know."

Neither did Socrates, as I understand him. What many call "Socratic irony" I think of as Socratic straightforwardness: when he said "I don't know," he meant, very simply and candidly, without a trace of irony, that he didn't know. That is, I think it was *not* the case, as is often meant by "Socratic irony," that Socrates was pretending ignorance as a means of eliciting some desired thought process from his interlocutor. He was simply ignorant, and he knew it and said it.

My take on where to go from here is to do more or less what (I think) Socrates did: try to figure out, with all the genuineness and sincerity we can muster, how to talk about things that are important, try to learn how to avoid saying things that are misleading or not true, in the hopes that tomorrow we will be better able to figure out what is important and more genuinely able to talk about those things and thus better able to avoid saying misleading or false things, in the hopes that the next day we will be better still. To try in that way, while perhaps difficult, is well within the human range of abilities. I don't know whether it is possible to attain the goal of perfection in knowing what is important and how to talk about it without misleading. As far as I can tell, Socrates didn't know that either, but that didn't stop him from trying. A foundational part of that trying is the recognition that at any given time on any given subject matter, one's view, which seems so obviously true as to be taken for granted, may be false (that is, I think, the heart of delusion). Therefore an important part of that trying probably has to involve enlisting others to attack the same subject matter from a different perspective. Such interlocutor-enlisted procedure provides no guarantees (shared delusion is obviously possible), but it can raise the stakes on particular details, thus providing the opportunity to refine the understanding of those details.

RE [106] Regarding the genie thought experiment: "I don't buy into the basic premise that we have to *choose* between pristine and nonpristine experience."

The genie's purpose was not so much to force a choice as to pry the two apart so as to tap into genuineness.

XI

ON THE ADULTERATION OF PRISTINE EXPERIENCE

March 22
Dear Russ,
Please see the comments below.
Marco

RE [107] "I . . . think the effectiveness of our ability to [make progress] depends on concrete examples."

You're perfectly right about this. This is a golden rule for literary theory, too: one should always anchor theoretical models to concrete examples and close readings, as I tried to do with the Joyce passage.

RE [108] "Pristine experience is *related to* worldly affordances . . . but it is not at all *limited* by worldly affordances."

I completely agree with you here. I was wrong to write that pristine experience is necessarily about actual worldly affordances. They do not have to be actual, because pristine experience is often about nonactual (remembered, imagined, etc.) events and existents. "Worldly" is problematic for the same reasons. These affordances remain, however, present to the senses—I think the difference between pristine and broad experience boils down to this.

RE [109] "The point is that a pristine experience is in absolutely no way the result of a passive perceiver being acted upon by environmental stimuli. Pristine experience, even when lying relatively tightly in the scope of worldly affordance, is an act of creation of the person."

Again, I entirely agree with this. Broad experience is an act of creation, too.

I guess you would argue that broad experience, unlike pristine experience, is co-created by the experiencer *and* by the situation in which he or she describes an experience. Perhaps that is another way of capturing the difference between pristine and broad experience: pristine experience is created by the interaction between a subject and a situation (be it actual, like seeing a honey-mustard dollop, or nonactual, like feeling an intense desire to go scuba diving); broad experience is created by the interaction between a subject, one or more past situations (the many situations I found myself in while traveling through India), and the situation in which I describe my "experience of traveling through India." Again, I believe this account shows that—while pristine and broad experience *are* different—they are not categorically different: broad experience adds one level of mediation, but the basic mechanism (the interaction between a subject and a situation) is there.

In my view, pristine and broad experience may be as different as McIntosh and Granny Smith apples, but not as apples and chocolate. [117]

RE [110] "I think your use of the word 'presuppositions' here is problematic and likely to lead to confusions."

In general terms, you are right about the usefulness of distinguishing between "presuppositions" and "tendencies."

I'm happy to use the term "tendencies," but I still think that there is a lot in common between presuppositions and tendencies, since they all form a backdrop to our engagement with the world, guiding and coloring it in various ways. Not all of them have the same importance, of course, and I agree with you that "Mike would be a *very* different person if his personal tendencies were different . . . , whereas Mike would be only a *somewhat* different person if he had a higher-fidelity view of his experience." However, it seems to me that what you call presuppositions tout court are actually presuppositions *about experience*—i.e., beliefs about how experience works or what it is like. [118]

To go further, if pristine experience is shaped by biological, cultural, and personal tendencies, then pristine experience has at least this in common with experience in the broad sense. Those tendencies will act on both my reports about pristine experience and on my descriptions of experiences in the broad sense. When I say that both of these kinds of experiences are "experiential," I am referring to the impact of these biological, cultural, and personal tendencies on people's interaction with the world. Of course, you could still say that descriptions of broad experience are *also* conditioned by our interlocutors and by the communicative situation, whereas descriptions of pristine experience are "unadulterated by anyone other than you." More about this in a moment.

RE [111] "I have not tried to say that you are *incapable* of understanding, only that you probably don't have the necessary facts at your disposal."

To me, this means that, given the necessary facts, experiences can be shared—even though I am ready to concede that they are not *genuinely* shared every time people say that they have shared an experience with someone else.

The difference between me and you seems to be that, for me, "the necessary facts" are usually much more easily accessible than they are for you (cf. your parallel with nuclear physics). Preverbal children and psychotic individuals are a somewhat extreme case, but in other scenarios I think we already possess most of the necessary facts for understanding others' experiences. But here, again, a lot depends on how similar experience A (undergone by one person) should be to experience B (undergone by another person) to qualify as a shared experience. I am ready to grant that experiences rendered at DES-level detail are almost impossible to share without *a lot* of "necessary facts" that we don't usually have at our disposal. Perhaps, then, what I am saying is that broad experiences are relatively easy to share, but that "sharing" would not stand up to closer, DES-level examination. However, I do think the sharing of broad experiences is (or can be) genuine sharing—it only has less rigorous standards than DES-level sharing. After all, DES is a scientific project, while broad experiences are usually shared in casual, everyday interaction. We can't expect those two activities to meet the same criteria.

RE [112] "I think it likely that Joyce's words do not effectively represent a 2-year-old's (or whatever age Stephen is taken to be) experience."

I think you've misunderstood my use of (or I've misspoken) the adjective "effective." To me, "effective" does not mean "scientifically accurate" or "veridical"—it means that Joyce created a representation of a young child's experience that strikes me as interesting, innovative, and convincing. (For more on this illusion, see my Caracciolo, 2014a.) Joyce succeeded in suspending my disbelief, but I doubt that this is what being a young child is really like. Thus, I completely agree with you that "Joyce did *not* claim (and he is under absolutely no obligation so to claim) that he was giving a veridical account of 2-year-old Stephen's experience." Unlike science, literary, fictional narrative does not make any truth claims about the world.

I think the illusion that literature can create of experiencing the world through a child's perspective is not without real-world consequences, however. It may invite me to reflect on the difference between my experience and other people's (including young children's). It may invite me to *value* this difference, and children's experience, more highly than if I observed them only from the outside. It may even encourage me to open a dialogue with a certain psychologist who scientifically investigates pristine experience. None of these things depend on the scientific accuracy of Joyce's text.

Further, I would insist that the *effectiveness* (in the sense defined above) of Joyce's text depends on its weaving a number of (apparently) pristine experiences into a temporal pattern. Thus, the result resembles more closely the description of an experience in the broad sense than a DES report (however referentially described). In my view, this shows that for all their constructedness, descriptions of broad experiences strike us as inherently experiential. But I think we've already agreed on this point. You're right to say that "The potential discontinuity between pristine experience and broad-sense experience is more or less like the 'discontinuity' between the rim and the floor of the Grand Canyon of Arizona: it's not *really* a discontinuity (there are trails back and forth), but it's a pretty darn big distinction, and failing to recognize the distinction might be fatal."

RE [113] "Pristine experience is unadulterated by anyone other than you."

It seems to me that this statement clashes with your claim that pristine experience is influenced by culture [at RE 101]. Insofar as a "person's language" and "cultural history" are shared with other people, acquired in intersubjective engagements, and co-constructed as joint human endeavors, our pristine experiences (and descriptions thereof) are *also* shaped by other people. You may be right to say that pristine experience is *less* adulterated by other people than is broad experience, but I still see that difference as a difference in degree, not in kind.

Take, for example, a paper in which Winawer, Witthoft, Frank, et al. (2007) showed that native speakers of Russian (a language that has two different words for "light blue" and "dark blue") perform better than native speakers of English on a color discrimination task—i.e., that they are quicker at distinguishing between the two shades of blue. This finding seems to suggest that people's perception is shaped by linguistic categories that are, in an important sense, shared—and that therefore there is no such thing as experience "unadulterated by anyone other than you."

RE [114] Your table.

I would edit it as shown in table 5. I think those are the most important considerations.

Table 5. Comparing pristine experience and broad experience (Marco's revision of table 4)

CONSIDERATION	PRISTINE EXPERIENCE	EXPERIENCE IN THE BROAD SENSE
Important (worthy of consideration)?	Yes	Yes
A phenomenon (present to the senses)?	Yes	No (but it typically involves phenomena)
Is an act of creation of the person?	Yes	Yes
Must be inferred or constructed?	No?	Yes
Shaped by ~~personal~~ tendencies?	Yes	Yes
Shaped by presuppositions about experience?	No	Yes
[122] Exists relatively independent of the interlocutor?	Yes (I would say no)	No
[123] Can be easily shared with others?	No	Yes
[124] Can training/method ~~substantially~~ improve the fidelity of apprehension?	Yes, substantially	No (I would say yes, marginally)

I agree that experience in the broad sense is not in itself a phenomenon—as we defined it a couple of emails ago—although I think it involves a number of phenomena (sensory imaginings and memories).

I'm not really clear on what you mean by "Must be inferred or constructed." If "training/method [can] substantially improve the fidelity of apprehension," then pristine experience can be said to be intersubjectively constructed (through the DES interview).

I would either add "biological" and "cultural" to "personal tendencies" or drop the "personal" altogether.

I would also add "about experience" after "shaped by presuppositions" to specify what we mean by "presuppositions."

As for "Exists relatively independent of the interlocutor," I have already said that some "tendencies" are acquired in intersubjectivity and shared with other people. However "private" pristine experience may appear, it cannot exist independently of other people. A further confirmation of this comes from the fact that the DES method is *based* on intersubjectivity (and *a fortiori* pristine experience cannot "exist relatively independent of the interlocutor"—depending on how much weight you attach to the "relatively," of course).

I do think training/method can improve the fidelity of the apprehension of experience in the broad sense, though perhaps not "substantially" (presuppositions about experience are difficult to eliminate in descriptions of broad experiences).

RE [115] "An investigation of pristine experience in all those places (which I would love to do) would be simultaneously an investigation of experience, of language, and of culture."

I agree that this would be an extremely worthwhile project. But, again, if you think cultural differences could have an impact on pristine experience, how can it be that "pristine experience is unadulterated by anyone other than you"?

[125]

RE [116] "An important part of that trying probably has to involve enlisting others to attack the same subject matter from a different perspective."

If this follows from being aware of our own delusions, then I agree that such awareness is an important—indeed, crucial—insight into the human condition.

XII

PHENOMENA, ADULTERATION, APPLES, AND TURKEY

March 28
Hi Marco—
I think we may have reduced our sauce down to three important themes: phenomenon, unadulterated, and language. But some more simmering seems required.
—Russ

RE [117] "In my view, pristine and broad experience may be as different as McIntosh and Granny Smith apples, but not as apples and chocolate."

I think pristine and broad experiences are *more* different than are apples and chocolate, and therefore *much more* different than are McIntosh and Granny Smith apples.

We have agreed, I think, that pristine experiences are phenomena whereas broad experiences are not phenomena. The phenomena/not-phenomena distinction is the defining difference between pristine and broad experiences: pristine experiences belong in the category *phenomena*; broad experiences do not belong in that category. Pristine experiences present themselves directly to a person; broad experiences do not.

I think that if we keep the phenomena/not-phenomena distinction firmly in view, then everything else is a detail. Whether either or both is an act of creation of a person is not consequential to the distinction between pristine and broad experience. That both *depend on* phenomena is not consequential to the definition of pristine and broad experience. Whether either or both are affected by language is not consequential to the definition of pristine and broad experience; whether either or both are created by interaction between subject and situation is not consequential; whether there are two or three levels is not consequential; and so on. Regardless of how, why, by whom, or where they are created, the fundamental difference between pristine experience and broad experience is that a pristine experience is a phenomenon, directly apprehended by a person, whereas a broad experience is not a phenomenon, is not directly apprehended by a person.

However, we apparently have not agreed on the importance of the phenomena/not-phenomena distinction. I hold, and will try to emphasize, that the phenomena/not-phenomena distinction is a *larger* difference than between apples and chocolate, whereas you hold it to be a similar difference as between McIntosh and Granny Smith apples and therefore a *much smaller* difference than between apples and chocolate.

To extend the metaphor, I think the difference between pristine experience and broad experience is roughly the same magnitude as the difference between the *taste* of apples and the *significance* of apples. The fundamental distinction is that taste is a phenomenon; significance is not a phenomenon. All other differences are secondary: That both taste and significance are created by a person is not consequential to the distinction between them; that significance *depends* to some degree on phenomena (if apples did not taste good, their significance would be different); that both depend to some extent on language (should a rose apple be considered an apple?) is not constitutive of the difference between taste and significance.

Taste does indeed depend on history, culture, and language: people who had two different words for sweet-like-a-McIntosh and tart-like-a-Granny-Smith would no doubt have somewhat different taste phenomena. But that is a detail in comparison to the main difference: taste is a phenomenon (directly apprehended by a person, albeit in private); significance is not a phenomenon. Significance fundamentally depends on the for-what: is our interest in the "An apple a day keeps the doctor away" significance? Is our interest in the "Apples as an antidote to obesity" significance? Is our interest in the "Apple pie as a mainstay of Marie Callender restaurants" significance? Is our interest in the "Apples as a factor in the economy of Washington State" significance?

You might say that significance and broad experience are not the same thing, and I agree, but I think they are similar. Significance, like broad experience, is not a phenomenon. Significance, like broad experience, derives from some complex judgments based on a variety of messy-or-impossible-to-specify factors, depends in some way on phenomena, depends fundamentally on the context. Therefore it seems to me that broad experience is *more similar to* significance than broad experience is to pristine experience.

[127]

More about phenomena below.

RE [125] "If you think cultural differences could have an impact on pristine experience, how can it be that 'pristine experience is unadulterated by anyone other than you'?"

A guy walks into a bar and says, "I'd like a drink of water, please." The bartender says, "With Scotch or bourbon?" The guy replies, "I'd like my water unadulterated," to which the bartender responds, "We don't have unadulterated water. Our water has calcium, sodium, iron, and lots of other trace minerals in it." The moral: we have to be careful not to confuse the magnitude of our adulterants.

[128] I accept that culture (including language) has an impact on pristine experience, but that adulteration is at a much smaller ("trace") magnitude than when I say "adulterated by someone other than you." Consider this new thought experiment. Scenario 1: Suppose you, Marco, are to create a movie where you, Marco, are the producer and also the writer and also the director, actor, cinematographer, and editor, and that your movie will be encrypted so that you can be confident that you, Marco, will be the lone projectionist and the lone member of the audience. That's a movie made by, of, and for Marco alone. Scenario 2: Suppose you, Marco, are to produce a movie where the writer is Adam, the director is Betty, the actor is Charles, the cinematographer is Delilah, the editor is Eli; and y'all will create a movie that will be shown by thousands of projectionists to millions of audience members. That is a movie made by Marco, Adam, Betty, Charles, Delilah, and Eli for many others.

I accept that the by-of-for-Marco-alone movie is impacted by the culture: the hardware is cultural, the potential topics are cultural, Marco's movie-making sensitivities are cultural, and so on. And yet I think there is an important way in which the by-of-for-Marco-alone movie-making situation is different from the by-Marco-Adam-Betty-Charles-Delilah-Eli-for-countless-unspecified-others movie-making situation. The viewer of the by-of-for-Marco-alone movie knows that every second of the movie reflects Marco's sensibilities in an important way (and also reflects the culture in an important way). By contrast, the viewer of the by-Marco-Adam-Betty-Charles-Delilah-Eli-for-countless-unspecified-others movie does not know at any second whether or to what extent the movie reflects Marco's, or Adam's, or Betty's, or Charles's, or Delilah's, or Eli's, or some-combination-thereof's sensibilities in an important way (and also reflects the culture in an important way). Do you agree that those situations are importantly different? If so, what term would you suggest to differentiate them? I have used "unadulterated by others" to refer to the by-of-for-Marco-alone movie, but I would be happy to hear alternatives.

Marco's pristine experience, I think, is by, of, and for Marco alone, unadulterated (or whatever substitute term you prefer) by anyone other than Marco, even though Marco's pristine experience is affected by the culture, language, and personal history.

RE [121] "This finding [by Winawer, Witthoft, Frank, et al., 2007] seems to suggest that people's perception is shaped by linguistic categories."

As I say, I have no doubt that people's perceptions are shaped to some degree by their linguistic categories. The question, as in our bar conversation about adulteration, is of the magnitude of that influence. Reconsider Melanie's body-bobbing-up-and-down and Mike's focus-on-the-spread-of-the-honey-mustard-dollop and the sing-song sound of his voice. I think the details of Melanie's language ability have little impact on her creation of the experience of bodily bobbing instead of creating a taste of the fettuccini she's eating, instead of creating a review of her schedule of tomorrow's activities, instead of creating a recollection of the cabin in the woods, instead of creating any of the millions of other potential experiences in the welter. And the same for Mike.

The Winawer et al. (2007) article provides an example of what fuels my interest in pristine experience. Winawer et al. found that Russian speakers, who have two separate words for light blue ("goluboy") and dark blue ("siniy"), are generally faster at discriminating two different colors of blue when one is goluboy and the other is siniy than when both are goluboy or when both are siniy. However, when subjects simultaneously performed a verbal interference task (silently rehearsing strings of digits), this cross-verbal-category advantage disappeared (actually, it worsened slightly, but that was not their main interest and they had difficulty explaining it). English speakers, who do not have this built-in language distinction, made distinctions at about the same rate regardless of the light-blue-ness or dark-blue-ness of the stimuli. Winawer et al. concluded that people's perceptions are shaped by linguistic categories.

However, and this is what fuels my interest, Winawer et al. fail to note the converse explanation: that linguistic categories are shaped by people's perceptions. This failure, I think, reflects the common presupposition that everyone's (here, Russian speakers' and English speakers') inner experience is the same. However, I think it is at least possible that there are basic differences in Russian vs. English inner experience that *lead the* Russian-speaking verbal community to create two words for blue and the English-speaking community to create only one. What are these differences? I don't know. Are they cultural or genetic or both? I don't know. But the Winawer et al. article, like most others, does not consider the *possibility of* such differences, does not note any experiential differences that might occur.

Here's a speculation. Suppose that for whatever reason (physiological, genetic, cultural, social, etc.) Russian speakers are more likely to have frequent visual sensory awareness (as I define the term, for example, applying it to Mike's visual focus on the spreading dollop) than are English speakers, and that that is a long-term fact (long enough to shape language). (I have no idea whether that is true, but it is at least a reasonable possibility that science has not investigated.) What effect would that have on language? I don't know that either, but I think it is at least possible that a culture that is preoccupied with visual sensory awareness is more likely to develop a language that is somewhat more differentiated with respect to visual characteristics such as color than is a culture that is preoccupied with, say, inner speaking. Winawer et al. make no mention of such a possibility. I speculate that the verbal interference task (rehearsing numbers) forces people to engage in verbal pristine experience. Being forced into verbal experience is (or at least may be) a substantial disadvantage for someone who is characteristically (and therefore skillfully) a visual sensory awareness person. If all that is true, the Russian speakers would be at more of a disadvantage than would be the English speakers, and that would account for the worsening that Winawer et al. were at a loss to explain. According to this explanation, the disappearance of the category advantage that Winawer et al. observed is not the result of *interference* in the making of linguistic discriminations but rather in the *potentiation* in the making of linguistic discriminations, but these linguistic discriminations are in a kind of pristine experience in which the Russian people are less skilled. I say again: I know nothing of Russian speakers' inner experience; but then neither does Winawer, I fear.

Recapitulating this speculative alternative interpretation of Winawer's results: (1) There are huge individual differences in pristine experience (I'm pretty sure that some people have sensory awareness almost all the time whereas others have sensory awareness never or almost never). (2) It seems reasonable to presume that such great differences have practical ramifications, such as, for example, the use of language about color. (3) There is no reason to assume that the distribution of varieties of pristine experience is the same across cultures (it is, of course, possible that the distribution is identical across cultures, but that would have to be shown by a mature science of inner experience). (4) Therefore differences between English and Russian speakers might be due to experiential differences (or a feedback loop thereupon), not language differences. (5) BUT THERE IS NO RECOGNITION OF (1)–(4) AMONG SCIENTISTS. (There again I am shouting—I wish I didn't have to do that!) Winawer and colleagues make no attempt to determine the individual differences in the characteristics of inner experience of their subjects (other than to determine the midpoint of their color definition), and do not express a hint of the possibility that they may be overlooking an important feature.

So when you say that the language influences the pristine experience, I wholeheartedly agree. I suspect such causation is circular: the hardwired experiential differences influence the language which influences the experiential differences which influence the language (across many generations). However, I say again that I think the effects such as Winawer et al. investigated are substantially smaller than non-language-based effects. Oversimplified: I don't think that having two words for blue would make it much more or less likely that Melanie would experience bodily bobbing instead of tasting fettuccini.

RE [118] "I still think that there is a lot in common between presuppositions and tendencies, since they all form a backdrop to our engagement with the world, guiding and coloring it in various ways. . . . What you call presuppositions tout court are actually presuppositions *about experience*—i.e., beliefs about how experience works or what it is like."

Most of what I write about is experience—that is my professional interest. But the Winawer example makes clear that the distinction between presuppositions and tendencies is broader than experience. Winawer and colleagues' *tendencies* lead them to engage in scientific behavior (were they apes, or horses, or cockroaches, they would have different tendencies and probably not be scientists). That is, if Winawer had different tendencies, he would be a very different entity. By contrast, Winawer and colleagues' *presuppositions* lead them to overlook individual differences. If they were to become convinced (say, by reading this) that it might be desirable to take individual differences into

[129]

account, their presuppositions would be changed while their tendencies would stay the same. Winawer would then become a *somewhat* different entity, but not a *very* different entity.

RE [120] "The illusion that literature can create of experiencing the world through a child's perspective is not without real-world consequences, however. It may invite me to reflect on the difference between my experience and other people's (including young children's)."

The consequences you list are positive (assuming the dialogue with the certain psychologist is positive), and I happily acknowledge and value those potentials. However, I also fear the negative: that you (or other readers) would be lulled into complacency by the false belief that Joyce has opened a veridical window into experience. That fear may reflect a certain negativity in my own personality, but it also reflects, I think, the widespread state of the culture: there are *very* few careful (in my view) investigations of experience, the result (I think) of the widespread being lulled into complacency.

RE [119] "Preverbal children and psychotic individuals are a somewhat extreme case, but in other scenarios I think we already possess most of the necessary facts for understanding others' experiences."

This is the kind of sentence that leads me to fear that you would be lulled into complacency by false beliefs. The chapter I referred you to in RE 86 (chapter 9 in Hurlburt, 2011a) was about mostly normal adolescents and the mostly normal elderly, not extreme cases. Most people are surprised by some or most of my speculations in that chapter (for example, that an elderly person's imagery is often in black and white, not color), which leads me to think that most people do *not* already possess the necessary facts. (I happily accept that I might be mistaken about some of the speculations in that chapter, but that proves the rule that there are very few high-quality studies of experience.)

RE [122] [In table 5] "Exists relatively independent of the interlocutor? I would say no."

What I meant by my Yes answer to that question is that once Melanie was trained to differentiate her pristine experience from (broadly speaking) all else, then at the moment of that beep she might have noticed her bodily bobbing regardless of whether she might talk to me about it, or to you about it, or to the Pope, or to the Devil incarnate.

Reprise: Phenomena, unadulterated, and language

In the spirit of continuing to simmer about why the distinction between pristine experience and broad experience is important, here is an example that draws on and extends my own early work (Hurlburt, 1993, 117).

During his first sampling interview, "John Michaels" said that at the moment of one beep he was thinking about how much he liked Farm Basket (a fast food restaurant) turkey sandwiches. I was the interviewer, and (as I usually do) I said, approximately, "Tell me exactly what this thinking was like." John said that he had an image of some turkey in the broiler at Farm Basket, so I asked him (as I usually do) to tell me exactly what he saw. He described innerly seeing an ugly green slimy gross-looking piece of breaded turkey boiling in grease. We recalled that he had said how much he liked Farm Basket turkey and this seeing seemed discrepant, but his description of his inner seeing was unshakable. At the conclusion of the interview he said that he finds Farm Basket turkey disgusting but his wife likes Farm Basket turkey, and when the beep occurred he was picking up the Farm Basket turkey for them at his wife's request.

It seems to me that *I like Farm Basket turkey* is an example (a small one, to be sure) of what you call a broad experience. So is *I find Farm Basket turkey disgusting but my wife likes it.* Had you asked John at the beginning of the interview about his experience of Farm Basket turkey, he would have enthusiastically and convincingly told you that he liked it. Had you asked John at the end of the interview about his experience of Farm Basket turkey, he would have enthusiastically and convincingly told you that he was disgusted by it but his wife liked it. I think both of those are good-faith accounts of broad experience, each in its own (implied, not explicit) manner-of-speaking way. That is, I think there is *not* an experience-of-Farm-Basket-turkey; instead, there is an experience-of-Farm-Basket-turkey-from-the-(unstated, inexplicit)-point-of-view-that-John-values-his-wife's-experience-over-his-own, and there is another (quite different) experience-of-Farm-Basket-turkey-from-the-(unstated, inexplicit)-point-of-view-that-John-is-discriminating-his-own-opinion-from-that-of-his-wife.

Note that the pristine experience of innerly seeing the disgusting turkey had taken place *prior to* both of these broad experiences. That is, John apparently overlooked, deflated, or denied his own inner seeing (even though he had made notes about it in his sampling notebook) when he created the broad experience of *I like Farm Basket Turkey*, but then focused on, valued, or inflated his inner seeing when he created the broad experience of *I find Farm Basket turkey disgusting but my wife likes it*.

The sampling interview changed the broad experience dramatically. By contrast, the phenomenon—the pristine experience—stayed pretty much the same throughout. He reported having seen an image of slimy turkey when he was describing his *I like Farm Basket turkey* broad experience, and he reported having seen an image of slimy turkey when he was describing his *Farm Basket turkey disgusts me* broad experience. That's what I mean to convey when I say that the pristine experience is pretty darn independent of language, pretty darn unadulterated by the audience. Pristine experience is a phenomenon, pretty much stubbornly what it is, regardless of wife-valuing or wife-caving-into or price or convenience.

RE [124] "Can training/method substantially improve the fidelity of apprehension [of broad experience]? I would say yes, marginally."

Is *I find Farm Basket turkey disgusting but my wife likes it* an improvement in fidelity over *I like Farm Basket turkey*? Years ago, I would have answered that question Yes, but now I would say No. Now I would say they are simply two different broad experiences, neither being more or less faithful to anything. One relies more heavily on recent pristine experience than does the other, but that doesn't make one better than the other. I think there is no method of getting more reliably or with higher fidelity to the broad experience of *Farm Basket turkey* because there is no broad experience of *Farm Basket turkey*. Broad experience always depends on what is taken for granted, what perspective is being considered, and that taking-for-granted and perspectival dependency can change (usually unnoticed) from one situation to another, leading to dramatically different (e.g., *like* vs. *disgust*) broad experiences. I have divided the original experience of Farm Basket turkey into two separate experiences (1 = valuing wife's experience; and 2 = discriminating wife's experience from mine), but this division is likely *not* the most faithful way of characterizing the two very different experiences—maybe John doesn't value his wife's experience; he just caves into it. And maybe the wife's experience is not really the most important feature—it's the price, or the convenience, or whatever. And there is no reason to presume a two-way division is best—maybe a three-way or five-way would be better. And each of the ways (whether two, three, or five) could doubtless be divided into sub-ways. Broad experience is fundamentally perspectival, and not merely perspectival [131] in its apprehension or description: broad experience is perspectival "all the way down." This perspectival-ness can lead to dramatically different takes (*I like* vs. *it disgusts me*) on broad experience.

I do not see how the fidelity of apprehension of broad experience [132] can be improved, even marginally, without changing the broad experience itself. For example, you might specify that you are interested in John's personal take on Farm Basket turkey and ask him therefore to ignore anyone else's take including his wife's. But I think that doesn't get you closer to John's experience of Farm Basket turkey: it asks him to describe a new broad experience of Farm-Basket-turkey-when-I'm-supposed-to-ignore-my-wife's-opinion-thereof.

One last observation about John: As you point out, broad experiences take phenomena into consideration, but their manner of taking-into-consideration is very different: they are devalued/denied in the *I like Farm Basket* case and centralized/enhanced in the *I find Farm Basket disgusting* case.

RE [123] "Can [broad experience] be easily shared with others? Yes."

I would answer Yes to the question, "Can [broad experience] *seem to* be easily shared with others?" To the extent that two people share the same unstated, inexplicit perspective, then broad experience as described is the same broad experience as understood—that is, broad experience can be shared. However, I think people often take for granted without warrant the similarity of their perspectives, often giving the illusion of shared experience rather than its actuality. Therefore I suspect that you think it is easier than I do.

I wish to reiterate that I happily accept that the attempt to share broad experience is often worthwhile. You say that you have a positive experience of *The Road*; that will factor into my real decision about whether to purchase *The Road*. Later, you and I may share our experiences of *The Road*, and that will doubtless feel to you like an elaboration of your original *The Road* experience. I would caution against taking that feeling to imply that you literally are referring to the same experience, but that wouldn't prevent our having an interesting conversation about *The Road* that might be useful to one or both of us.

I also reiterate that my aim here is to distinguish plainly between pristine experience and broad experience. I am not attempting to devalue broad experience. It may be valuable for John to work through his takes on Farm Basket turkey (and what they say about his relationship with his wife, for example). But I do not think it will be productive for John to try to work through his *experience of Farm Basket turkey* as if that were an existing entity. I am also not attempting to overvalue pristine experience. I am attempting to think clearly about both, and that requires (as it seems to me) pulling back on broad experience and pushing forward on pristine experience until each occupies its rightful space. I am not claiming that pristine experience is the true North of the human condition, but *from here on,* I think it needs to be moved northward. So I hope I can be forgiven for my repetitive go north. Go North! GO NORTH!! Maybe when it is investigated adequately it will be discovered that pristine experience is unimportant, epiphenomenal, a mere scientific curio. I'd bet against that conclusion, but would happily accept it. To reach that conclusion requires, of course, adequate investigation, so I say GO NORTH!!!

I critique broad experience not because I think it is worthless but because it is, in my view, often (as in nearly always) confused with pristine experience, giving the false impression that our knowledge of pristine experience is farther north than it is. So I am at pains to extricate pristine experience from the experiential jungle that includes broad experience.

XIII

PRISTINE EXPERIENCE : BROAD EXPERIENCE :: PHENOMENA : NOT PHENOMENA

NOTE: Not all rounds of a heavyweight fight are equally interesting to the casual spectator: some rounds seem to be trading punches with little progress being made. But to the fighters themselves, and to the knowledgeable observer, those "little progress" rounds are often of great consequence: it is there that the fighters discover their own and their opponent's strengths and limitations.

Some might say that chapter XIII is a little-progress round, but we disagree. To be sure, the confrontation becomes bloodier a few pages into chapter XIV and even more personal in part 3 (chapter XV and beyond), but that is possible only because of the clarifying punches that we trade here in chapter XIII. So we urge you to hang with us through chapter XIII as we refine some crucial distinctions about phenomena, and as we continue to hone the distinctions among pristine experience, mental states, mentalisms, and broad experience. The payoff is coming, but we still need to pound away.

March 31
Dear Russ,
Please find below the result of some further simmering.
All the best,
Marco

RE [126] "The phenomena/not-phenomena distinction is the defining difference between pristine and broad experiences: pristine experiences belong in the category *phenomena*; broad experiences do not belong in that category."

I think you're going too fast here. First, I'm not sure "phenomena" is really a category. What else is in the category "phenomena" apart from pristine experience? Second, I find that the distinction you trace between

[133]

[134]

pristine and broad experience lacks in subtlety. "Pristine experiences present themselves directly to a person; broad experiences do not": sure, but when John says "I like Farm Basket turkey" (a description of a broad experience, according to your discussion), he is talking about something that presents itself directly to the senses. Maybe John is lying, or unaware of what he really likes or dislikes, but his utterance is still directed toward something that can be apprehended through the senses. So my solution is: broad experience may be very different from pristine experience, but it is at least entangled with pristine experiences in many ways. I take it that you're saying something along these lines when you write: "broad experiences take phenomena into consideration."

Thus, the important fact for me is not whether pristine and broad experiences are as different as McIntosh and Granny Smith apples or as chocolate and apples or as solar wind and a pair of flip-flops: as you say, broad experience is not an object, so I don't think that comparison really works. Rather, my claim is that broad experience is a composite entity which involves, at some level, pristine experiences. To put it otherwise, pristine experience is an *ingredient* of broad experience. The difference between the ingredient and the product (but again, I am skeptical about this kind of talk, because I agree that broad experience is not object-like) may be large: think about the difference between wheat and bread. And the difference *is there*; I'm not denying that, and I'm not denying that it is crucial for the scientific investigation of experience to acknowledge it. Yet I believe it would be harmful for this project *not* to acknowledge that there is a relationship between pristine and broad experience. Even if they fall into different categories, they are importantly related.

You may reply: that relationship is messy, and part of the challenge of studying pristine experience is that it is extremely difficult to do so *through* broad experience. I agree with this, and I agree that—methodologically—investigating pristine and broad experience may involve different kinds of expertise and procedures. Perhaps pristine and broad experience are not scientifically knowable through the same route; perhaps broad experience is not even scientifically knowable. But, in my view, none of these things warrants the conclusion that the epistemological difference between pristine and broad experience extends into the ontological realm, as if they were completely different—and unrelated—entities.

RE [127] "You might say that significance and broad experience are not the same thing."

Actually, I would say that significance is an important part of broad experience. Whether we eat an apple because we are starving, because it is an antidote to obesity, or because we want to support the Washington State economy is anything but irrelevant to experience. These motivations may emerge in pristine experience, and are likely to emerge in descriptions of experiences in the broad sense. Significance may not be apprehended through the senses, but evacuating it from experience (pristine or broad) is misguided.

RE [128] "Suppose you, Marco, are to create a movie where you, Marco, are the producer and also the writer and also the director, actor, cinematographer, and editor, and that your movie will be encrypted so that you can be confident that you, Marco, will be the lone projectionist and the lone member of the audience. That's a movie made by, of, and for Marco alone."

Again, I think the comparison is problematic. Pristine experience is not made or created for anyone, including the experiencer. Pristine experience exists, as a result of our interaction with the world, and most of the time we neither pay close attention to it nor use it for a particular purpose. But there is more. I think your comparison between pristine experience and making a movie for oneself shows why even pristine experience is (in one sense of the term) adulterated by other people. Even if I make a movie for myself, I will be drawing on my familiarity with stories, genres, techniques that I will have learned from other movies. If I know what a movie is, it is only through the movie expertise that I have acquired in social interaction. All in all, pristine experience may be (relatively) invisible to other people, but the tendencies and presuppositions that underlie it—and the language with which we talk about it—are inherently, and irreducibly, intersubjective. This doesn't mean that pristine and broad experience are affected by social parameters to the same extent; I agree with you that they are not. I agree with you that my pristine experience is mine, and no one else's. But I would still insist that, on these grounds, we can trace a difference only in degree, not one in kind, between pristine and broad experience.

[135]

RE [129] "Winawer and colleagues' *tendencies* lead them to engage in scientific behavior. . . . That is, if Winawer had different tendencies, he would be a very different entity. By contrast, Winawer and colleagues' *presuppositions* lead them to overlook individual differences."

I don't object to this, but I would argue that your distinction between tendencies and presuppositions is based on two criteria, only the first of which is spelled out in your account: (1) tendencies are more important, and more central to one's identity, than presuppositions; (2) tendencies are axiologically neutral, whereas presuppositions are axiologically negative (they are always undesirable, and should be eliminated). In both cases, I think it's important to stress that "being a presupposition" depends on an evaluation: thus, it is inherently subjective and perspectival. What looks like a presupposition to you may seem a tendency to me (and vice versa).

RE [130] "Once Melanie was trained to differentiate her pristine experience from (broadly speaking) all else, then at the moment of that beep she might have noticed her bodily bobbing regardless of whether she might talk to me about it, or to you about it, or to the Pope, or to the Devil incarnate."

When I took issue with your statement that pristine experience "exists relatively independent of the interlocutor," I didn't take the term "interlocutor" in the narrow sense. Of course, the interlocutor may change, and Melanie may still be able to pay attention to her pristine experience, and the experience may still be the same. But consider this: would Melanie be able to do this without some kind of training? Maybe she could teach herself to concentrate on pristine experience. Would the results of this be reliable from a DES perspective? I doubt it: a lot of presuppositions would creep in, and pristine experience would become broad experience. The point is the following: if we take the property "to exist independent of the interlocutor" to mean that an experience can be privately apprehended, then I don't see how we could distinguish between pristine and broad experience on these grounds. If I tell myself a story about my travel through India, then my (broad) experience exists independent of the interlocutor too. If what you mean is that the *description* of an experience is relatively independent of the context in which we offer it, then I agree that there is indeed a difference between pristine and broad experience: the former appears to be *less* affected by contextual parameters. But even in that case I would deny that DES reports about pristine experience are completely independent of the context: DES (the beep, the interview) provides a context that cannot but affect—perhaps subtly, but significantly—the report. In other words: the particular interlocutor may not influence the report, but the context does (as a matter of fact, it creates the possibility for the report)—and the DES context is still a human-made practice that relies on intersubjectivity. This is what my concern about the idea that pristine experience "exists relatively independent of the interlocutor" boils down to.

RE [132] "I do not see how the fidelity of apprehension of broad experience can be improved, even marginally, without changing the broad experience itself."

I do think we can do our best to remove elements that could lead people to respond in one way rather than another, therefore distorting the report. If we asked John "Do you like Farm Basket turkey?" in front of his wife, he's very likely to say yes and stop there.

Let me point out two things here. First, I don't agree that John's statement is not "more or less faithful to anything." Insofar as broad experiences involve pristine experiences, we can say that John's report is less faithful to his pristine experience of Farm Basket turkey than the statement that "he finds it disgusting but his wife likes it." Second, I agree that John's statement—even if it contradicts his pristine experience—can still be seen as an experience in the broad sense. Perhaps you're right to say that the "fidelity of apprehension of broad experience [cannot] be improved, even marginally." However, I don't think this makes the investigation of broad experience inherently worthless, or flawed. We can adopt strategies to improve the methodological rigor of the investigation even if we don't improve the fidelity of apprehension itself (this is what I meant when I said that such apprehension can be improved "marginally"). For instance, we may compare John's statement with statements produced in similar situations, and draw some kind of conclusion from there—even if we have no way to ascertain whether those statements are accurate or inaccurate with respect to the participants' pristine experiences.

RE [131] "Broad experience is fundamentally perspectival, and not merely perspectival in its apprehension or description: broad experience is perspectival 'all the way down.' This perspectival-ness can lead to dramatically different takes (*I like* vs. *it disgusts me*) on broad experience."

But isn't pristine experience perspectival, too? To summarize (what I take to be) our disagreement: you argue that broad experience is perspectival because every time people describe an experience, they *create* or *recreate* such experience in a way that crucially depends on the context. By contrast, pristine experience is thought to be context-independent: the same pristine experience is described in the same way,

[138] no matter the context (or the interlocutor). My sense is that you're overlooking the ways in which your method can shape people's reports about (what you consider to be) pristine experience: DES is, in itself, a context, and what people say (and what you call pristine experience) is in fact the product of the experience itself *and* of the context in which you ask people to describe it. DES encourages participants to adopt a perspective on their own engagement with the world—it asks them to value the pristine, the unadulterated, the prereflective. These normative assumptions do not disqualify the method, of course; yet drawing attention to them suggests that descriptions of pristine experience are dependent on the communicative situation—and therefore, in one sense, on the interlocutors—in the same way (but maybe not to the same extent) as broad experiences. The only way to prove that I'm wrong would be, I think, to demonstrate that participants' reports are relatively independent of the DES method itself: that is, that a substantially different method could deliver approximately the same results.

April 9
Hi Marco—
I think we've boiled it down to one central lump in the soup: "phenomena."
—Russ

RE [133] "I'm not sure 'phenomena' is really a category. What else is in the category 'phenomena' apart from pristine experience?"

Probably nothing. That's what is important about pristine experience.

RE [134] "When John says 'I like Farm Basket turkey' (a description of a broad experience, according to your discussion), he is talking about something that presents itself directly to the senses. Maybe John is lying, or unaware of what he really likes or dislikes, but his utterance is still directed toward something that can be apprehended through the senses."

This seems to be the heart of our discussion, but first we need to be unambiguous about your referent. I take it that you intend your word "something" (which occurs twice in this passage) to refer to John's broad experience of liking Farm Basket turkey (and not to the turkey itself). So I understand that you intend, "when John says 'I like Farm

Basket turkey' (a description of a broad experience, according to your discussion) he is talking about ~~something~~ the broad experience of liking Farm Basket turkey that presents itself directly to the senses."

I think you voice a commonly (perhaps nearly universally) held view that is, nonetheless, incorrect. "I like Farm Basket turkey" is *not* talk about something that presents itself directly to the senses. John may taste Farm Basket turkey, but he does *not* taste his *liking of* Farm Basket turkey. He may see, smell, or touch Farm Basket turkey, but he does *not* see, smell, or touch his *liking of* Farm Basket turkey. The turkey (or a tasting/inner seeing/feeling/touching thereof) may present itself directly to the senses, but his *liking of* Farm Basket turkey does not present itself directly to any of his senses.

Liking is a judgment of some sort (about which I know very little), which may involve some set of sensations—phenomena that are now or have been directly present to the senses. But how that judgment operates (what set of sensations are involved, what that "involvement" actually is) is unknown to me, to John, to you, or to anyone else, as it seems to me. I think the act of judgment is not directly present to the senses. For example, we have agreed that John has two judgments (broad experiences) regarding the turkey: *I like Farm Basket Turkey* and *Farm Basket turkey disgusts me*. And we know of at least one pristine experience (innerly seeing green turkey) that precedes both of those judgments. That pristine experience is consistent with one of the broad experiences but inconsistent with the other. You might say, the judgment *I like Farm Basket Turkey* does not involve the inner seeing of the green turkey, whereas the judgment *Farm Basket turkey disgusts me* does involve the inner seeing of the green turkey. But the basis on which you would make that distinction is post hoc, not phenomenal: the green turkey is inconsistent with *I like*, and therefore *must not have* been involved in the judgment, whereas the green turkey is consistent with *it disgusts me*, and therefore *must have* been included in that judgment. In neither case did John's including or excluding process "present itself directly to the senses"—John did not, for example, directly apprehend himself as excluding the green-turkey inner seeing from his *I like* judgment.

So judgment (whatever that is) does not depend directly on vision, because the (inner or outer) sight of the green turkey apparently is excluded in the judgment *I like* but included in the judgment *It disgusts me*. And the judgment process (whatever that is) is not itself seen—that is, the judgment itself does not present itself directly to the sense of

[139]

vision. Thus vision is not an essential part of judgment, either as an input or as giving evidence that the process has taken place. And the same is true for all the other senses. Thus no phenomenon (that which directly presents itself to the senses) is an essential or apprehendable part of judgment (including broad experience and significance).

So I think it is not true that "when John says 'I like Farm Basket turkey' he is talking about something (some broad experience) that presents itself directly to the senses." In general, I think it is not true that broad experience presents itself directly to the senses. Experience in the broad sense is, I think, an instance of the kind of "mentalism" that B. F. Skinner spent his entire career disparaging (e.g., *Science and Human Behavior*, 1953; *Beyond Freedom and Dignity*, 1971; *About Behaviorism*, 1974; his well-known paper "Why I Am Not a Cognitive Psychologist," 1977; etc.). I'll leave to Skinner the thorough exposition of why mentalisms are problematic (I recommend *About Behaviorism* and "Why I Am Not a Cognitive Psychologist"), but here is a brief account (cf. Hurlburt and Heavey, 2001). Skinner says that "We eat because we are hungry" *seems* to offer an experience (hunger) as an explanation for our behavior (eating)—*of course* we eat because we experience hunger. But this putative state called "hunger" turns out to be quite elusive. Many methods have been advanced to measure hunger: self-report, time since last meal, blood-sugar level, weight as a percentage of free-feeding weight, amount of saliva secreted at the sight of food, amount of electrical shock that will be endured to gain access to food, amount of (bitter) quinine that can lace the food before the food is rejected, and so on. It turns out that these "measures of hunger" are not strongly correlated with each other. Why not? Probably because hunger as a state does not exist. "Hunger" is a mentalism—a reference to a supposed internal state that seems to have explanatory power but is elusive at best.

Skinner was opposed to mentalisms (1) because the putative states probably don't exist; and (2) because even if they do exist, they discourage clear thinking. If I say "Of course I eat because I'm hungry," that's the end of the story—why should I search for additional explanation if we have already "explained" an outer behavior by referring to a (supposed) inner state? But actually we have explained nothing—we have just given up the urge to explain.

I think it is useful to think of mentalisms as metaphors: "we eat because we are hungry" unpacks to read "we eat *as if* there were a mental state of hunger which drives our external eating behavior."

Being explicit about the metaphor calls attention to the fact that a mental state of hunger probably does not (or at least may not) exist—that there are probably many different orthogonal physiological subprocesses, any one of which deserves equally (which is to say, weakly) to be called hunger.

Thus being explicit about our metaphors may keep us on the right track. I agree with Aristotle (*Poetics*, 1459a5–8; 1967) that "The greatest thing by far is to be a master of metaphor. It is the one thing that cannot be learnt from others; and it is also a sign of genius, since a good metaphor implies an intuitive perception of the similarity in dissimilars." But mastering metaphor requires recognizing their metaphoricity and not confusing it with reality. When Jaques in *As You Like It* says "All the world's a stage, and all the men and women merely players," it would be a mistake to look too hard for the world's playwright or its curtain.

[142]

I think it is useful to think of the broad experience of traveling through India as being a metaphor: It is *as if* there is an inner state of experience-of-traveling-through-India that drives our talk about India. But a mental state of experience-of-traveling-through-India probably does not exist—there are probably many different orthogonal substates, any one of which deserves equally (which is to say, weakly) to be called the experience-of-traveling-through-India.

I say again that I am not criticizing the use of metaphor. I just don't want us to be kidnapped by metaphors.

In broad strokes, Skinner's career presents two themes: (1) that mentalisms are fictions that seem to have explanatory power but in actuality impede the progress of understanding; and (2) that contingencies of reinforcement in the environment are the most desirable explanations of behavior. Skinner's views have lost much of their influence because (I think) he overemphasized the explanatory power of contingencies of reinforcement (theme 2). As collateral damage of science's reaction to that overemphasis, the anti-mentalism theme (1) also lost its influence. However, Skinner's critique of mentalisms is as trenchant now as it was 50 years ago. His critique of mentalisms has never been refuted, but as people came to see Skinner's emphasis on external contingencies as too restrictive, they turned their attention inward without solving (or attempting to solve, or noticing that they were not attempting to solve) the problems of mentalistic pseudo-explanations. (I think Skinner saw that coming, as his article "Why I Am Not a Cognitive Psychologist" demonstrates.)

One might fairly say that DES is my strategy of recognizing that Skinner's emphasis on external contingencies was too restrictive and that turning attention inward was a good idea *while at the same time continuing to recognize* the problems of mentalisms and striving to avoid those problems. That is, DES can be fairly described in five words: look inward but remain mentalism-free. That requires distinguishing consistently between phenomena that present themselves directly (those are not mentalisms), and concepts/explanations about those phenomena (which are mentalisms). Pristine experience is *not* mentalistic—pristine experience is indeed directly apprehended (albeit privately).

Let me personalize the statements that we have just been discussing, because as a general rule I find that such personalization helps to clarify thinking. Suppose that you've just said: "*Juanita's* hunger is *Juanita's* physiological state—or rather a set of physiological parameters—that have a phenomenal quality *to Juanita*." The physiological state is Juanita's; the mentalism is Marco's. Juanita's neurons, blood, and endocrine glands and whatever else are doing what they do. (I have no strong objection to calling that totality "Juanita's physiological state," as long as it is clear that we do not know specifically what we are talking about and therefore are not in a position to use physiological state as an explanation of anything.) The mentalism (which is problematic for Skinner and me) is when *Marco* pretends to know what that state is and what phenomenal qualities it has, when *Marco* uses one figment of Marco's imagination (knowledge about Juanita's physiological state) to explain another figment of Marco's imagination (Juanita's phenomenal quality). The mentalisms are *Marco's*; the physiological/mental states are *Juanita's*. Mentalisms and physiological/mental states are fundamentally different. Table 6 presents a schematic of those relationships.

Let's apply these distinctions to *The Metamorphosis* example. When Lynn innerly sees a dimly lit room with a bat (perhaps a foot tall) hanging from the ceiling over a bed with white sheets, that inner seeing is *not* a mentalism—it is a description of directly apprehended (inner) experience. Despite its privacy and its innerness, Lynn's seeing a bat is no more a mentalism than, for example, Lynn's external behavior while reading *The Metamorphosis* of turning from page 24 to page 25.

By contrast, broad experience is a mentalism. For example, your questionnaire asked Lynn, "Did you visualize Gregor's body? *never/*

TABLE 6. Discriminating among phenomena, mental states, and mentalisms

WHAT	HOW	WHOM	APPREHENDABLE?
Phenomenon	Directly presents itself	to Juanita	Yes
Mental state	Presumed underlying entity	in Juanita	No
Mentalism	Fictional explanation	by Marco	No

occasionally/fairly often/quite often/very often. If you can, describe how you visualized Gregor." Lynn circled *very often* and wrote "I visualized Gregor as a giant spider; lots of legs, crawling, grayish color, dirty, covered in a sticky, gray, liquid substance." Your instruction ("describe how you visualized Gregor") invites, and Lynn's response is, a mentalism: Lynn is required to provide a self-referential generalization of a kind that she is not likely to be able to make. She did not write "I usually visualized Gregor as a giant spider but on at least one occasion I visualized him as a bat," despite the fact that our interview had made her visualization of Gregor-as-bat absolutely explicit throughout an extended conversation. Your instruction requires (or at least strongly suggests) that Lynn (and probably you) blur the distinction between mentalisms and direct observation: it seems to ask for a generalization about a series of pristine experiences, but that is not how such a question is actually understood. In response to such questions people give what I have called *faux generalizations* (Hurlburt, 2009b, 2011a) about their behavior; such faux generalizations are mentalisms. Lynn doubtless answered your question in a heuristic way, which involved responding to your instruction by currently seeing Gregor and then (mentalistically and incorrectly) faux-inferring that that was how she had seen him throughout.

You could have given a nonmentalistic instruction had you so desired (say, "Try now to visualize Gregor, and if you are successful, please describe what you see"). I think it likely that Lynn would have written exactly the same thing ("I visualized Gregor as a giant spider . . ."). The difference is that your original question/Lynn's answer is a collusion: you asked an impossible question and she misrepresented her experience with the tacit understanding that you both will not notice the other's breaches. You might ask, What difference does it make if the answers are the same? The answers use the same words, but they are not the same answers. In your original question, Lynn's "I visualized" refers to a faux-series of events that she claims (incorrectly, or at least incompletely) took place while reading; in the nonmentalistic version, "I visualized" refers to one actual event that that is taking place right now (or very recently).

Broad experience is of the nature of mentalism. Pristine experience is of the nature of phenomenon. I harp because I think it is crucial. One important strand in the history of the last century and a half of civilization is the rise of the importance of mental life (think Freud, Wundt, James, etc.). But the rise of interest in mental life was brutally smacked down, and pinned down for over half a century, by the behaviorists. I think the interest in inner life deserved (at least in part) its smacking because it claimed more than was warranted. Freud, for example, started out (as I read the beginning of *Interpretation of Dreams*) with a metaphorical account of mental processes but gradually morphed his account into a science of putatively actual mental structures of id, ego, and superego. However, those structures don't actually exist and therefore deserved their eventual comeuppance. Freud's defense-as-metaphor is quite perceptive—it is indeed *as if* one part of the psyche is suppressing another part. Furthermore, that metaphor can be quite useful—it calls attention to the fact that people are not single minded or coherent, that people do not necessarily know their own motives, and so on. But to go beyond the metaphor and believe that a defense exists as a mental structure (for example, that its strength and scope can be measured) is misguided and will, sooner or later, be smacked down.

The same is true of broad experience. Broad experience as metaphor can be quite useful: I am interested in your broad experience of traveling through India. But to believe that broad experience exists as a mental structure, whose strength or scope can be measured, is misguided and will sooner or later earn its comeuppance.

It may seem that I am defending the desirability of DES as a way of investigating experience, but that is backwards, as it seems to me. I see myself as defending the desirability of investigating experience *period*, regardless of manner. DES is the *result* of defending that desirability, which must acknowledge Skinner's critique of mentalisms. If one is serious about the desirability of knowing something about experience, then the question becomes, How can one be interested in inner experience without falling into the snares of mentalism? My answer to that question has come to be known as DES: pristine experience is inner but not mentalistic, and DES is my way of investigating pristine experience. DES avoids mentalisms not because it is good for DES but because experience is interesting/important and Skinner was right. As a result, DES does *not* investigate mental states—any talk of mental states is mentalistic; DES does *not* investigate how experience causes behavior—attributing causation is mentalistic. So when I say that "DES investigates pristine experience and nothing else," that could rightly be translated as "DES avoids mentalisms."

[145]

ROAD MAP: *Russ's comments in the previous RE introduce themes (f) (do judgments always involve pristine experience?) and (g) (mentalism and pristine experience).*

RE [135] "Most of the time we [do not] pay close attention to [pristine experience]."

I disagree. We typically pay 100% of our conscious attention to our pristine experience. When John innerly saw the green turkey he paid close attention to it, to the exclusion of all else in the inner and outer world. A few moments later he may have forgotten entirely that he had paid attention to it, like a dream on waking, but that is a very different thing from not paying attention to it in the first place (the dream is vivid; the immediate recollection of it is vivid; a few minutes later it is "gone").

RE [137] "I don't think this makes the investigation of broad experience inherently worthless, or flawed."

Neither do I, and I have tried to say that consistently throughout our interchanges. I think broad experience does not exist as a state, probably does not exist as a coherent entity of any sort, but that does not make it inherently worthless or flawed. My aim is *not* to say that broad experience is worthless or flawed. My aim is to explore the differences between pristine experience and broad experience, so that one who is interested in broad experience does not fall into the trap of believing that methods and conclusions that are (or should be) based on pristine experience can be automatically and unthinkingly applied to broad experience, and vice versa. In particular, my aim is to recognize that pristine experiences are directly apprehended phenomena, whereas broad experiences are not. That has no implication whatsoever for the value of either pristine experience or broad experience.

[146]

RE [136] "This is what my concern about the idea that pristine experience 'exists relatively independent of the interlocutor' boils down to."

Perhaps I should say "depends minimally on" rather than "is independent of." What I am trying to convey is that the pristine experience phenomenon is stubborn—it bears phenomenal scrutiny, it resists being bullied out of being what it is. A typical DES interview, recreated for John, is:

> RUSS: When you say "green" do you mean to be taken literally—that is, are you actually innerly seeing something green?
>
> JOHN: Yes.
>
> R: And what shade of green do you see? Green like a traffic signal? Green like a 7-Up can? Green like the jacket at the Masters?
>
> J: No, not like any of those. More green like the Grinch's face in the movie.
>
> R: And when we are saying "like" here, do you mean that metaphorically, as if . . .
>
> J: I know what a metaphor is! No, I do not mean that metaphorically. I *saw* the turkey (in my imagination, of course). The turkey *was green*. The green *was about the same color* as the Grinch's face.

At the specified moment, John was innerly seeing turkey, was not innerly seeing a Cadillac Escalade, was not outerly seeing the kitchen table, was not sensing his body position, was not recalling the invasion of Iraq, was not tasting a margarita, and so on. There was one particular experience, no other, regardless of context or interlocutor. The seen turkey was the Grinch's particular shade of green, and no other shade of green (not that of a 7-Up can or a Masters jacket), regardless of context or interlocutor. I accept that the seeing of turkey was influenced by John's history—had he never visited the Farm Basket restaurant, for example, he would not have been seeing Farm Basket turkey. All that is a specific example of the general principle: pristine experience stubbornly presents itself as itself, mostly regardless of context or interlocutor.

By contrast, John's broad experience is highly dependent on the interlocutor. If his wife asks him about his experience of Farm Basket turkey, he will in all honesty say he likes it. But if I ask him about his experience of Farm Basket turkey, he will in all honesty say it disgusts him. Thus the broad experience of Farm Basket turkey depends greatly on context and interlocutor.

RE [138] "My sense is that you're overlooking the ways in which your method can shape people's reports about (what you consider to be) pristine experience. . . . The only way to prove that I'm wrong would be, I think, to demonstrate that participants' reports are relatively independent of the DES method itself: that is, that a substantially different method could deliver approximately the same results."

I don't think I overlook the fact that DES shapes people's reports. (1) I work hard to minimize that shaping. (2) I have written about the effects of subtle pressures on interviews (in Hurlburt and Schwitzgebel, 2007, 285–89), where I maintain that what are typically called subtle pressures are not at all subtle and that DES effectively avoids those pressures. (3) I heartily agree with the desirability of investigating whether substantially different methods could deliver approximately the same results. I would greatly value such studies, which should be commonplace in a mature science of experience. I myself cannot perform such studies because I would be (or at least would be understood to be) tainted by the DES perspective.

Reprise: The big picture [147]

I have said (harped) that pristine experience and broad experience are very different from each other, that the heart of the difference is that pristine experience is of phenomena whereas broad experience is not. That is, I think, true, but in the distinguishing/clarifying, we may have lost the big picture of why this distinction is of vital importance, so I offer the following example.

My first "thought sampling" paper (Hurlburt and Sipprelle, 1978) was a case study of "Donald," a university professor who suffered from anxiety so extreme that he no longer drove his car because he was afraid his anxiety would cause him to black out and kill somebody or himself. The source of his anxiety was a mystery to him: he was tenured, was successful, and had a loving wife and family. His life was perfect except for the bouts of anxiety that came "out of the blue."

We gave him a random beeper with instructions to write down his thoughts and come back in a couple of days. He did so, saying, "I've got really terrible handwriting so I've transcribed my thoughts for you," and he gave us a typescript. We took a glance at this typescript and said, "There's an obvious theme here." He said, "I didn't see a theme!" He looked again, and still maintained that there was no theme to be seen in the transcript. We said, "The theme is that you're frequently angry with your kids." He looked again and said, "No, I'm not angry with my kids, and you're mistaken about that being a theme here."

We went through his thoughts with him one by one. "Here you said you were thinking that Johnny's got the radio turned up too loud; were you angry then?" He said, "Yeah, I was." "And here you're thinking that Billy got ice cream on his shirt again. Were you angry then?" "Yeah, I was." It turned out that about a third of his thoughts (one third is a huge percentage for any content theme) involved anger at his kids. As we inquired about his anger sample by sample, one pristine experience at a time, it was easy for Donald to acknowledge that yes, he had in fact been angry in that sample. By the time we had finished the series of such samples, he had come to realize, to his great surprise, that he was in fact frequently angry. We reassured him that anger at kids is not uncommon, and as long as it is not acted upon it is not a problem. Donald's anxiety disappeared in what he viewed as a miracle.

In our present terminology, prior to sampling, Donald would have said that his broad experience was *I experience only loving and positive feelings toward my children*. After sampling, he would have said that his broad experience was *I am frequently angry toward my children*. The distinction between these two broad experiences is *not* merely some idiosyncratic meaning of words such as "angry." We used *Donald's* understanding of "angry" throughout. By his own (new) understanding, he was indeed angry at moments where he had originally denied the existence of anger. These two broad experiences (*I experience only loving and positive feelings* and *I am frequently angry*) are not equal: the first did not conform to the facts of Donald's own experience.

[148]   This example highlights why the distinction between pristine experience and broad experience is vital. Donald's commitment to his *I experience only loving and positive feelings* broad experience had hugely negative consequences for him. It is important to recognize that Donald's commitment to his broad experience was *not altered by a suggestion of an alternative broad experience*. When we suggested that the typescript had lots of anger toward his children (the alternative broad experience), that did not in the slightest alter his commitment to his broad experience—he looked at the typescript and said *Nope! No anger here!* However, when we looked at one pristine experience at a time (and pristine experience is always one at a time), Donald could easily realize, by his own definition, that *Yep! This singular pristine experience*

involved anger! That's a hugely different response, which I think should be understood as deriving from the fact that broad experience does not have any essential dependence on phenomena, whereas pristine experience has phenomena at its heart.

After examining a series of pristine experiences, Donald was able to create a real generalization: I do indeed have frequent anger toward my kids. A real generalization is a faithful characterization of an explicit series of real phenomena. A faux generalization might use the same words as a real generalization, but it does not characterize an explicit series of real phenomena. *I experience only loving and positive feelings toward my children* sounds like a generalization about phenomena, but it is not. It is a fiction.

Donald's anxiety largely disappeared after discovering his angry experience. A cognitive psychologist might explain that Donald's altered broad experience transformed his behavior (eliminated his anxiety). I don't think that is correct. What changed is Donald's skillful apprehension of his pristine experience. Prior to sampling, he skillfully *avoided* his own pristine experience, to the extent that he occasionally blacked out (the ultimate avoidance of pristine experience). After sampling, his pristine-experience-apprehending skill allowed him to experience his anger without turning away from it so dramatically. His change in broad experience had nothing to do with it.

You might ask how this anger-avoiding skill works. I don't really know, but here's a speculation. Suppose that anger has a rise time—first there is a little bit of anger; later there is a lot of anger. (That's in accord with the physiology, but that is not my point.) Donald's skill (prior to sampling) is to be sensitive to the very beginning of this rise-in-anger, and then immediately to do what it takes to derail the experience of anger. Perhaps at the first hint of anger he digs his fingernails into his palms; perhaps at the first hint he holds his breath; perhaps he visualizes naked women. I don't know what he does; the point is that people can learn the skill of altering their own experience, that that skill (constructive or otherwise) might be invoked early in the anger process. That skill is not the result of some broad experience; it is a skilled reaction to the situation.

So Donald "gets a whiff of" the beginnings of anger, and he adjusts himself (digs his nails or whatever) to control that experience. If Donald's usual anger-experience-avoiding skills don't work, then he might invoke a more extreme skill aspect such as blacking out (just as in tennis if the backhand won't reach, you might invoke the more extreme diving-for-the-ball skill aspect). Donald's transformation ("miracle") resulted from our teaching him (not on purpose) a new skill—together we looked situation (1), and he experienced his anger without fingernail digging or naked-lady picturing; together we looked situation (2), and he again experienced his anger without fingernail digging or naked-lady picturing; and also in situation (3); and also in situation (4). As a result, Donald learned a new (for him) skill of experiencing anger without (minorly or heroically) distracting himself. Altering broad experience had no more to do with it than broad experience has to do with diving for the just-too-distant-for-the-normal-backhand tennis ball.

(I have made similar speculations about "Fran" in Hurlburt and Schwitzgebel, 2007, 32–35.)

Contrary to cognitive psychology, it's not the broad experience itself or its change that is important in this story. It is Donald's quintessentially skilled but counterproductive behavioral response to his pristine experience. To the extent that he bought into (was committed to) the broad experience of successful career/loving wife/perfect family/perfect life, he did not seek to improve/hone/accurately target the skills with which he really deals with his environment. Skinner was right: mentalisms are problematic because they seem (incorrectly) to offer explanations and thereby stultify the urge to search for real explanations. The stakes (as for Donald) can be high. But you don't get over mentalisms by invoking other mentalisms; you get over mentalisms by paying attention to phenomena.

April 13
Dear Russ,
Many thanks for your further comments. I agree that the concepts of "phenomenon" and "direct apprehension" are at the heart of our discussion. See my responses below.
All the best,
Marco

RE [139] "His *liking of* Farm Basket turkey does not present itself directly to any of his senses"; and

RE [140] "No phenomenon . . . is an essential or apprehendable part of judgment."

I agree that liking or disliking Farm Basket turkey is a matter of judgment, but I would insist that those judgments are based on (or in some way related to) pristine experience. I accept that John may be wrong about his pristine experience of Farm Basket turkey (e.g., John may be induced by situational pressures and demands to say that he likes Farm Basket turkey even if this statement conflicts with his pristine experience of Farm Basket turkey). Still, my sense is that arguing that "no phenomenon . . . is an essential or apprehendable part of judgment" is too strong. To me, this sounds like denying any continuity between pristine and broad experience.[1]

[149]

[150]

RE [141] "Experience in the broad sense is, I think, an instance of the kind of 'mentalism' that B. F. Skinner spent his entire career disparaging."

Your (and Skinner's) use of the phrase "mental state" in this discussion strikes me as potentially problematic. First of all, Skinner is often understood as being interested in mental states only insofar as they play a causal role in triggering behavior. Is that how you understand Skinner? In this sense, it may well be that "hunger" is a mentalism because it does not lead to consistent (i.e., entirely predictable) behavior. But of course hunger is a physiological state—or rather a set of physiological parameters—that have a phenomenal quality. Whether it is a mental state or not, there is a way it is like to feel hunger.

[151]

[152]

Building on Skinner, you argue that talk about "broad experience" is a mentalism because broad experience is not directly apprehensible. Note that you're already redefining Skinner's "mentalism," from the realm of causation and external behavior to the realm of direct internal observation: for you, something is *not* a mentalism when it can be directly observed by a subject. And hunger, it seems to me, *can* be directly observed by a subject. In this sense, this discussion merges with the previous discussion about whether broad experience is a phenomenon. I have already said that broad experience is *not* a phenomenon (as you define it) since it cannot be directly apprehended; but it involves phenomena to the extent that it is always in a (perhaps indirect) relation with phenomena.

[153]

A lot depends on how we define "mental state" here—whether in cognitive terms, in terms of neural correlates, or otherwise. I'm not sure I understand the definition that you're adopting in this discussion.

---

1. This discussion is abridged. The unabridged discussion is on the Companion Website.

RE [143] "In response to such questions people give what I have called *faux generalizations* about their behavior; such faux generalizations are mentalisms."

I wouldn't object to this. Yet it's important to keep in mind that people routinely use generalizations and faux generalizations when talking about experience: these strategies are phenomena in the sense that they "naturally" appear in social exchanges and interactions. I agree that they are ways of talking about (reflecting on, interpreting, etc.) past events, and that they should not be equated with a mental state. But I don't think this mentalistic stance is necessarily implied by references to broad experiences such as "traveling through India."

RE [145] "As a result, DES does *not* investigate mental states—any talk of mental states is mentalistic; DES does *not* investigate how experience causes behavior—attributing causation is mentalistic."

[154] I'm not sure I follow here. If pristine experiences are inner without being mental states, what are they? Or, to put the question otherwise, how would you characterize the difference between mental states and pristine experience? More generally: are you distinguishing between references to "fictional" mental states (mentalisms) and nonfictional mental states, or are you rather saying that *any* reference to mental states is flawed? See also my following comment.

RE [142] "Mastering metaphor requires recognizing their metaphoricity and not confusing it with reality."

[155] I entirely agree here. As far as I can tell, the phrase "mental state" has a metaphorical flavor too. Unless you come up with a convincing theory about how mental states are related to electro-neuro-biological states of the brain (which I don't think anyone has done), any reference to a mental state is at best an abstraction, and at worst a metaphor. Thus, I think you're on the right track when you write that "all language is metaphorical to some degree." But it is crucial to (1) be aware of the metaphorical nature of language; and (2) be aware that there are different degrees of metaphoricity (i.e., different kinds of "fits" between metaphors and the world).

Still, I doubt that talk about broad experience is committed to men-
[156] talism in any relevant sense. Since descriptions of broad experiences are produced in social interaction, they are behavioral patterns that seem to be *less* suspect of mentalism than pristine experience.

ROAD MAP: Marco's remarks in the previous RE anticipate our later discussion of the role of metaphor in conveying experience (theme h).

RE [144] "In your original question, Lynn's 'I visualized' refers to a faux-series of events that she claims (incorrectly, or at least incompletely) took place while reading."

Maybe, but again you're using pristine experience as a touchstone for Lynn's broad experiential report. Incidentally, this shows that broad experience is not completely unrelated to pristine experience, because there does seem to be a continuity between Lynn's pristine experience and her later report. Further, even if I agree with you that Lynn's report is "incorrect, or at least incomplete" with respect to her pristine experience, I think her description is interesting in its own right. Maybe it tells us something about Lynn (compare the detail of her description with the brevity of Alex's "like a giant brownish black beetle"); maybe it tells us something about Kafka's text (the vagueness of Kafka's characterization of Gregor). In any case: if, as you say, you are "not attempting to devalue broad experience," the logical move is to try to evaluate it without contrasting it with pristine experience.

RE [146] "My aim is to explore the differences between pristine experience and broad experience, so that one who is interested in broad experience does not fall into the trap of believing that methods and conclusions that are (or should be) based on pristine experience can be automatically and unthinkingly applied to broad experience, and vice versa. In particular, my aim is to recognize that pristine experiences are directly apprehended phenomena, whereas broad experiences are not."

We're in complete agreement here. To the question "what are broad experiences?" I would respond the following: broad experiences are context-sensitive reflections on and generalizations about events and existents (people, objects, etc.) that have been directly apprehended in the past, and which now are only—and at best—*indirectly* apprehended. Here "indirectly" means: through the mediation not only of a context, but also of an experiential background of tendencies and presuppositions. [157]

RE [148] Donald's anxiety "example highlights why the distinction between pristine experience and broad experience is vital."

Very interesting example. I agree with you that it shows how attachment to broad experience (that is, to particular interpretations of one's life) can prove harmful in some situations. It also demonstrates the benefits of "paying closer attention" to pristine experience. I wonder if Donald couldn't have come to the same conclusion through other means—for instance, by reflecting or being invited to reflect on his life without any kind of experience sampling. I have the sense that broad experience, too, can have beneficial effects, especially when it is discussed in dialogue with someone who knows what he or she is doing. But I take your point about pristine experience and its distinction from broad experience.

By the way, in chapter 8 of my *The Experientiality of Narrative* (Caracciolo, 2014b) I offer an interpretation of Vladimir Nabokov's novel *The Defense* that reminds me of Donald's story. In case you're not familiar with the novel: its protagonist—Luzhin—is a chess player who becomes increasingly obsessed with chess. He starts to see chess patterns everywhere: in garden decorations, tablecloths, the frosting of a cake, people's behavior. Ultimately, his obsession reaches a point where he sees his own life—including his final suicide—in terms of chess moves. My interpretation is that chess "blocks out" Luzhin's consciousness, so that he is no longer able to reflectively attend to his experience of the world around him: he becomes "experience blind" because of the pervasiveness of chess. I guess today I would write that chapter differently: maybe it's his broad experience ("my life is a chess game") that acts as a presupposition, preventing him from recognizing the *difference* between his interpretation of events and pristine experience. Maybe Luzhin would have benefited from experience sampling!

RE [147] "The big picture."

I also think it's important to keep in mind why I am "defending" broad experience here. My point of departure was that pristine experience is not enough to do justice to the ways in which people experience (i.e., respond to and interact with) literary narratives. In this respect, my position hasn't changed: I'm still convinced that reflections and interpretations are a crucial part of people's narrative experiences, and these modes of engagement—while being in an important sense experiential—are difficult to pin down in pristine experience and/or capture through DES.

XIV

PHENOMENA, MENTAL STATES, JUDGMENTS, AND HUNGER

April 16
Hi Marco—
Here's my next shot.
—Russ

RE [149] "John may be induced by situational pressures and demands to say that he likes Farm Basket turkey even if this statement conflicts with his pristine experience of Farm Basket turkey."

I understand you to be saying throughout our correspondence that broad experience is not merely the *speaking about* broad experience. That is, I understand you to be saying that your broad experience of traveling through India somehow exists whether or not you are talking about it or explicitly thinking about it. So when you say "John may be induced by situational pressures and demands *to say* that he likes Farm Basket turkey," I understand you to be conveying that the situational pressure is on the *saying*, not on the *broad experience*. [160]

People can have broad experiences about things that they have no pristine experiences about. One dramatic example that comes to mind is false memory syndrome, but more mundane examples abound. False memory syndrome is a condition where a person strongly *believes* in a memory of a traumatic experience which objectively did not occur (see McHugh, 2008, 67–68). I'm not taking sides on the frequency of false memory syndrome (which is controversial), but false memory syndrome seems to be an example of a (strong) broad experience that incorrectly believes itself to be based on pristine experience. Furthermore many people (Donald, for example) have broad experiences that forget, overlook, or deny pristine experience.

Those examples demonstrate that judgments can be quite distant from pristine experience, so I think "those judgments are based on (or in some way related to) pristine experience" is not (necessarily) true unless one has a *very* broad understanding of "in some way related to." I accept that judgments are *sometimes, probably often, maybe usually* based on (or in some way related to) pristine experience. But I also think that judgments are *sometimes, probably often, maybe usually* based on (or in some way related to) *something that is not closely related to or that substantially distorts* pristine experience. Furthermore, I think that most people most of the time are not good judges of the extent to which their judgments are or are not related to pristine experience. As you yourself, here (to my ear) exemplify, people often (if not generally) substantially overestimate the extent to which their judgments accurately portray their pristine experience.

RE [150] "Still, my sense is that arguing that 'no phenomenon . . . is an essential or apprehendable part of judgment' is too strong."

Regarding "essential": I agree that judgments *can be* (and often are) based on (or in some way related to) pristine experience. However, I don't think pristine experience is an *essential* part of judgment. In your bread metaphor, bread *can* be based on wheat, but wheat is not an essential part of bread (there is potato bread, oat bread, corn bread, etc.). I happily accept that pristine experience *can* inform judgments, but judgments can be made without pristine experience or contrary to pristine experience. You might ask, "Would judgment[(s) made without pristine experience] be worth anything?" Your answer would be "I don't think so," and I would agree. But as we have noted, a worthless judgment is a judgment, nonetheless. And this is, I think, important: there are very many worthless judgments, very often held by the judger as being true or as being the Truth.

Regarding "apprehendable": First, we should agree that apprehending an ingredient is not the same thing as apprehending the process of using the ingredient: seeing (or tasting or smelling or touching) the wheat is not the same thing as seeing the baking. The process of arriving at a judgment (whatever that is) is not directly apprehendable. Skinner is one among many who make this point. At best, you can apprehend a small part of the judgment process; much of (probably most of) the judgment process takes place out of sight. For example, William (a racist person) sees Henry (a minority person) make a mistake. William forms the judgment: Henry is a stupid <insert racial slur here>. William's judgment arises from his seeing (pristine experience) Henry's behavior and a whole lot of other factors impossible to specify, no doubt including patterns of activity in the amygdala, dorsolateral prefrontal cortex, and who knows what else. William does *not* apprehend the activity of his amygdala, etc., even though science has (tentatively) shown that amygdala patterns might be important to racist judgments (e.g., Phelps, Cannistraci, and Cunningham, 2003). (I am not claiming to know how judgments are made, only that judgments are complex processes.) At best Henry's (apprehendable by William) behavior is an ingredient in William's judgment; how that ingredient is used in William's judgment-making process is not directly apprehended by William or anyone else.

So I think that phenomena are neither essential nor an apprehendable part of judgment. As to whether it "sounds like denying *any* continuity between pristine and broad experience," I've tried to be pretty clear about that: pristine experience and broad experience are very different but not necessarily discontinuous, like the rim and the floor of the Grand Canyon, with a few tortuous paths in between.

[161]

RE [151] "Your (and Skinner's) use of the phrase 'mental state' in this discussion strikes me as potentially problematic. . . . Skinner is often understood as being interested in mental states only insofar as they play a causal role in triggering behavior. Is that how you understand Skinner?"

No! That understanding of Skinner, although common, is not correct. Skinner and I avoid speaking about mental states because they may not exist, and if they do exist they are probably impossible to specify, and if they are possible to specify, they are not possible to specify *in the universe as it has currently evolved*. Worse, the use of putative mental states as explanations for behavior (or for anything else) is problematic because it lulls one into complacency, gives the false sense that something has been explained, and therefore inhibits the urge to find real explanations and contributes to the obstruction of others who are trying to find real relationships and/or explanations.

RE [152] "But of course hunger is a physiological state—or rather a set of physiological parameters—that have a phenomenal quality."

Regarding the upcoming, I apologize if I am mistaken, and I would be happy to have you show me my mistakes. That said, I think your of-course-hunger-is-physiological statement is quintessential mentalism: you speak as if you know what you're talking about but you don't; you seem to have unwarranted, unquestioned confidence in your view (as reflected in "of course"); and as a result you discourage yourself from your own and impede others' potentially important investigations. That is, your statement says, to my ear, "*Of course* we all know what hunger is: it's a state with such-and-such properties. Therefore *we have no further need* to investigate what hunger is—at most all we need to do is investigate its phenomenal qualities." That is exactly the kind of thing that Skinner (assuming I understand him aright) and I oppose.

(Skinner and) I think you don't know a thing about what you're talking about here. To specify a physiological state is to specify the state of 20 billion neurons and their interconnections, and to specify the chemistry of the blood at every artery, vein, and capillary, and to specify the secretion and readiness of each endocrine and ducted gland, and to. . . . If not that, then what do you mean by "physiological state"? Perhaps you would prefer to specify exactly what is contained in the set of physiological parameters? That specification would have to be complete and based on a complete understanding of those parameters' actions and interactions. I therefore think you cannot do either one; that your reference to "physiological state" gives the appearance but not the reality of a known referent. If that is correct, on what grounds does it make sense to say that this impossible-to-specify-state-or-set has a phenomenal quality? And what about that phenomenal quality itself? Your statement implies that hunger has *one* phenomenal quality, the same for all people (young/old, thin/fat, industrialized/aboriginal, etc.), the same in all situations (when dinner at a five-star restaurant is delayed by 15 minutes, a pot smoker's munchies, in a concentration camp, in the Congo). I doubt that that is true. And if it isn't, then you haven't explained anything about how the variation in phenomenal quality across person or situation is connected to the state or parameters. That is, you haven't explained anything.

I accept that there is physiology, and that physiology involves ingestion and glucose and osmotic pressure and lots of other stuff. I accept that sometimes I feel hungry—that there is sometimes a pristine experience on which the word "hunger" rests easily. I accept that physiology and hunger are probably related (in probably a very complex way), but I'm pretty sure that science doesn't know much more about it than that. I think the relationship between physiology and pristine experience is worthy of investigation, and I think I know what it would take to do such an investigation well (it would require DES or something as good or better). I'm pretty sure such investigations have not been done. Why not? Because you (and most others) believe that you already know what you actually don't know—that is the curse of mentalism. (Either that or I am substantially mistaken.)

RE [153] "And hunger, it seems to me, *can* be directly observed by a subject."

No, it cannot. Hunger does not exist as a phenomenon. Some particular sensations when dinner at the five-star restaurant is 15 minutes late exist as a phenomena; I might say "I'm hungry" in that situation. Some particular sensations occur when the pot smoker reaches for the Pop Tarts: he might say "I'm hungry." The inmate of the concentration camp or the child in the Congo might say "I'm hungry." None of them "observed hunger." Was there something similar across the phenomena present to the diner, smoker, inmate, starving child? Perhaps so, but even if so (which I think is questionable), that similarity, which might be called the "phenomenal quality of hunger" is not apprehended by the diner/smoker/inmate/child; it would be *induced* by a careful researcher. [162]

Perhaps (in a hyperbolic kind of way) our difference is this: you feel your stomach growl and say (without much thought) "I'm hungry." Your wife says "I'm hungry too" and you presume (without much thought) that she experiences the same thing that you do. You extrapolate that to a general experience of hunger. By contrast, I encounter DES subject Abel who says, "At the moment of the beep I felt hungry." I (with a lot of thought) ask him exactly what he intends to convey by "I felt hungry" and he describes his experience carefully. Sometime later I encounter another DES subject, Baker, who says, "At the moment of the beep I felt hungry." I (with a lot of thought) ask him exactly what he intends to convey by "I felt hungry" and he describes his experience carefully. And the same for Charlie, Delta, and many others. I then compare what Abel, Baker, Charlie, and the others have said about their "I felt hungry" experience, and discover (on the basis of real induction) that they have described different phenomenology. So I conclude (with much thought) that the phenomena of hunger differ from one person/situation to another.

Then I describe these results to you, and you say, "But of course hunger is a physiological state—or rather a set of physiological parameters—that have a phenomenal quality." And then I feel the need to harp.

NOTE: Russ sent this addendum the following morning:

In the light of day, the previous two paragraphs seem unfairly glib, and I apologize for that. The point I was trying to make, too heavy-handedly, was that the exploration of pristine experience is often taken to be easier than I think it actually is (see my "crossfire" comment below [in the section called Reprise]). Most people with whom I discuss inner experience give every indication of believing that they know far more about inner experience than do I, and not just about their own inner experience but about inner experience in general. I find it remarkable that most people would rather tell me about the general characteristics of inner experience than ask me about it, despite the fact that I am a pretty smart guy who has spent 30+ years exploring it carefully. When I suggest to them that many people are mistaken about important features of their own experience, I can watch those words zip past them without the slightest hint of penetration, especially without a hint of recognition of the possibility that the words apply to them.

[163]   But all that provides no excuse for the way I expressed that in the previous two paragraphs, which overlook the important fact that you (unlike my typical correspondent) are indeed committed to trying to figure this stuff out. If I could retract those paragraphs I would. Sorry.

RE [154] "If pristine experiences are inner without being mental states, what are they? Or, to put the question otherwise, how would you characterize the difference between mental states and pristine experience?"

Pristine experiences are phenomena—they present themselves directly to a particular person at a particular time. At some specific moment, Lynn innerly saw Gregor-as-bat. Gregor-as-bat (and all the other details of that experience—lighting, bedding, etc.) were directly, unambiguously, experienced: Gregor was a bat, not a bug; the bedding was white, not blue; the lighting was dim, not bright; and so on. There was nothing (or at most very little) inferential about Lynn's seeing of Gregor-as-bat. Was Lynn's Gregor-as-bat experience a mental state? I don't know. I know nothing about the mental state that led Lynn to see Gregor as being a bat, not a bug, or the bedding white, or the light dim. By distinct contrast, I do know something of Lynn's pristine experience. Lynn directly apprehended the pristine experience (she innerly saw bat/bed/lighting/etc.) and described it to me in a way that I find, on the basis of rationally conceived and skillfully executed probing, believable. Might Lynn be mistaken about her seeing of the bat? Of course. Might I be mistaken in believing that Lynn saw a bat? Of course. But that potential mistakenness is not at all the same as the mistakenness about Lynn's mental state. Neither I, Lynn, nor you know anything about her mental state. I've never seen or otherwise directly apprehended a mental state, and neither has Lynn nor you (as it seems to me).

So I characterize the difference between mental states and pristine experience this way: a mental state is what I and no one else ever directly apprehends (at best must be inferred, but more often merely asserted without foundation); pristine experience is what some particular person at some particular time directly apprehends.

RE [155] "The phrase 'mental state' has a metaphorical flavor too."

I agree. That is why it is crucial to distinguish between mental states and phenomena. And I accept that everything said about a phenomenon has a metaphorical flavor. When Lynn says "I saw a bat," the concept *bat* has metaphorical significance—Lynn's concept of bat doubtless differs somewhat from mine or yours. And the same goes for the "I saw" part. But the "distance" (another metaphor, to be sure) from "I saw a bat" to Lynn's phenomenon is far smaller than is the distance from "hunger is a physiological state" to any phenomenon whatsoever.

RE [156] "Since descriptions of broad experiences are produced in social interaction, they are behavioral patterns that seem to be *less* suspect of mentalism than pristine experience."

That is indeed the way it seems to most commentators, but I think it is not true. That is the mistake on which much of cognitive psychology rests. People believe and give all sorts of broadly experiential descriptions of and explanations for their behavior; some of those beliefs/descriptions/explanations are partially true, some are mostly false, few if any are totally true, nearly all are held/given with conviction (as fervent for the mostly false as for the partially true), most if not all are produced in social interaction (some more than others).

"But of course hunger is a physiological state—or rather a set of physiological parameters—that have a phenomenal quality" is a broad experience produced in social interaction: most people, including most cognitive psychologists, would say the same thing and would reinforce you when you say it. Ubiquity has nothing to do with mentalism. The question is whether you know what you're talking about, not whether others say the same thing.

RE [157] "Broad experiences are context-sensitive reflections on and generalizations about events and existents (people, objects, etc.) that have been directly apprehended in the past, and which now are only—and at best—*indirectly* apprehended."

I agree, if we can edit that sentence to read (underlining my additions):

"Broad experiences are context-sensitive reflections on and (perhaps faux) generalizations about putative events and existents (people, objects, etc.) that may or may not have actually existed and may or may *not* have been directly apprehended in the past, and which now are only—and at best—*indirectly* apprehended."

My additions are intended to weaken the connection between actual events and existents and broad experiences. False memory syndrome is an extreme example in which broad experience refers at least in part to events that didn't take place and to people who didn't exist. Furthermore, if something didn't exist, it is not possible to generalize about it, which is why I inserted "(perhaps faux)."

RE [158] "I wonder if Donald couldn't have come to the same conclusion through other means—for instance, by reflecting or being invited to reflect on his life without any kind of experience sampling."

Yes, I think that is possible. Much of psychotherapy depends on that kind of invitation to reflect. I am not opposed to that—it is often useful, and often the only possible way. On the other hand, there are (or at least may be) situations, including psychotherapeutic situations, where experience sampling would be beneficial, perhaps more beneficial than standard psychotherapy. A mature science of experience would investigate those situations.

For example, chapter 2 of my 2011 book (discussing work that Sharon Jones-Forrester, Stephanie Doucette, and I performed) discussed the pristine experience of women with bulimia nervosa, concluding that multiple fragmented experience was a common denominator. Let me substitute "bulimic women" for "Donald" and "their" for "his" into your statement, giving: "I wonder if bulimic women couldn't have come to the same conclusion [that multiple fragmented experience is important] through other means—for instance, by reflecting or being invited to reflect on their life without any kind of experience sampling." We have sampled with 24 women with bulimia nervosa; all had fragmented multiple experience to some degree; prior to sampling *none of them* was aware of the fragmented nature of her own inner experience. There are perhaps 50,000 articles about bulimia nervosa, and *none of them* (as far as we have found) mentions, much less stresses, the importance of fragmentedly multiple inner experience. So: perhaps the individual women (and the science thereof) *could have* come to the same conclusion, but they *have not* come to that conclusion, given many, many, many opportunities. (In Hurlburt [2011a, chapter 2] I presented six potential explanations for this shared oversight.)

RE [159] "I'm still convinced that reflections and interpretations are a crucial part of people's narrative experiences, and these modes of engagement—while being in an important sense experiential—are difficult to pin down in pristine experience and/or capture through DES."

I agree. My harping to the contrary notwithstanding, I do not think that DES is the only solution, or always the best solution, or even necessarily a good solution. A mature science of experience would sort that out. I harp because DES is often not seen as a solution at all, because DES is often misunderstood, and because I think the distinctions between broad experience and pristine experience are worth exploring and explicitizing. I don't want to discourage you or others from thinking about broad experience; I do want you and others to be clear about the distinctions between broad experience and pristine experience.

[164]

Reprise: Another stab at the big picture

I think, on the basis of my years of investigations, that at least sometimes the careful apprehension of pristine experience is a worthwhile endeavor. How often, and for whom, and under what conditions has yet to be determined, but my opinion (rightly or wrongly) is that there is substantial importance to apprehending pristine experience.

I have, throughout our interchanges, tried to distinguish carefully pristine experience from all else, particularly from broad experience. I have tried, probably not always with success, to draw that distinction brightly without criticizing broad experience per se. There are many important situations where broad experience is of vital importance, so I have no wish to criticize broad experience. But cleanly, clearly, relentlessly distinguishing between pristine experience and broad experience is of enormous importance to the investigation of pristine experience for two very different reasons, which I might call the interference and the contribution reasons.

Interference: it is an empirical fact of our research that most DES subjects come into their participation with strongly held broad experiences about a variety of issues. They are, typically, attached to those broad experiences and are highly practiced at telling those broad experiences to family, friends, bar mates, fellow travelers, and so on. (Think about your tellings about experiences in India, for example.) That is, their linguistic skills were honed in large measure to support the speaking about broad experiences. DES asks subjects to report pristine experiences and nothing else; DES subjects are (initially) prepared to talk about broad experiences (or some impure mixture of broad experiences and pristine experiences). Therefore, one of the primary DES interviewer skills (perhaps *the* primary skill) is the consistent, relentless, supportive discrimination of pristine experience from broad experience, helping subjects distinguish between what was directly before the footlights of consciousness at the moment of the beep and all else (which is primarily broad experience). In an important way, the DES interviewer says, over and over, something like "That is interesting and doubtless important. What of that, if anything, was directly present to you at the moment of the beep?" The response, typically, is something like, "Well, nothing. At the moment of the beep I was actually. . . ." That happens repeatedly, until the subject internalizes the distinction between phenomena and broad experience, at which time she stops reporting broad experiences and cleaves to phenomena. In a nutshell: I spend much of my professional life distinguishing between pristine experience and broad experience and helping others to do the same.

Contribution: DES has revealed some (I think) important results, and I would like to make those results available and to encourage others' explorations (that is, I would like to contribute to a mature science of experience). But making that contribution has not been easy, doubtless to some extent because of my own personal inadequacies but more importantly (I think) because the science of pristine experience is caught in the crossfire between two deeply entrenched and energetically defended positions. There are those who think all reports of experience are "subjective" and therefore impossible to pin down, and therefore should be excluded from science; and there are those who think subjective reports of experience are important, easy to accumulate (just ask), and that much is already known about them (as in "Of course hunger is . . ."). That crossfire has been bloody (as in the beginning and middle of the 20th century); the bloodletting is currently lessened but the differences have never been resolved.

I think both sides are right, but not completely right (see Hurlburt and Heavey, 2001), and a possible way toward resolution is to distinguish between pristine experience and other (e.g., broad) experience. Both sides have lumped pristine experience in with other kinds of experience, and I think that is not constructive on either side. I have discussed why pristine experience should not be dismissed as "subjective" in Hurlburt (2011a, chap. 17). I have discussed in many places why it is a mistake to think that people know about their pristine experience, including Hurlburt (2011a, chap. 2) and here.

However, as our interchanges have demonstrated, it is very difficult to extricate pristine experience from broad experience.

Where to go from here [165]

We have batted back and forth the distinctions between pristine experience and broad experience, and the potential importance thereof, for quite some time. One could say that our discussion has been conceptual: we have tried to help each other refine, revise, discard, reinvent our conceptualizations of pristine experience and broad experience. Perhaps it is now time to move our interaction from the arena of the conceptual to the arena of the concrete. I could send you a beeper and treat you like a DES subject (well, not really like a typical DES subject because we have had extensive conversations about inner experience, whereas the typical DES subject comes in pretty "cold"). You would wear the beeper and jot down some notes about whatever experience was ongoing at the moment of the beep; after collecting a half dozen such experiences, we would discuss them (perhaps using Skype). And we would repeat that process across several days. That is the crucible in which the distinction between pristine experience and broad experience exists or doesn't exist; we might learn something from that concreteness.

If in a preliminary way that prospect appeals to you, we should discuss the rules of engagement, confidentiality, etc. Then if we still think it is a good idea, we can proceed.

ROAD MAP: Russ's invitation to move from the conceptual to the concrete opens the discussion of why the personal is important (theme i).

THIRD PART
PERSONAL

XV

GETTING EVEN MORE PERSONAL

April 21
Dear Russ,
Many thanks for your insightful comments—I think we've reached a point where it would be indeed important to move beyond the conceptual domain. Please find my responses below.
All the best,
Marco

RE [161] "I think that phenomena are neither essential nor an apprehendable part of judgment."

    I don't know or understand how phenomena could not be an essential part of judgments about phenomena. If John says that he likes the taste of Farm Basket turkey without having ever tasted Farm Basket turkey, then his statement is more (or less) than worthless: it has the appearance of a judgment without being, in effect, a judgment. In this scenario, John is *not* talking about a broad experience. He's not talking about experience at all. He's just saying something to please his interlocutor, or otherwise giving in to situational pressures.

[166]

RE [160] "I understand you to be saying throughout our correspondence that broad experience is not merely the *speaking about* broad experience. That is, I understand you to be saying that your broad experience of traveling through India somehow exists whether or not you are talking about it or explicitly thinking about it."

    I think you've put your finger on a key issue. I would argue that broad experience *is* a way of speaking or thinking about experience. This is because—we should probably agree to disagree here—I cannot accept that experience falls into two categories, one being "pristine" experience, the other being "broad" experience. I don't think that "experience" has two different referents in the phrases "pristine experience"

[167]

183

and "broad experience." Experience is experience: what we're conscious of at any given moment and how we respond to or interact with it. Some ways of describing or reporting experience may be rather loose, context-dependent, and shot through with presuppositions (hence broad experience) while others may meet DES-like standards of fidelity and presuppositionlessness (hence what you call "pristine experience"). If, based on the figures you provide near marginal 113, we have about 19,000 experiences per day, some ways of reporting experience may target *a lot* of experiences, organizing them according to their emotional salience, temporal ordering, or otherwise (broad experience), while others may target only single or few experiences (pristine experience).

The key question is whether a report involving a large number of experiences (say, my telling you about my trip to India) is, or references, an experience. As things stand—and I recognize that this may contradict some of my previous statements—I would say that such report is experiential without *being* or *referencing* a stand-alone experience. There is no such thing as *the* experience of traveling to India, or *the* experience of reading *David Copperfield*. There is a report in which someone generalizes about a number of experiences he or she has gone through while traveling through India or reading *David Copperfield*. Sometimes these reports bring to light patterns or structures that would be difficult to discover or describe if we focused only on *single* experiences. Such patterns or structures may show how (people think that) their experiences are interconnected, temporally, thematically, or otherwise.

Now to your objections about broad experiences (broad experiential reports) that are uncoupled from pristine experiences. I accept that this may happen, and that it probably happens more often than we think. The case of false memory syndrome is interesting. The fact that a person's memory is "objectively false" does not mean that that person has no experience of the memory itself, however. On the contrary, the memory is a phenomenon (it is, as a memory, directly apprehendable), and as such it may emerge in pristine experience. Thus, I would rewrite your sentence "false memory syndrome seems to be an example of a (strong) broad experience that incorrectly believes itself to be based on pristine experience" in the following way: "false memory syndrome seems to be an example of an experience that incorrectly believes itself to be based on a specific, prior pristine experience." This experience has important consequences for broad experiential reports, because it seems to orient the person's self-concept and worldview.

I like your metaphor of the *distance* of experiential descriptions from phenomena. Right now I would put it like this: the experiential reports obtained through DES are extremely close to phenomena, perhaps as close as it gets; the experiential reports that we've called "broad experiences" so far ("traveling through India") are relatively far from phenomena, but still directed *to* series or sequences of (putative) phenomena; predispositions and presuppositions can be inherent in our experience of phenomena, but they are in themselves very distant from phenomena.

Finally, one note on broad experiences. I agree with you that generalizing about phenomena carries a considerable risk of distortion or falsification. But I don't think I have remarked on how important and useful this kind of generalization can be. Storytelling is a powerful instrument for compressing experience (see, e.g., Herman, 2003). If we lived immersed in phenomena, if we weren't able to generalize (and, surely, distort and falsify) our past experiences, we'd lose much of what makes us human.

ROAD MAP: *Note that Marco's comments on pristine and broad experience conclude the discussion of the status of pristine experience vis-à-vis broad experience (theme a). Marco argues that the experiential descriptions obtained through DES are indeed much closer to phenomena than broad experience, but they should not be confused with phenomena themselves. However, he agrees with Russ that DES reports are high-fidelity with respect to phenomena, and he will reiterate that view when discussing his own DES samples (see, e.g., RE 225).*

RE [162] "No, [hunger] cannot be [directly observed by a subject]. Hunger does not exist as a phenomenon."

As I've already pointed out, this kind of statement sounds tendentious to me. It's like saying: "You never owned a car. You only owned a 2003 red Honda Civic and a 2009 blue Ford Focus." Concepts always subsume a number of different referents and situations—otherwise what would be the use of a concept? When I say "hunger can be directly apprehended," all I'm saying is that the situations to which the concept "hunger" can be applied have a phenomenal quality. It may well be that there is no single, universal hunger-quality that recurs in all situations. But, as far as I can see, this is in no way implied by saying that "hunger

[170]

[171]

can be directly apprehended." Thus, I think you're arguing (or harping!) against a straw man when you point out that "the phenomena of hunger differ from one person/situation to another." Who said that they are the same? I've just used a concept, which—like all concepts—works by generalizing across a range of (more or less different) situations.

This does not mean that it is pointless to show that different people experience hunger in radically different ways. Like you, I think there is much to discover in the process.

ROAD MAP: *Here begins the discussion of the relationship between concepts and experience (theme j).*

RE [163] "But all that provides no excuse for the way I expressed that in the previous two paragraphs, which overlook the important fact that you (unlike my typical correspondent) are indeed committed to trying to figure this stuff out. If I could retract those paragraphs I would."

Yes, I am indeed committed to this project, and you don't have to apologize about anything.

RE [164] "I harp because DES is often not seen as a solution at all, because DES is often misunderstood, and because I think the distinctions between broad experience and pristine experience are worth exploring and explicitizing. I don't want to discourage you or others from thinking about broad experience; I do want you and others to be clear about the distinctions between broad experience and pristine experience."

I entirely agree with all this.

RE [165] "Where to go from here."

Yes, sampling my own experiences through DES sounds like an interesting, and useful, experiment. I'm willing to try.

April 23
Hi Marco—
I'm still working on a reply. In the meantime, I think we have agreed that I should send you a beeper. If you will tell me the address, I'll get that process started—it may take a couple of weeks to get it there.
—Russ

April 26
Hi Marco—
Please see the comments below.
—Russ

RE [171] "When I say 'hunger can be directly apprehended,' all I'm saying is that the situations to which the concept 'hunger' can be applied have a phenomenal quality."

Thought experiment: Before you proceed further, jot down on a piece of paper (or computer) what counts as a situation to which the concept "hunger" can be applied. Also, jot down what counts as a phenomenal quality for the hunger concept. Seriously, I mean jot it down. I'll wait! The jottings are notes from you to yourself—I will not ask to see them.

NOTE: *We recommend that the reader engage in this thought experiment.*

RE [166] "If John says that he likes the taste of Farm Basket turkey without having ever tasted Farm Basket turkey, then his statement is more (or less) than worthless: it has the appearance of a judgment without being, in effect, a judgment. In this scenario, John is *not* talking about a broad experience. He's not talking about experience at all. He's just saying something to please his interlocutor, or otherwise giving in to situational pressures."

I use the term "faux X" to refer to that which has the appearance of an X without being an X. (E.g., "I always do R in situations like S" is a faux generalization unless the person saying it has indeed made a complete or at least representative accounting of his responses in S situations.) So I would say that John is giving a faux judgment. I suspect you agree with that.

Where we may disagree is the frequency of faux judgments, which I think are very frequent, and mostly made without much inkling of their "fauxity."

"Faux" as I use the term is or may be something of an oversimplification. Webster's *faux* is all or nothing—either something is real or it is an imitation—but judgments or generalizations exist on some sort of continuum of fauxity. If John never tasted Farm Basket turkey, his *I like* judgment is entirely faux. But there may well have been, over

[173]

the course of John's life, a few Farm Basket turkey taste experiences that were pleasant (along with those that were disgusting), so his *I like* judgment is not 100% faux—it is 99.44% faux, or 73% faux, or some other impossible-to-specify percentage faux. I suspect you agree with that, also.

[174]   When most people (including John) give faux generalizations, they do not have any explicit understanding of the degree of fauxity of their expressions. I suspect you agree with that, as well.

ROAD MAP: Note that Marco and Russ have reached an agreement on the relationship between judgments and pristine experience (theme f).

RE [168] "There is no such thing as *the* experience of traveling to India.... There is a report in which someone generalizes about a number of experiences he or she has gone through while traveling through India."

Your way of describing the situation is too clean, in my view. It unquestioningly presumes the existence of the experiences and the adequacy of the generalization about them. I would recast that sentence to read (underlining my additions): "There is a report in which someone faux-generalizes about a number of experiences he or she has or may have gone through while traveling through India, where the degree of fauxity is difficult or impossible to specify by either the reporter or the recipient, and where that degree might be small or large or anywhere in between." I think that recasting is neither unquestioningly naive nor desperately cynical. On the contrary, it is humanistic—it is open to the possibility of 0% faux or 100% faux or anywhere in between; that is, it faithfully reflects the human condition.

RE [170] "It's like saying: 'You never owned a car. You only owned a 2003 red Honda Civic and a 2009 blue Ford Focus.' Concepts always subsume a number of different referents and situations—otherwise what would be the use of a concept?"

I accept that concepts are necessary and useful. So, for example, if I point at a 2003 red Civic and say, "Is that a car?" you will say Yes. And if I point at a Caterpillar D9 and say, "Is that a car?" you will say "No. That is a bulldozer—cars have wheels, bulldozers have tracks." And if I point at a bottle of Heineken and say, "Is that a car?" you will say "No. That is a beer—cars are for driving, beer is for drinking." We share the concept *car*.

Willy walks into a bar and says, "I need a drink but I don't have any money. I'll sell this for $100." He holds up a photo of a 2003 red Civic and says "This is not a bulldozer or a Heineken." Hugo lurches to his feet and says "I'll buy it!" and produces a hundred-dollar bill. Willy pockets the cash, gives Hugo the photo, and walks out. Willy is happy; Hugo not so much.

Hugo was swindled not because of a failure of his concepts, but because of his failure to appreciate that the same words can apply to very different concepts (it is absolutely true that a photo of a 2003 red Civic is not a bulldozer or a Heineken). [175]

So . . . concepts are necessary and useful, but that utility can lull one into complacency. Willy's scam involved constructing a situation where Hugo would apply the concept *car* while simultaneously (and with the same words) Willy applied the concept *photo of car*.

You may think the scammer is an extreme example, but I think not, and will provide an example below (see the discussion of "Tim" in the next section).

RE [171] "When I say 'hunger can be directly apprehended,' all I'm saying is that the situations to which the concept 'hunger' can be applied have a phenomenal quality."

I think you are implying something about the *sameness* of the phenomenal quality of hunger—that is, that we all have more or less (not necessarily exactly) similar phenomenology when it makes sense to apply the concept *hunger* to ourselves. I think that is probably not true, which was also the point of my five-star restaurant, post-toke, concentration camp, and Congo example.

As we have agreed, concreteness is desirable, so I went looking for my most recent "hunger" sample. Here it is:

> At the moment of the beep, "Dennis" was innerly seeing himself from a third-person perspective, looking down at himself from slightly above and to the right of his actual position. The innerly-seen-Dennis had an exaggerated hungry/sick/stomachache facial expression. Simultaneously, Dennis was also innerly seeing his stomach and several (approximately four) other organs, seen blue/green/black like a colorized x-ray. The seen stomach was pinched together, understood to be indicating that it was very empty. Simultaneously, Dennis was

also innerly seeing liquid acid, which was understood to be characterizing his stomach as being acidy. Dennis also had an acidy sensation in his stomach.

In the thought experiment at the beginning of this email, I asked you to jot down some features of hunger and its phenomena. Does this sample fit your expectations? Did you jot something like *part of the phenomenology of hunger is that people innerly see themselves with exaggerated facial expressions of hunger?* For your information, Dennis had very frequent inner seeings of himself, and those inner seeings often conveyed something about his state, as here: his innerly seen face had an exaggerated hungry/sick expression. But that's pretty unusual—most people do not routinely (or ever) innerly see themselves, and most people do not visually display their state as a facial expression. So I'm guessing that this experience is not in the center of the target of what you would expect hunger phenomena to be.

I think it is not safe to assume that "hunger" is a concept that is always applied in more or less the same way; and I think it is not safe to assume that we know very much about the phenomenology of hunger, even if we could be sure that the concept *hunger* is applied in the same way.

While looking for the most recent hunger sample, I came across this other recent sample, which is about thirst rather than hunger, but that may be close enough to be informative for our discussion.

> Joan (a graduate student trainee) and I were interviewing "Tim" about a DES sample. Joan began the interview, finding that at the moment of the beep Tim was thirsty and was thinking about making some iced tea. This "thinking" involved innerly seeing five jars of ice tea, clear glass/screw-top jars of tea that his wife had made, sitting on the top shelf of the refrigerator door. Then it was my turn. I discovered that the "thirst" that Joan and Tim had been discussing was actually a metallic taste in his mouth (the result of a medication he was taking); Tim understood that drinking the tea would make the metallic taste go away.

Joan and Tim had not discovered this metallic-taste aspect, which had been prominent in Tim's experience, because Joan and Tim employed different concepts of *thirsty*. Joan used something akin to

Merriam-Webster's definition ("being deficient in moisture"), and she assumed that Tim did the same. Tim used a behavioral definition of thirst (some sort of mental state that is reliably followed by drinking behavior) and assumed that Joan did the same. As a result, Joan and Tim overlooked an important (arguably the most important) feature of Tim's pristine experience—the strong metallic taste. Perhaps Tim was not thirsty at all (by Joan's, Marco's, and Webster's definition)— he just had a bad taste in his mouth. Or perhaps he was thirsty (by Joan's, Marco's, Webster's, *and Tim's* definition)—that is, Tim was moisture-depleted but his way of experiencing that is to have a bad taste in his mouth. Either way, it illustrates the risk of assuming that one knows what phenomena are being invoked by the word "thirst."

Joan and Tim are like Willy and Hugo: the concepts they employed were different in important ways, but the words they used were consonant with both discrepant concepts. Willy was a conman, purposefully duping Hugo. Joan and Tim were just as much duped but it wasn't intentional by either party.

Regarding the personal and the conceptual

Marco, you and I have spent a lot of time and effort clarifying concepts like "broad experience" and "pristine experience" and "phenomenon," and so on, and that has been time and effort well spent. But I think we have to recognize the limitations of the clarifying of concepts. No amount of clarifying what is generally meant by "car" would have saved Hugo from Willy's con; no amount of clarifying what is generally meant by "thirst" would have helped Joan understand Tim. In fact, the opposite is doubtless true: the more Hugo had explored the definition of "car" the *more* likely he would have been duped by Willy; the more Joan had explored what is meant by "thirst" the *more* likely she would have been duped by Tim. And most importantly, the more Marco believes he understands what "hunger" is, the *more* likely he is to *overlook* important phenomena in the vicinity. Presuppositions, suppositions, and concepts in general are the enemy of phenomena.

So in an important sense, from my view, I have not aimed our conversations primarily at the clarification of general distinctions about broad experience, or hunger, or traveling through India. I have aimed *at you,* Marco, trying to undermine your delusions so that you might be more open to phenomena. That is, our conversation has not been primarily conceptual; it has been primarily personal. A conceptual conversation would have been:

> MARCO: I know what broad experience is. It is like this. . . .
> RUSS: No, *I* know what broad experience is. It is like this other. . . .

A personal conversation is:

> MARCO: I know what broad experience is. It is like this. . . .
> RUSS: I don't know what broad experience is, but it doesn't seem that you do, either; or if you do, it probably isn't good for you.

The conceptual conversation would aim at clarifying the general concept *broad experience*. The personal conversation is aimed at *Marco*—weakening Marco's attachment to Marco's general concept of broad experience so that Marco might apprehend phenomena with higher fidelity. The personal conversation is also aimed at Russ—weakening any unwarranted attachment that can be discovered there.

You may ask, What right does Russ have to aim at Marco in this way? To which I answer: I have no right to diagnose your delusions, no right to impose my views, no right to take personal aim at you. And I would go further than that: I have no right to feel certain that I have diagnosed your delusions correctly, no right to feel certain that it would be good for you to alter your stance toward phenomena as I have suggested. I acutely feel my limitations in this regard. There is a chasm betwixt thee and me: not only do I have no right to cross to your side of the chasm, I have no ability to cross even if I so desired. I have tried to be forthcomingly transparent on my side of the chasm; you may choose to look across and be influenced by what happens on my side, or not. And the relationship is symmetrical: I can look across and choose to be influenced, or not.

I have commented at length about broad experience because I think (rightly or wrongly) that your view of broad experience interferes with your apprehension of phenomena. I fear that had you been Tim's interviewer, believing that you know something about thirst and its phenomena, you would have heard Tim's opening description that he was thirsty and was thinking about making some iced tea *and that would have been the end of the story for you.*

The bottom line: If you are interested in phenomena, then you have sincerely to act as if mental or brain states don't (or at least may not) exist, as if apparent generalizations are actually (or at least possibly) faux generalizations, as if every word that is spoken has the potential of being used in an idiosyncratic way, as if you know nothing about the phenomena that should be expected. And all that is about Marco, not about concepts.

You may say that it is not possible to act as if every word that is spoken has the potential of being used in an idiosyncratic way. I think that view is mistaken. I did not single out "thirst" as being the one word that might be idiosyncratic; I hold that *all* words might be idiosyncratic, and therefore am always on the lookout for any evidence that says that any word is or is not idiosyncratic. Then I follow up. If you say thirsty but scowl when you say it, then I ask what you mean by "thirsty." If you say "I like it" but you look disgusted, then I ask what you mean by "I like it." If you say "I rushed" but speak slowly, then I inquire what "rushed" means. I don't presume to know what a gesture or expression conveys; instead I inquire whenever I detect any hint of discrepancy.

To the extent that you think that you know what "thirst" or any other word means, then you will be deaf to hints that suggest an alternative. It is really quite simple in conception (although substantial practice is required to be skillful). If you want to know about phenomena, you have to be on the alert for hints that suggest an alternative understanding to the one you currently hold, and then check it out.

RE [167] "I don't think that 'experience' has two different referents in the phrases 'pristine experience' and 'broad experience.' Experience is experience: what we're conscious of at any given moment and how we respond to or interact with it."

I fear that if *you think* that pristine experience and broad experience are the same, or are essentially two points on a continuum, then *you* will not be available to the pristine experiences that try to present themselves to you (that is, you would likely not discover that "thirst" means "metallic taste"). Therefore, I must repeatedly challenge your conviction that "experience" has the same referent in the phrases "pristine experience" and "broad experience."

RE [169] "Memory is a phenomenon (it is, as a memory, directly apprehendable), and as such it may emerge in pristine experience."

Memory is *not* a phenomenon, is not part of pristine experience. What-is-<remembered> may well be a phenomenon or pristine experience.

"Memory" is a putative process that "retrieves memories." You have never seen, felt, tasted, or otherwise directly apprehended your memory process. You may well have apprehended some correlate of the putative process (waiting for a missing word, etc.) but you have no more apprehended the process itself than you have apprehended the combustion process in your Civic. You put the gasoline in; you got burned by the hot engine; you smelled the exhaust. Those are correlates of combustion, not combustion.

I put the term "<remembered>" in angle brackets to emphasize the fact that what is <remembered> is *not* really remembered in the sense that it is retrieved from some memory bank. What is <remembered> is actually created in the present with the understanding that it is of a past event.

Memory, like hunger and thirst, is a mentalism: it invokes as mental process that seems to explain something, when actually it merely dulls the urge to explore.

RE [172] "Yes, sampling my own experiences through DES sounds like an interesting, and useful, experiment. I'm willing to try."

[176]   A beeper is in the mail. Here are the instructions for the project, as I see it—I'd be open to discuss any modification. We can talk about the operation of the beeper itself via Skype.

DES instructions

Wear the beeper in your everyday environments and engage in whatever activities you would usually do (short of swimming, which would be hard on the electronics!). Use the earphone, not the onboard speaker.

When the beep occurs, "freeze" your experience, interrupt your activity (whatever it is), and jot down a few notes about your experience in a notebook. Collect about six beeps, which is likely to take three or four hours; within about 24 hours we should discuss each beep in detail via Skype.

I'd like you to write in the notebook whatever it takes for you to recall in detail what the experience was like at the moment it was occurring. I don't want to tell you what to write. I want you to convey the features of your experience as they occur to you—in your words, your way—and what you choose to write is up to you. I will not ask to see what you write—think of it as a message from you to you. It may develop, as we get more experience together, that I'll ask you to pay particular attention to some kind of detail and make some notes about that particular detail, but that is fairly unusual.

Our discussion of six beeps is likely to take about an hour, and I'd like it to take place within 24 hours of the beeps, either later that same day or the next day. I like "fresh beeps"! The shorter the time between the beeps and the interview the better, but one overnight seems in general to be OK. I don't particularly care when you wear the beeper, although I do request that you wear it at times that you are engaged in different activities. If you always wear it when you're watching TV, for example, the results are likely to be somewhat one-sided.

I'd like to be perfectly clear that you have total control over this project. If you agree to participate today, you can change your mind tomorrow. Sooner or later, we or I might want to tell others or write about what we have found, but before I do that I'll ask for your permission, and you should feel free to give or to decline to give permission at that time. You have no obligation to anything at any time.

I fully recognize that we would be exploring something that is by its very nature absolutely private, and that I have no right to view your experience unless you invite me to do so. I will do all I can to honor that privacy.

It may happen that the beep occurs when you are doing something or thinking something that you would prefer not to discuss. In that case you should feel free to tell me that something occurred that is none of my business, and I'll respect that. I have things that are none of your business, and I presume that you have things that are none of mine.

If a particular beep is none of my business, please tell me that explicitly rather than simply trying to omit talking about the sensitive portion of that experience. I make this request for practical reasons. When we discuss a sample, I will keep questioning until I feel that I have a clear understanding of your experience. If you are holding something back, I'm likely to feel that my understanding is somehow incomplete, so I'll keep questioning and questioning, trying to understand it fully. It's just easier if you say right off, "Some or all of this beep is none of your business."

I'd like you to be absolutely comfortable, with no reluctance, in saying, "That's none of your business." If I can trust you to tell me that something is none of my business when that is the case, then I can feel free to ask whatever I might wish to ask in order to understand some aspect of your experience.

Actually, I might say, it's fairly rare that people invoke this none-of-your-business privilege, because it turns out that most experiences are fairly mundane or prosaic (as judged by the people themselves, not by me). But I want you fully to appreciate the privilege so that our conversations can be candid and complete.

It is *always* OK to say that you couldn't respond to the beep—because it was too loud, or you were engaged in an activity that you didn't want to interrupt, etc.

Don't try to make something up just to answer a question. It may well be that I ask questions that are impossible to answer, that don't apply to you, or that you don't understand. Simply say "I don't know" or something like that. Our task is to describe accurately your inner experience, and we'll accomplish that most efficiently if we're honest with each other about what was happening at the moment of the beep and how well we understand it. If a question is impossible to answer, then it's impossible, and that's OK.

When the beep comes, I'd like you to focus on the very moment that the beep occurred, that microsecond just before your awareness was disturbed by the beep. I'm not interested in what your reaction to the beep was—I'm interested in your experience just at that instant that the beep began. It's rather like a flash photograph. The very beginning of the beep is the flash. I'm interested in what was ongoing right at the moment of the flash. The flash very often makes you blink, but the photo records your face immediately prior to the blink. Just like the flash photo, I wish our research to record the experience that was ongoing immediately *prior* to your reaction to the beep.

I'm not particularly interested in *why* your experience was the way it was. Sometimes you'll need to give such an explanation so that we can have effective communication about your experience, but I'm primarily interested in *what* the experience was like, *not* in *why* it had the content or features it had. Furthermore, I'm not interested in whether a particular sample is typical or unusual for you. The random method will tell us whether something is usual or unusual. If a kind of experience is typical, then we'll see many of them, and if not, not.

I'll be interested in the content of the experience—what you were thinking about or how you were feeling, for example. But I will also be interested (actually, probably more interested) in the phenomenon of the experience itself—how this particular thought or feeling was experienced.

Prior to sampling, most people think sampling will be difficult, but most people have little difficulty once sampling begins.

Furthermore, the method will evolve as we do it—that's part of the reason we meet repeatedly over several or many days. During the first few days you will come to understand the kinds of questions I ask, and as a result you will probably become better able to answer them. At the same time, I will come to understand the kinds of experiences you have, and as a result I will probably become better at asking good questions.

I'd actually prefer that our first few sessions seem like something of a struggle. We will be struggling in parallel to find the best way to explore and describe something (your experience) that I have never seen before and you have probably never tried to describe before.

I could, of course, give you a list of the kinds of questions I sometimes ask, but I'd rather not do that. I want us to approach your experience in whatever way seems most natural for you. I want to color your expectations as little as possible. That may lead to some challenging moments in the first few sessions, but that's just part of the game. [These instructions are adapted from Hurlburt and Heavey, 2006, chap. 6.]

XVI

SIMILARITY AND FAMILIARITY, SCAMS, AND THE FIGHT TO THE DEATH

April 27
Dear Russ,
Great, I'll let you know when I receive the beeper and we'll arrange a Skype call.
    Many thanks for your comments—my responses are below.
All the best,
Marco

RE [173] "Judgments or generalizations exist on some sort of continuum of fauxity"; and

RE [174] "When most people (including John) give faux generalizations, they do not have any explicit understanding of the degree of fauxity of their expressions. I suspect you agree with that."
    You suspect well, since I agree with all this. Generalizations and judgments are inherently faux, and that seems to reflect what you called a few emails back the "perspectival" nature of broad experience. I am slightly suspicious about the negative connotations of the adjective "faux," however: "faux" is, of course, French for "false." A faux generalization is not useless or uninteresting because it is faux. And while some generalizations are indeed fully faux (e.g., I claim that I like Farm Basket turkey without ever having tasted it), most of them fall on a continuum of increasing "fidelity" to pristine experience. I think metaphors such as fidelity and closeness might be more neutral ways of expressing this idea. But that's just a terminological point.

[177]
[178]

RE [175] "Hugo was swindled not because of a failure of his concepts, but because of his failure to appreciate that the same words can apply to very different concepts (it is absolutely true that a photo of a 2003 red Civic is not a bulldozer or a Heineken)."

I completely agree with you that words can be misleading. Maybe they are more often misleading than I—or most people—think. And yet, judging from how people use words in their everyday life (Willy's scam worked because he correctly *guessed* that Hugo would interpret the statement as saying that Willy wanted to sell his car, not the photo), one can conclude that words and concepts are not employed in an arbitrary, haphazard manner either.

If a child says "I feel hungry," it is because he or she has learned that this phrase is bound up with a certain inner feeling, whatever the exact characteristics of that feeling. When I say "I feel hungry" I recognize hunger even if I don't stop to dissect its phenomenal qualities. I could, of course, say it for a number of other reasons—maybe I don't feel hungry at all and I want to cut short a conversation. But there are at least *some* cases in which I say it and I really feel hungry. Maybe feeling hungry for me is different from feeling hungry for you. Maybe my feeling hungry when I wake up is different from my feeling hungry after work. Why not? Maybe my feeling hungry after work yesterday is different from my feeling hungry after work today. Continuing like this, the phrase "feeling hungry" will be completely deprived of any meaning. We will only have countless (virtually infinite) states to which the phrase "feeling hungry" can be applied, without any shared phenomenal quality. I do think it is at least possible that "feeling hungry" works only at the behavioral level, signaling that the speaker wants to get some food (in most scenarios) without implying any underlying shared phenomenal quality. I do think it is possible, in other words, that in all these situations in which the phrase "feeling hungry" is used, those who utter it have radically different phenomenologies. It is possible, but it is unlikely, given the similarities in the way human beings are wired up. Moreover, I'm not saying that people's hunger-phenomenologies are *very* similar. I'm just saying that they should be similar enough for people to (roughly) understand what another person means when he or she claims to feel hungry. In your example, Dennis's hunger sample, it is hardly surprising that Dennis feels a sensation in his stomach. It is hardly surprising that he characterizes his stomach as empty and acidy. All this resonates with my own experience of hunger (at least as apprehended in broad experience!). It is surprising, of course, that Dennis saw himself from a third-person perspective, that he innerly saw (rather than just felt) his stomach as in an x-ray, and so on.

All these discoveries are extremely interesting. They are much more interesting than the sensations of emptiness and acidity. If all you're saying is "look, there's so much to be discovered by exploring people's experience beyond the words and concepts that they generally use, and by inviting them carefully to articulate what they mean by those words and concepts!" then I couldn't agree more. In this sense, and for whatever my opinion counts, I think you've been successful in convincing me of the importance of going beyond words and concepts. I only wonder, since our conversation is personal, if claims like "Hunger does not exist as a phenomenon" are helpful in conveying this much more modest—and yet extremely challenging—invitation to go beyond the façade of concepts and words. You've gone through this argument many more times than I have, of course, but I have the sense that denying the obvious, or what people tend to take for granted (hunger-qualities are similar) might not always be the best conversational strategy for getting the invitation across. I think denying the *similarities* between people's experiences is likely to get you into trouble. In broad terms, there is no doubt that I recognize Dennis's experience of hunger as one that is familiar to me.

[183]

[184]
[185]

I trust you when you say that "To the extent that you think that you know what 'thirst' or any other word means, then you will be deaf to hints that suggest an alternative." But again this is no either/or phenomenon, where one either thinks he knows or he doesn't. I think I know what thirst is like, but I would have difficulties enumerating the qualities of thirst here, probably because my familiarity with thirst does not (usually) involve words and concepts. For this reason, I believe I can be open to other people's descriptions of thirst without starting from the premise that other people's experiences of thirst are necessarily, and radically, different from mine. Again, I may be wrong here. Yet this default assumption of human difference sets off alarm bells for me. It may have heuristic validity in the DES context, but it seems undesirable, and even dangerous, to deny that such difference can be comprehended only against a background of similarity.

[186]

[187]

RE [176] "The instructions for the project."
All clear, we can go ahead.

NOTE: During their first Skype conversation, Marco and Russ agree that their first sampling day would be May 8.

May 7
Hi Marco—
Looking forward to the beeps tomorrow! Please see below.
—Russ

RE [184] "I think denying the *similarities* between people's experiences is likely to get you into trouble"; and

RE [187] "This default assumption of human difference sets off alarm bells for me."

I don't think I denied (and I certainly didn't *intend* to deny) that there sometimes are similarities in experience across people. And I did not intend to assert or by default assume that people are indeed very different from each other. My intention was to assert that if and when one wishes to apprehend phenomena with fidelity, it is probably desirable, and perhaps necessary, to *act as if* people's experiences were (or at least might be) very different from each other's. If one starts from the standpoint of probable difference, it is relatively easy to overturn that standpoint and discover similarities. However, if one starts from the standpoint of probable similarity, it is very difficult and perhaps impossible to overturn that standpoint and discover differences. This asymmetry is, first of all, an empirical observation, the result of having tried to train dozens of people in the DES interviewing skills: trainees (nearly) always naturally assume that they know the features of others' experience (and have great difficulty breaking that assumption down), but they never naturally assume their own ignorance about others' experience. That is, I didn't have a theoretical perspective that predicted that asymmetry—the asymmetry was forced on me by my DES training experiences. [188]

That said, I can speculate three reasons that the asymmetry exists: First, everyone throughout their lifetimes has seen thousands of examples of inner experience, and they are all indeed very similar to their own (in fact they *are* their own!). Until they meet me, they have probably never had the occasion to challenge the assumption of similarity across people. Second, people are *attached* to their supposed similarities, because the alternative to potential dissimilarity is recognizing their own ignorance, which most people do not easily do. Third, there is lots of psychological evidence in all sorts of situations (and everyday observation) that shows that people are much more likely to ask [189] questions that confirm beliefs rather than disconfirm them (the effect generally known as "confirmation bias").

The existence of the asymmetry is important. If one starts from the premise that "I don't know what this experience will be," the amount of evidence/time/energy necessary to arrive at a high-fidelity description (regardless of how you define "high fidelity") is simply the amount of evidence/time/energy necessary to apprehend/describe the phenomenon. However, if one starts from the premise that "I know what experience will be," the amount of evidence/time/energy necessary to arrive at a high-fidelity description is (a) the amount of evidence/time/energy necessary to apprehend/describe the phenomenon plus (or maybe it's *times* or maybe *to the power of*—I'm not advancing a mathematical model here) (b) the amount of evidence/time/energy necessary to weaken/abandon/bracket one's cherished beliefs/presumed prior knowledge. That is a serious problem (if one's aim is to apprehend phenomena) because the amount (b) is very high because those attachments are (mini or maxi) delusions, and escaping one's delusions is difficult.

You may find the following "escape velocity" metaphor a bit of a stretch, but I present it on the possibility that it may be helpful. If you fire a rocket at 25,000 mph from the earth's surface into space, it will leave the earth's gravity and continue forever. Once free of the earth, it requires very little energy (tiny rockets will do) to direct it to the moon, or to Mars, or to Venus, or to any other target. If you fire it at 10,000 mph or 18,247 mph or 23,419 mph or any velocity less than 25,000 mph, the rocket will fall back to earth. Thus hitting a target out in space requires providing a very large chunk of energy necessary to escape the earth's relentless attraction (which is metaphorically like (b) of the preceding paragraph), but then only a very small amount of energy is necessary to aim at the target (and to adjust course if necessary) once you've escaped (that's (a) of the previous paragraph). So, according to this metaphor, one's attachment to the supposition of similarity is like the earth's gravity: it pulls and pulls, wherever you go, back to where you started from, unless you can provide enough energy (successfully bracket the presuppositions) to escape. But once you have neutralized gravity, fidelity to the desired course is easy.

It required about a million pounds of fuel to get the Mars Science Laboratory out of the earth's gravity. It required only about a thousand pounds of fuel to guide the spacecraft to its position and land on Mars. Applying that to presuppositions is just metaphor, of course. But the point is that it is far more difficult to overcome one's own initial presuppositions than it is to hear another's experience in high fidelity once one has successfully escaped one's own presuppositions.

RE [186] "I believe I can be open to other people's descriptions of thirst without starting from the premise that other people's experiences of thirst are necessarily, and radically, different from mine."

First, as I have said, I have not recommended "starting from the premise that other people's experiences of thirst are *necessarily, and radically, different* from mine." I have recommended starting from the premise that *you don't know* whether other people's experiences of thirst are similar to or different (perhaps radically different) from yours.

Second, I think you dramatically underestimate the difficulty of being open to other people's experiences if you start with the premise of similarity. You have to radically excise the premise of similarity (reach escape velocity), so that then it requires only a little energy to attend to the actual phenomena. Note again that excising the premise of similarity is *not at all* the same thing as assuming everyone is necessarily and radically different from you.

You are saying in effect, to my ear, "I don't have to radically excise my preconceptions—I can apprehend other's experience just the way I am, thank you very much." (Please pardon my slight hyperbole; I've found that casting things in the least favorable light is often a useful tool in the abrading of presuppositions.) From my point of view, you are fighting strenuously, to the death almost, against the very thing that I'm pretty sure you have to do if you are going to be good at attending to phenomena.

This fighting-against is both Marco's personal failing and not Marco's personal failing. It *is* Marco's personal failing because Marco's presuppositions are idiosyncratically Marco's, and because no one besides Marco can fight or is fighting against Marco's presuppositions. On the other hand, it is *not* Marco's personal failing because nearly everyone says, "I don't have to radically excise my preconceptions—I can apprehend other's experience just the way I am, thank you very much." That's the way presuppositions are for everyone, not just for Marco. Nearly everyone thinks that their own presuppositions are not problematic. In fact, nearly everyone thinks of their own presuppositions as virtues, rather than impediments. Everyone thinks that it is easy to set aside their own presuppositions and see the world accurately. I'm pretty sure that everyone is wrong on all counts. Everyone's presuppositions fight to the death.

RE [179] "One can conclude that words and concepts are not employed in an arbitrary, haphazard manner either."

[190] I think you do not distinguish carefully enough between words and concepts that apply to the external world and words and concepts that apply to inner experience. Words and concepts about the external world can be shaped with precision by the verbal community; words and concepts about inner experience can*not* be easily shaped with precision by the verbal community, and are therefore not typically shaped with anything that approaches precision (this is Skinner's main point; see also Hurlburt and Heavey, 2001). Willy's scam worked because the concepts were about the external world, and there is, as you say, typically relatively little disagreement about external-world concepts.

But the situation is entirely different with respect to inner experience. Here's a passage from my 2007 book with Eric Schwitzgebel where I discuss the polysemy of the word "thinking":

> Russ: With striking regularity, subjects early in their sampling refer to their own most-frequent kind of inner experience as "thinking," saying things like, "At the moment of the beep I was thinking that I don't want to take that exam." Carefully examining the details of those experiences reveals that people differ substantially in what they mean by "thinking." When Alice says "I was thinking . . . ," she means that she was saying something to herself in her own naturally inflected inner voice. When Betty says "I was thinking . . . ," she means that she was seeing a visual image of something. When Carol says "I was thinking . . . ," she means that she was feeling some sensation in her heart or stomach and that she had no awareness of cognition whatsoever.
>
> "Thinking" refers to cognition in its dictionary definition, but it is decidedly not necessarily used that way in DES self-descriptions, even by sophisticated subjects. My sense is that this is an unsurprising result of the way children learn language. Children observe adults say "I'm thinking . . ." and gradually realize that this utterance "thinking" must refer to whatever is going on in the adult out of direct sight of the child. Children then, on this understanding, use the utterance "thinking" to refer to whatever is most frequently going on

inside them, out of sight of others. Those whose principal inner experience is inner speech will come to use "thinking" to refer to inner speech; those whose principal inner experience is emotion will come to use "thinking" to refer to emotion. (Hurlburt and Schwitzgebel, 2007, 61)

That passage is, in my opinion, an entirely straightforward example of Skinner's point: the word "thinking," because it refers to a private event, is not adequately shaped by the verbal community, and therefore people almost always believe they know what the other means when they say "I'm thinking," but they are frequently, probably usually, wrong, and frequently, probably often, dramatically wrong.

I was sampling yesterday with Joanna in her first DES interview. She said, sincerely and earnestly, that at the moment of the beep she was "saying to herself" that X, but she could not remember, she added, the words she was saying. I'd say the odds are that at the moment of the beep she was not *saying* anything—that is, at the moment of the beep there were no words in her experience (inner or outer) whatsoever. She was not merely slightly mischaracterizing her experience; she was mistaken about its core. And she is by no means unusual in this regard.

(It is worth a parenthetical paragraph to explain how I will come to believe—or reject—what I said in the previous paragraph. Joanna said she was "saying to herself." As of the end of the first sampling day, I don't know (and she cannot be expected to know) whether that characterization is true or false. So at the end of the first sampling day, I encouraged her on subsequent sampling days to pay attention to the features of that saying: features of voice if any, exact words if any, and so on. If subsequent sampling days do not produce any sayings-to-herself, then I think we can be confident that there were no sayings-to-herself on the first day either—that her first-day *report* of saying was driven by presupposition, not phenomena. As I write this, there has not yet been a second sampling day with Joanna, so I don't know how this will turn out.)

Q: *Russ, I tend to agree with Marco on this. I find it hard to believe that people use words like "thinking" with the variety of meanings you described in Hurlburt and Schwitzgebel (2011). Every adult knows the dictionary definition of "thinking" and uses the term accordingly.*

RUSS: You voice a common concern, but one that follows, I fear, from not listening carefully enough. We shall soon see that Marco himself used "thinking" in an idiosyncratic way. Early in his DES sampling, the first round of which took place later on this day, Marco frequently called "thinking" experiences that were actually (as became evident later) the particular awareness of some sensory aspect. For example, he said in the first DES interview that at one beep he was thinking about scratching his beard when subsequent sampling makes it far more likely that he was feeling the bristliness of his beard without any cognitive experience whatsoever.

RE [181] "I do think it is possible, in other words, that in all these situations in which the phrase 'feeling hungry' is used, those who utter it have radically different phenomenologies. It is possible, but it is unlikely, given the similarities in the way human beings are wired up."

You voice a commonly held but I think dramatically untrue opinion. As we have seen, people who utter "thinking" or "saying" have radically different phenomenologies, and they presumably belong to your similar-wired-up-human-being category. Really! Their phenomenologies are about as different as is possible to get! There's very little doubt about it!

If that's true for thinking and saying, I think it is likely to be true about some other or perhaps all aspects of inner experience. That does not imply that everyone is radically different; it implies that it is not safe to assume that radical differences are "unlikely."

RE [185] "There is no doubt that I recognize Dennis's experience of hunger as one that is familiar to me."

Yes, and that's the problem. You have no doubt that you recognize Dennis's hunger as familiar to you, even though his hunger experience itself may not be familiar to you. Your lack of doubt is, I think, likely to make you insensitive to Dennis's phenomena if they do happen to be unfamiliar.

I accept that Dennis's experience of hunger may be similar to yours. *But it may not be similar to yours,* and if you want to be able to hear that, you have to create a level playing field, level equally for similarity and dissimilarity.

Q: *Russ, Marco said there is no doubt! Can't you just accept that?*

RUSS: *I have toyed with the notion of writing a paper that combs the scientific literature for the phrase "there is no doubt" and makes the case that the use of that phrase is usually mistaken. The logic is this: If there really is no doubt, then it would not occur to you to say "there is no doubt." For example, it would not occur to you to say "There is no doubt that when I walk my head is usually higher than my feet." So people usually use the phrase "there is no doubt" to signal that there is a doubt but they wish or hope or mistakenly believe that there is no doubt.*

This is a big deal because if you (or I) want to be good at the bracketing of presuppositions, then whenever you (or I) hear yourself (myself) say "there is no doubt," you (or I) should rewind the conversation and search for a possible presupposition.

RE [180] "If a child says 'I feel hungry,' it is because he or she has learned that this phrase is bound up with a certain inner feeling, whatever the exact characteristics of that feeling."

I accept that that is the usual opinion, including among developmental psychologists, but I think there is reason to believe that it is mistaken. You imply that the feeling exists first, and then the words are applied. I suspect that that is not true. I suspect that what you would call "a certain inner feeling" does not really exist for many (perhaps most, perhaps all) children until late childhood (see chap. 9 of Hurlburt 2011a.).

RE [182] "If all you're saying is 'look, there's so much to be discovered by exploring people's experience beyond the words and concepts that they generally use, and by inviting them to carefully articulate what they mean by those words and concepts!' then I couldn't agree more."

This is indeed the heart of it, because that is exactly what I would like to convey. But there is a rub (and it is a serious rub); see next.

RE [183] "I have the sense that denying the obvious, or what people tend to take for granted (hunger-qualities are similar) might not always be the best conversational strategy for getting the invitation across"; and

RE [186] "I believe I can be open to other people's descriptions of thirst without starting from the premise that other people's experiences of thirst are necessarily, and radically, different from mine. Again, I may be wrong here. Yet this default assumption of human difference sets off alarm bells for me."

Your worry about my conversational strategy is important—most of my friends agree with you. I accept the possibility that it is a self-defeating strategy of my own personality, to which I would of course, but no less unfortunately, be blind. But to the extent that I have access to my own broad experiences, here is why I take this tack:

I am convinced, rightly or wrongly, on the basis of my repeated attempts to train people, that the apprehension of phenomena in high fidelity is not an easily acquired skill. Most people, when they hear about DES, think, "Ah! I can do that! I'll just read *Moments of Truth*, get a beeper, and try to be open to experience!" They think that will be good enough, but I'm pretty sure they are mistaken. I don't think it is possible to "ease into" the high-fidelity apprehension of phenomena. So I am not interested in a "conversational strategy for getting the invitation across" unless I can at the same time get across the notion that there is some radical effort required. A lot of people doing DES badly (by my lights) might be worse than a few people doing it well.

You would like me to say, "Look, there's so much to be discovered by exploring people's experience beyond the words and concepts that they generally use, and by inviting them to carefully articulate what they mean by those words and concepts!" I fear (with what I think is good reason) that "inviting people to carefully articulate" is a recipe for disaster. Every scientist (or literary scholar) thinks they carefully articulate! So the invitation you suggest will almost always be understood to mean, Do what you already do, and apply it to exploring inner experience. That is simply not good enough. For example, this is from the abstract of one of the top consciousness journals: "The present article reports the development and psychometric validation of a novel instrument, the Varieties of Inner Speech Questionnaire (VISQ), *designed to assess the phenomenological properties of inner speech*" (McCarthy-Jones and Fernyhough, 2011; my italics). The VISQ does not (I think) assess phenomenological properties. The VISQ is a one-shot questionnaire with items such as "I think to myself in words using brief phrases and single words rather than full sentences." As I have said above, people do not use phrases like "think to myself" in consistent ways, and in fact people do not know how they themselves use phrases like "think to myself," and for sure the questionnaire item interpreters cannot know what a checkmark of 5 on that item means. Therefore, I think a questionnaire item like this cannot be expected to reveal the phenomenological properties of inner speech. And I do not think the aggregating of items can overcome the problem. I don't single out the VISQ because it is a *bad* questionnaire; it is a state-of-the-art questionnaire. In particular I do not criticize the authors, because the editors and the readership are equally involved. Psychological science does not adequately distinguish between the exploration of phenomena and all else. (Sound familiar?) Hurlburt and Heavey (2015) make a similar argument.

RE [177] "I am slightly suspicious about the negative connotations of the adjective 'faux,' however: 'faux' is, of course, French for 'false.'"

By using "faux" I intend the connotation "false," along with the connotations of "imitation" and "pretend." The heart of my (metaphorical) use of "faux" is as in "faux fur." A *faux leopard fur jacket* is truly a *jacket,* and as such has many of the characteristics of real jackets: warmth, fashion, etc. But it is falsely a *leopard fur* jacket because it does *not* have many of the characteristics of real leopard skin: it is not as warm or insulating; it does not breathe; it does not have the ability to keep snow from melting and re-freezing; and it did not come from a leopard.

So I think "faux" has partially true and partially false connotations, and that is exactly my aim. I emphasize (harp) on the false connotation because nearly everyone overlooks it (or argues vehemently against its falseness).

RE [178] "A faux generalization is not useless or uninteresting because it is faux."

I agree, and I think I have said as much on many occasions in our correspondence. But I must harp: The fact that a faux generalization may be useful or interesting *does not make it any less false, does not make it a real generalization,* just as the fact that a faux leopard jacket is warm and beautiful does not make it real leopard.

XVII

MARCO WEARS THE BEEPER

NOTE: Marco's first day (of six) of DES sampling, with Russ as interviewer over Skype, took place at this point. Russ wrote contemporaneous descriptions of each of Marco's samples, but for reasons that will become clearer in a few pages, we did not discuss those descriptions until Marco's sampling was complete. We will therefore present those descriptions in chapter XVIII.

May 8

Hi Marco—

I attach my descriptions of this morning's samples. Please let me know if I have overlooked anything, distorted anything, or otherwise missed the high-fidelity experiential target.

I also attach the audio recording of today's Skype conversation. No need to listen if you don't want to; I send it so that if for whatever reason you do want to refer to it, you have it.

In most samplings I would not give subjects the written descriptions as I am doing now, because of the risk that the written descriptions would tend to "reify" patterns—influence subjects to report similar things in subsequent sampling days. That is a risk with you, as well, but our "rules of engagement" are somewhat different than is typical for me. So I'll just explicitly encourage you: please recognize that the samples on your second sampling day may be much different from what is written here, both because it is a different day and your experiences may be different, and because you will be a more experienced sampler on your second day. In short, your task is to bracket any impressions you might have about any of these beeps.

Alternatively, you may decide that you would prefer not to read these beep descriptions now. That would be fine as well.

—Russ

May 9
Dear Russ,
Many thanks for the descriptions and the recording, I've downloaded both files. I appreciate your giving me the chance to review the descriptions, but on the whole I think I'd prefer to stick to the normal DES procedure, so I won't open your document for now. I'm sure that it will prove useful as we discuss the results of our samples, but at this early stage I'm concerned—as you are—that my reading the descriptions might influence the next sampling days.

Going through the DES in a first-person way makes me fully understand what you say about the importance of not taking for granted the meaning of words, so I'm really glad that we've started this new phase in our conversation. I'm looking forward to Day 2.
All the best,
Marco

NOTE: *Because Marco decided not to look at the sample descriptions until the conclusion of sampling, we will present the written descriptions after Marco's final (sixth) sampling day (see chapter XVIII).*

May 10
Hi Marco—
I think that's a good decision, but I wanted it to be yours to make.

By the way, I sent those now so as to be entirely unambiguous that I wrote those descriptions immediately following the first interview. Then there will be no doubt that what is written about a beeped experience is how I apprehended it contemporaneously, not colored or influenced by what might transpire in future interviews. That is the heart (in my view) of real (as opposed to faux) generalization: the data points that might be generalized about have to be independently existing entities not shaped or colored by subsequent interactions (as far as that is possible in human interchange).

I'm looking forward to Day 2 as well.
—Russ

May 11
Dear Russ,
Many thanks for your May 7 comments and thoughts.

You'll find my responses below. At this stage in our conversation I feel that it would be useful for me to slow down the theoretical back-and-forth and focus on the sampling instead. Feel free to reply, of course—I may just want to wait until the sampling is over before picking up the conversation again. This is in the interest of not letting my presuppositions about DES get (too much) in the way, so that I may have a fresh look at the theoretical issues when I go back to the conceptual discussion. Let me know if this sounds okay to you.
All the best,
Marco

RE [188] "If one starts from the standpoint of probable similarity, it is very difficult and perhaps impossible to overturn that standpoint and discover differences."

I accept that this might be true for the DES method, and probably for every empirical method that makes a serious attempt at capturing pristine experience. I trust you when you say that there is a huge amount of work required in becoming a skilled DES interviewer, and that a major part of that work is devoted to abandoning presuppositions, including the presupposition that others' experiences are necessarily similar to one's own. I also have no doubt that good will is *not* sufficient to reach this goal, and that delusions are hard to kill.

[192] However, all this seems to presuppose that the question that we're trying to address in this conversation is: how can Marco learn to skillfully and effectively apprehend pristine experience? I don't deny that such question may have been on the horizon of our exchanges, especially at the beginning, but I have the impression that that is only one facet of [193] what we're trying to figure out here. When you write that "you [have] sincerely to act *as if you know nothing about* similarities between people" (in the "Regarding the personal and the conceptual" section of chapter XV), I wonder what exactly the scope of application of this principle is. I think you've shown conclusively that it works in the DES setting. I have reason to think—and so, I imagine, have you—that any kind of faithful apprehension of pristine experience would have to use this idea as a point [194] of departure. But apprehending pristine experience is not everything. And when I say this I don't mean to diminish DES in any way—I'm only

saying that what you would call a "mature science of experience" has to rely on experience samples, but it cannot stop there.

First of all, I'm tempted to ask: can a mature science of experience be a purely empirical, inductivist endeavor, in the sense that you would approach not only the sampling activity (where presuppositionlessness is essential) but your *analysis* of the samples without "a theoretical perspective"? In other words, does the need to eliminate presuppositions carry over into the analysis phase? I know too little about empirical science (or the philosophy of science) to claim any authority here, but I have the sense that such pre- or perhaps a-theoretical way of analyzing and modeling experience might be full of pitfalls. Phenomenologists from Husserl onwards have offered some pretty interesting insights into experience. What's the relationship between your science of experience and the work of these philosophers? Can one really afford to ignore them?

Second, after years spent on sampling and studying experiences, can you still claim that you "know nothing about similarities between people"? I doubt it. Maybe the knowledge you have is provisional, maybe it only scratches the surface of a "mature science of experience," but even now it would be absurd to say that you "know nothing about experience" when you proceed to analyze experience samples after having done so for decades. Aren't we allowed to draw some kind of preliminary conclusion or at least hypothesis—on the issue of similarity, for instance? Take, for example, the following comment: "I accept that Dennis's experience of hunger may be similar to yours. *But it may not be similar to yours,* and if you want to be able to hear that, you have to create a level playing field, level equally for similarity and dissimilarity" [from RE 185]. This seems to presuppose that I know nothing about Dennis's experience of hunger, whereas that is simply not true: I'm saying that his experience sounds familiar after reading an elaborate description of his faithfully apprehended experience of hunger. Of course, for the comparison to be valid one would have to start from my pristine experience rather than from my broad experience of hunger. Perhaps my impression of similarity is just a presupposition. Yet I would be *very* surprised if my typical pristine experience of hunger didn't involve at least one or more sensations localized in my stomach. If this could be proven in pristine experience sampling, then there would be grounds for claiming (beyond any presupposition) that my and Dennis's experiences of hunger are partially similar. I don't want to exaggerate the similarity, of course; when I talk about similarity, I really mean "similarity-in-difference." Moreover, I believe I was creating "a level playing field, level equally for similarity and dissimilarity" when I originally wrote that "It is surprising, of course, that Dennis saw himself from a third-person perspective, that he innerly saw (rather than just felt) his stomach as in an x-ray, and so on."

I'm saying all this because I think that the conceptual matters we've been debating here (for example, the distinction between pristine and broad experience) go far beyond the question: "how does one apprehend experience faithfully?" They have to do with how experience can be conceptualized and modeled *after* the apprehension phase. And here, I think, your objections and caveats about the inherent delusionality of the human condition or (especially) the difficulty of acquiring DES expertise are somewhat less forceful. Despite your claims to the contrary, you seem—at times—to consider DES a one-size-fits-all solution to the questions raised by experience, but I think that view can be problematic. It is at least a theoretical possibility that the skills acquired in DES training are different from those required to analyze the results of experience sampling, and more generally to build a mature science of experience.

RE [189] "Until they meet me, they have probably never had the occasion to challenge the assumption of similarity across people."

Isn't this an important fact? Doesn't this tell us something that a mature science of experience should acknowledge and explain rather than explain away? I don't think that the similarity assumption is *just* a matter of presupposition. Surely, it may become a presupposition in the DES setting, but the fact that people can go about interacting with others (and others' experiences, however broadly and fauxly reported) for years and years without suspecting that others' experiences are significantly different from their own is, it seems to me, *evidence* that there is a background of similarity against which experiential differences can be comprehended. The similarity assumption just works, and there are relatively few situations in daily life in which we ask: "Wait, what do you mean by 'hunger'? What do you mean by 'saying to yourself'?"

This comment goes in the same direction as the previous one (and many other comments I have made in our conversation): it seems unreasonable to assume that DES should be the only standard for judging how experiences are described, referenced, or even studied. I remain convinced that sharing experiences is an important—indeed, essential—component of intersubjectivity (whatever the degree of fauxity of those shared experiences); a mature science of experience should be able to address that issue and explain why that illusion of shareability (if it is an illusion) exists.

RE [190] "Words and concepts about the external world can be shaped with precision by the verbal community; words and concepts about inner experience can*not* be easily shaped with precision by the verbal community, and are therefore not typically shaped with anything that approaches precision (this is Skinner's main point; see also Hurlburt and Heavey, 2001)."

I think you're raising a very interesting point here, and I accept that words and concepts referring to internal events may be less precise—and precisely employed—than words and concepts referring to the public world. I wonder why that is the case, however. Is that because we don't spend enough time talking about inner events? Is that because of some characteristics of inner experience, which make it difficult to capture via words and concepts? Further, don't philosophers and in part also literary texts—at least those that focus on the representation of (fictional) consciousnesses—give us a vocabulary to talk about inner lives? It seems plausible that such vocabulary may be useful, if not in the apprehension, at least in the analysis of DES reports. In my view, this points back to the need for integrating theoretical models and concepts into a science of experience rather than building it from scratch, in a purely bottom-up, inductivist way. [200]

RE [191] "If subsequent sampling days do not produce any sayings-to-herself, then I think we can be confident that there were not sayings-to-herself on the first day either—that her first-day *report* of saying was driven by presupposition, not phenomena."

This line of reasoning is based on the assumption that people's experiences are always somewhat similar to themselves. You spell out this assumption when you write [at marginal 189]: "everyone throughout their lifetimes has seen thousands of examples of inner experience, and they are all indeed very similar to their own (in fact they *are* their own)." So, if Joanna has experience A1 which she describes as "thinking with words," and later has experience A2, which is superficially similar to A1 but is found out to be "thinking without words," then the discovery that A2 is without words applies back to A1. But isn't this a presupposition in itself? You've convinced me that people's experiences are more different than we usually think they are. But why should broad similarity be [201] posited at the individual level? You may argue that this is what DES findings show, but isn't this rather the result of a bias that is built into the method itself?

May 12
Hi Marco—
I look forward to reading your comments, but in the meantime I absolutely agree about the desirability of slowing the theoretical while we focus on the concrete, particularly if you keep some sort of journal/notes/questions/comments/reactions about the concrete so that later (when the concrete dust has settled) we can hash out anything that might have arisen. So I will plan not to reply unless I see something that I think will affect the sampling itself.
—Russ

XVIII

ULTIMATELY PERSONAL: TWENTY-FOUR MOMENTS OF MARCO'S PRISTINE EXPERIENCE

NOTE: Marco's second through sixth days of DES sampling, with Russ as interviewer over Skype, take place at this point (between May 13 and 26). At the end of each sampling day Russ sends Marco a document that contains the sampling descriptions from that day, which Marco saves but does not review while he continues to sample. Here, now that the six days of sampling are complete, are the descriptions of Marco's experience at each sample. These descriptions are written by Russ from Marco's point of view. Audio of the DES interviews can be found on the Companion Website.

Day 1

Sample 1.1. [first day, first sample] I had just sat down, looking at the computer screen preparing to read but not yet reading. In my experience is the white space between two words—not of the words themselves but of the white space between them, and I'm more drawn to the whiteness of the space than to the shape of it. (The words may have been where I was going to begin to read, but I'm not sure.) I'm also somehow thinking about being slightly self-conscious that the beep might occur; also thinking about having just scratched my beard (that if put into words would be "I've just scratched my beard," but there were no words, or if there were words I'm not sure what they were); and also thinking about having just sat down. These three thinkings (self-conscious, beard, just sat) are simultaneous, and the strength or focus was most on the self-conscious, least on the having just sat down. The three thinkings are more cognitive than sensory events (perhaps 70–30, although they may have been closer to being entirely cognitive). The thinkings are quite specific (as I've just scratched my beard, *not* I've just scratched my neck).

NOTE: *This description (like each of the descriptions in this chapter) is contemporaneous—written within a few hours of the interview. As we remarked above (see Russ's response in chapter XVI at marginal 190 and the box near marginal 191), Marco's use of the term "thinking" in this sample should not necessarily be understood to refer to a cognitive event. Later we will discover that Marco uses "thinking" to refer to what DES calls "sensory awareness," but at the beginning of the sampling we did not yet know that.*

Sample 1.2. [first day, second sample] I'm in a restaurant with my friend Paolo, who is speaking. I can't remember Paolo's words—I'm not sure whether what he is saying is in my direct experience (although I do not doubt that I am somehow, perhaps not experientially, tracking his meaning). I am re-experiencing the chewing movement in my jaws, particularly inside my left jaw. This is apparently a recollection (or re-experiencing in imagination) of the chewing of a sandwich bite that had just been finished, but I don't re-experience the sandwich bite or the teeth portion of the original experience—I am now experiencing just the movement of the left jaw. I am not at the moment of the beep actually chewing—the re-experiencing is a sensory (perhaps mostly muscular) recollection of a motion that no longer exists. I also experience the shift in visual field from left to right and from bottom to center, as if my eyes had moved (which probably they had, but my experience was not of the eyes themselves). I'm not sure whether this movement was in response to the beep.

Sample 1.3. Still in the restaurant. Paolo is speaking, and I hear Paolo say the (Italian) word "saltavi" with some emphasis. That is, my experience is of Paolo speaking a sentence: word word word *saltavi* word word word. (Saltavi means "you skipped.") I am attending more to the word *saltavi* and to its emphasis than to the meaning that Paolo is transmitting. (In retrospect I have some sense that perhaps I myself, not Paolo, have created the emphasis, but at the moment of the beep I was merely hearing the emphasized word. Whether created by Paolo or by me, I'm pretty sure that the emphasis was naturally ongoing in the last undisturbed moment before the beep—that is, I did not create the emphasis *because* that word was interrupted by the beep.) I'm also seeing Paolo's face—no particular aspect thereof, but his face is in my experience (that is, it is not merely that my eyes are aimed at his face; I'm experientially seeing his face).

Q: Marco's word—word—saltavi—word—word reminds me of the beginning of this project when you asked Alex to read *The Metamorphosis*. You described his fourth beep (see table 2 in chapter II) as "Alex is speaking the word and then the next word and then the next word, and the beep happens to catch 'cleaner.' That is, it seems more a word—word—word experience than a speaking-a-sentence experience." Alex's and Marco's experiences seem very similar. But Marco received Alex's word—word—word report with shock and disbelief—he said at marginal 10, "Should I really understand him to be experiencing merely one word after the other, each word with no experienced meaning? That doesn't seem possible." Are you really saying that Marco was shocked and disbelieving about aspects of Alex's experience that were, it turned out, remarkably similar to his own experience?

RUSS AND MARCO: Yes! In an important way, this encapsulates the heart of this book. We make these observations:

1) Like many others (including, very likely, you, dear reader), in this regard Marco was ignorant of important aspects of his own experience. Russ and his colleagues have very frequently observed such ignorance.
2) Presuppositions are affectively powerful, not merely cognitively distorting. Marco was not dispassionately skeptical about Alex's word—word—word experience; he was passionately dubious.
3) People often passionately find impossible precisely those things that they themselves frequently do.
4) The strength of one's conviction is often not necessarily related to the truth of that conviction.
5) This example illustrates why DES is a powerful tool. Its focus on randomly selected moments allowed Marco to report in high fidelity an experience (word—word—word) that he would otherwise have passionately denied.

Sample 1.4. Paolo and I have left the restaurant and we are standing while we talk. Paolo is speaking and I'm trying to follow (or maybe I'm just following) the conversation. (Now, during the interview, I don't know to what "trying to" refers. I wrote down "trying to," but I don't recall what I meant, so maybe those words are slightly off target). The center of my focus is on my shoes: the leather, its color and texture, and (perhaps mostly) that the right shoe is forward of the left. (It is the shoes that I attend to, not to my feet.) I also see my legs and that the right leg is slightly forward of the left. I also have some kinesthetic sense of motion in my legs, perhaps more in the right leg—a kinesthetic sense of my right leg's moving forward.

NOTE: *Marco had collected two additional samples, but we didn't have time to discuss them.*

Day 2

Sample 2.1. I'm walking with my wife. She has said or is still saying something like, "I won't have time for lunch," to which I am replying, "Yes you'll have time to" <beep> [have lunch]. I experience a slight fastness of the speaking, slightly faster than is comfortable. I am walking, and I experience the walking as slightly faster than is comfortable. I am slightly irritated. There is no specific irritation present, but everything is somehow irritated—the fastness of the speaking and the walking is irritation. It is as if all aspects of my experience are pervaded or perfused by a slight irritation.

I can't be confident about how my wife's talk is present to me: maybe she is still speaking in actuality; maybe I still hear an inner copy of her voice; maybe the meaning or sense of what she has said is somehow present to me. I'm not sure.

My eyes are open, but I don't experience myself as seeing what my eyes are pointing at.

Sample 2.2. I'm looking at the computer screen and just pressed a button on the keyboard. There are three aspects of my experience. First, I feel a downward pressure on the outside of my eyelids, as if there is an external force pressing down (there is in reality no such force, but the pressure is experienced as coming from a real force outside of me). I don't feel it in my eyeballs—just the eyelids.

Second, I'm thinking that I should find that file. It somehow seems like there are or should be words present in this thinking, but I can't say what the words were, whether they were voiced, or even what language they were in (I could speculate that they were in English [Marco speaks several languages], but that would come from my knowledge of the task, not recollection of the phenomenon). This is a pretty specific thought process that is not exactly in sync with what I am doing—that is, I am *not* looking for the file at the moment of the beep; I am performing another task, so the desire to find the file is not directly tied to the ongoing task.

Third, I feel slightly anxious—which, like the irritation of sample 2.1, does not have a directly experienced aspect (no sweaty palms, no heart racing, no shortness of breath, etc.) but seems a part of all aspects of the experience. For example, the eyelid pressure seems anxious.

The relative intensities are (very roughly) 40% (eyelid)—40% (find file)—20% (irritation), but that makes it seem that the three things were separate, which does not do justice to my experience.

Sample 2.3. I'm typing on the computer ". . . of" <beep> [reader]. I'm focused on the screen (40%) and on my body being moved left to right (40%) and the tactile sensation of the keyboard slightly but distinctly under my fingers (20%).

Later in the interview I came to wonder whether I was actually focused on the screen.

My shoulders and arms felt like they were moving or being moved from left to right, in the same direction as the text on the screen. It is a sense of movement but there is no real movement. It doesn't seem like I am doing the moving, but it does not seem like the movement is being done by an external force (unlike in sample 2.2 where the eyelid pressure seemed distinctly as if being created by an external force). I used the metaphor of a "spring" to describe this, but Russ is not confident that he entirely understood it—the spring somehow conveyed that the experienced agent was not external or internal but both, Russ thinks.

Sample 2.4. I am "taken by" the word "project" in English in my own voice (in no particular location). The particular single word "project" stands out (which is what I mean by "taken by") in my experience. That is, this is the experience of hearing a single word, not a sentence. I am at the computer, paused, perhaps seeking the next thing to write (I'm not sure); the word "project" appears. I innerly hear it rather than innerly speak it. I also have a feeling of the positioning of my fingertips on the keyboard. The division of my attention is roughly 70% ("position")—30% (fingertips).

Q: *Russ, I understand that you said that these descriptions were "written by Russ from Marco's point of view," but it seems weird for you to write things like "I'm walking with my wife" when your first-person "I" refers to Marco, not you. Why do you do that?*

RUSS: The most straightforward answer is that it feels natural to me to write like that. Moreover, it similarly feels natural to me to adopt the other's first-person viewpoint in the interview itself, asking Marco such questions as "How does my wife's speaking sound to me?" As an empirical fact, I can confidently say that subjects are never startled or confused by such unusual pronoun usage; instead, I believe most subjects recognize and accept it as a natural part of my authentic attempt to apprehend their experience from their own point of view. Furthermore, when I make notes about a subject's experience I generally continue in the subject's first-person—that is, after all, the point of view I was trying to apprehend during the interview, and continue that into the written description of the samples.

Often when I write for publication I transform those descriptions into the third person, because that is what most readers expect. But I did not do that when I sent them to Marco, preferring to stay in the more intimate (it seems to me) first person.

By the way, I make no claim that such first-person interviewing/writing is desirable for all interviewers. I claim only that it seems natural for me, so I do it.

Day 3

Sample 3.1. I'm eating cereal, attending to the sweetness and the hard/stiffness of the cereal. I'm also seeing the black/white color and the shape of the man on my computer screen. It's a TV show, and the guy is an actor playing a role, but I'm not at all attending to the action or plot or significance of the scene, other than the color and shape of the guy. The color (which is actually black and white) of the guy seems most salient to me. (As far as I know, this is just a random feature of the visual display—that is, I don't think there was anything particularly objectively salient about the black/white color—for whatever reason I was attending to it.) My attention seemed about 50%—50% on the sweet/hard and on the color/shape.

Sample 3.2. I am moving the cursor on my laptop computer screen using the pointing stick, and I have just removed some yellow highlighting from a passage. I feel the pointing stick, its edges and hardness with my index finger (but the sensation is more of the stick than the finger) as I push it to the left and up. I am also watching the cursor move across the screen. Furthermore, I'm somehow aware of the close connection between my moving the pointing stick and the movement of the cursor. That is, it is not merely a fact of the universe that the two are closely connected; somehow I am at the moment of the beep experiencing the close connection. Also simultaneously I am seeing the white space where the yellow highlighting had been, and also (in my imagination continuing) seeing the yellow highlighting in the same space. That is, I am seeing two things in the same place—the real white space and the imagined yellow highlighting. There is no thought process involved, no label of any kind in my experience that identifies the yellow highlighting as being imagined, and yet I have no confusion about it—the white is real and the yellow in created by my imagination. The relative intensities of these experiential aspects are 40% (pointing stick) 40% (seeing the cursor) 20% seeing the yellow/white. The awareness of the connection between stick and cursor seems to be somehow part of the first two 40%—40%, rather than its own thing.

Sample 3.3. I'm reading or scanning text on computer screen looking for something related to "life world." There are three aspects ongoing at the moment of the beep. First, I "perceive my eyes move downward." We worked hard at clarifying this, and eventually understood this to mean that I am now taking a new point of focus on the screen at a point that is lower than it was previously. That is, the sensation is not in the eyes, nor in the movement or trajectory of the visual scan down the screen. We agreed not to be too confident about the description of this aspect (see also sample 3.4). Second, I feel stiff hairs as I idly play with my beard with the thumb and forefinger of my left hand. I feel the stiffness; this is not a thought process. Third, I am somehow looking for something related to "life world." There is or may be something of the concept of life world present as I look, but I am not at all confident about that. I can confidently say that the words "life world" are neither spoken nor heard nor seen; perhaps there is some sense of the concept of *things related to life world* present to me, but I am not at all confident about that.

Sample 3.4. I had received an email, had opened it and now I'm scanning through it. I experience my eyes moving downward, or perhaps more accurately I experience the downward-moving path or trajectory that my eyes take on the page. I'm not sure whether I experienced anything physical in my eyes. I initially said that this was pretty similar to sample 3.3, but we eventually arrived at a different conclusion: here we concluded that the motion of the point of focus was in experience; in sample 3.3 we had concluded that it was merely the coming to attention of the new position. [Russ encouraged us to leave whether this is the same or different as unsettled—perhaps later samples will shed light on this issue.] I also am apprehensively questioning whether I have done the right thing, experienced as a cognitive and affective questioning/apprehension. The overall target of this questioning is that I have just signed a contract to rent a house and am now questioning whether it is the right house, too much money, etc., but none of that specificity is present in the questioning. The email I am scanning is offering a different house available to rent, but I am not thinking about that house; in fact I am also not thinking about the house I have contracted to rent. I am questioning whether I have done the right thing without explicit content about the thing that I have done (but understanding that it is the house that I am questioning). The apprehension is felt at least in part on the surface of my chest, or perhaps on the surface and down a few millimeters. That is, the apprehension is in my chest but not down deep. The chesty apprehension has no particular characteristics (not pressure, not tension, not tingling or tickling, etc.). My chest makes itself present to me, more present that usual, but beyond that I can't be more specific.

Q: *Sometimes I feel overwhelmed by the insignificant details you describe. Who really cares, for example, whether the point of focus was in Marco's experience or whether he was merely attending to a new position?*

RUSS: *That is an important question, for which I have two answers.*

First, recall from our epigraph that the novelist Philip Roth said that "it is from a scrupulous fidelity to the blizzard of specific data that is a personal life, it is from the force of its uncompromising particularity, its physicalness, that the realistic novel . . . derives its ruthless intimacy." If uncompromising particularity is important in fiction, it is probably also important in fact.

Second, I like to say that in a fundamental sense the DES process never knows what is important until it is too late. What will eventually emerge as a salient characteristic may not be recognized on its first or second appearance. When we begin to notice a pattern of characteristics, we go back to the details of earlier interviews to see whether the pattern applied there as well. At that point it is too late to create the necessary details—those had to have been noted in the contemporaneous interview and described in the contemporaneous write-ups. As a result, we have to apprehend all details in as high fidelity as possible.

Maybe Marco's attending to position will emerge as important; maybe it won't. We have to get it right in the one chance we have.

Day 4

Sample 4.1. I'm sitting at my computer and had just finished drinking from my water bottle and set it back down on my desk. I'm moving my arm from the bottle to my face. I feel the movement/tension in my left upper arm as it moves. This is more a muscular tension and the change in muscular tension than a feeling of translation of the arm in space.

Sample 4.2. I am drinking from a glass, and (1) I feel the pressure of the glass against my lips. This is primarily a sensation of pressure in my lips rather than a sensing of the glass itself. (2) I feel the shape of the interior of my mouth as it is prepared to receive the drink. This is a sensory apprehension. And (3) I hear my wife talking to me. I hear her voice, but at the moment of the beep I don't experience the words or the meaning of what she is saying. (I am doubtless processing the words and meaning at some level—I respond appropriately a few seconds later) but at the moment of the beep I am not aware of the meaning. These are all simultaneous and roughly 50%—25%—25%.

Sample 4.3. (1) I am playing with the cap of the water bottle and feel it with my fingers. This is primarily a sensation of the cap (it is of course the fingers that feel it, but my experience is of the cap; this is different from sample 4.2(1) where the experience is of my body (lips), not the object (glass); see also sample 4.6, which is like sample 4.2 but not sample 4.3). (2) I am speaking aloud to my wife and I hear myself utter "speciale" ("special" in Italian). I do *not* hear myself speak the entire sentence of which one word is "speciale"; I hear only that word. (I don't know whether had the beep come a few seconds later I would have been focused on a word later in the sentence, or whether there was some aspect of that word that drew my attention.) I am hearing the aural characteristics of the word, rather than hearing its meaning. (3) I'm feeling sad because I couldn't make the special meal that I'd like to make (that's the meaning of the sentence I'm uttering.) It is difficult to describe the sadness other than to say it seems to color everything or is like a layer on everything. It is not bodily—I do not feel a heaviness in my heart, or a weight on my shoulders, or a tear in my eye, or anything like that. Rather, everything seems to have a sad resonance. For example, the word "speciale" has a sad resonance, even though its objective characteristics (tone, emphasis, etc.) are not sad. The bottle cap, the word, and the sadness are all simultaneous and roughly 40%—40%—20%.

Sample 4.4. I'm walking into a store and (1) I am noticing the obliqueness and red-brownness of the tiles that form the pavement. The obliqueness is relative to me—I am looking at them at an angle to me (in reality, the tiles are set perpendicular to the wall, and I am moving obliquely across them, but the experience is of the tiles' obliqueness, not my oblique path). (2) I have a bodily sense of moving—my whole body moving. This movement is in the direction of into the store, but the into-the-storeness direction is not in my experience. It is my whole body that is moving all in the same direction, even though in reality parts of my body are swinging in the opposite direction, etc. The obliqueness and bodily moving are simultaneous and roughly 60%—40%.

Sample 4.5. (1) I'm walking briskly, energetically, and I feel a tension in my legs. The tension is experienced as muscular tension, but it is steady and equal throughout both my lower legs from knee to ankle (and perhaps less so but present in my upper leg). (That is, the tension does not reflect the rhythmic waxing/waning of actual muscle tension while walking.) The tension somehow reflects the second aspect of my experience. (2) A sense of busyness, of having things to do. This is more a felt movement; it is not a cognitive knowing or listing of the things I have to do. I immediately recognize the tension in my legs as reflecting the sense of busyness. (3) I am innerly seeing clearly the Dutch word "wereld" in yellow letters. I had seen this word in a storefront advertisement a few seconds earlier—now I see the same word innerly. I don't see the rest of the sentence (something about travel); I don't see the cardboard sign that held the real words. I see just the yellow letters and their shape. I recognize the word-ness of the seen display, and the meaning (world) is somehow present to me. That is, this experience is *not* merely of seeing letters; it is of seeing the word "wereld." The walking briskly/tension is the largest portion of my experience; the busyness and inner seeing less strong.

Sample 4.6. I'm typing on my laptop. I innerly say/hear the sentence "Because of the cognitive basicness" as I type that sentence. At the same time I feel the sensation of keys in my fingertips—this is a tactile sensation rather than a feeling of the keys (that is, I feel my fingertips like sample 4.2; I do not feel the keys like sample 4.3). Although this feels like my fingertips being impacted by the keys, it is a steady pressure, not tied to the pressure of one key after the other. My eyes are aimed at the computer monitor, but I don't experience it. The inner saying is stronger than the fingertip sensation, perhaps 60%—40%.

Day 5

Sample 5.1. I'm stirring tea in a cup. Three things are in my experience 40%—40%—20%. (1) I'm feeling the motion on the skin or surface of my thumb and forefinger and to a lesser extent the rest of my hand. This is a circular motion; I feel the motion, not the kinesthetics of making the motion. This is felt as a slight pressure on the skin or surface of my hand, as if a handkerchief rests lightly on my hand and weighs it down slightly. I feel my hand and this pressure make a circular motion. Note that I do *not* feel the spoon in my thumb and forefinger, even though I am in reality holding the spoon there and stirring with it. (2) I see the bright-metallic-coloredness of the spoon. I see the entire spoon, even that portion that is obscured in reality by my hand and the tea. It is the bright-metallic-coloredness that draws my attention, not the shape or design of the spoon. (3) I hear a voice to my front right. It is my wife's voice, and she is speaking "piacere" (Italian for "pleasure"), but experientially I am not relating to the content or the source. Rather, this is an aural experience—I hear a sound (which in reality is my wife's voice). The content or meaning of what she is saying is not in my direct experience, even though I am at some level processing what she is saying (and could respond appropriately a few seconds later).

Sample 5.2. I'm reading an article on my computer screen. At the moment of the beep I am reading "criticism voiced by readers." There are two aspects of my experience, about 50%—50%. (1) I am "scanning," by which I mean I see a rectangular area moving from left to right as I read. This area is roughly .5 or 1 cm high and 5 or 6 cm wide. I see it to be rectangular in that is has straight sides and square corners, but I'm not sure how the rectangle-ness presents itself. That is, the rectangle does not have a border (or if it does, it is very vague); the rectangle does not have a different color (or if it does, it is very subtle), and yet I see a rectangle moving left to right as I read. I don't feel eye movements—this is an on-the-screen experience, not an in-the-eye experience. The rectangle height seems slightly less than the line height. The text within the rectangle is *not* more clear than the surrounding text—that is, it is the rectangle itself that draws my attention, not the text within it. (2) I am innerly speaking "criticism voiced by readers" in my own voice, with a relaxed pace (relatively slow) and relatively little inflection. The inner speaking seems to have the same characteristics as my exterior voice had I spoken those words aloud. I experience this as more a speaking than a hearing, but I believe I hear the words as well as speak them. The speaking seems to be located (even though this may sound crazy) inside my head on the upper right side, sort of in front and above the temple.

Sample 5.3. I'm walking and looking through a glass door. My experience is divided roughly 60%—40% between (1) a seeing and (2) a feeling. (1) I am seeing blueness with white above it. I of course know that the blue is carpet on a corridor that extends beyond the glass door and the white is the walls of the corridor, but my experience is of blueness with white above it, not corridor-ness or wall-ness. Simultaneously (as part of the 60% seeing experience) I am seeing the stuck-on-ness and the light coloring (white or light yellow) of the lettering on the door. The lettering says "Language Center," but I am not attending to the meaning of the words. (2) I am feeling a slight apprehension that I can't find the place I'm looking for. This apprehension is felt primarily on the surface of my chest, a slight pressure on the skin. The pressure is directed inward and is small but stronger than the pressure on my hand of sample 5.1. There is something of the *I can't find it* that is present in this experience, but I am not able to describe it. The chest pressure does not exhaust the experience of apprehension—the best I can say is that perhaps it is like a color that suffuses everything as I have described feelings in sample 4.3.

Day 6

Marco collected only three beeps this day.

Sample 6.1. I'm reading an email, looking at the word "Utrecht." My experience is split about 50%—50% between (1) the sensory characteristic of the word and (2) the desire to find the names that will be listed farther down in the email. (1) I see the black letters of the word "Utrecht" surrounded by a white rectangle. The white rectangle is created by my imagination (that is, an external observer would not see it). Its edges are straight but the corners are slightly rounded, and it extends a millimeter or two beyond the word in all directions. The word "Utrecht" is seen clearly as it appears on the computer monitor (unlike sample 5.2 where the letters/words inside the rectangle are seen indistinctly, and unlike sample 6.3 where the words are seen clearly but the letters/words themselves have been massed together). (2) I originally referred to this as "cognitive," but it seems more a combination of cognitive and sensory or perceptual and perhaps emotional. The sensory/perceptual part is that I observe myself to be reading quicker than usual, and immediately recognize the quickness to be the attempt to reach the goal quickly. That is, I am not merely reading quickly; I *notice* that I am reading quickly. At the same time, the cognitive part is that I am looking for the names that I expect to find in the email. This is an expectation of discovering names, not of discovering people who happen to have those names. At the same time there may be (but probably is not) an emotional tinge to this experience—an eagerness or something like that. But if this is present at all, it is very faint.

Sample 6.2. I'm at the computer. I have three simultaneous experiences: (1) wondering why the beeper hasn't beeped; (2) feeling myself running out of time; and (3) feeling the mouse beneath my fingers and my hand moving; approximately 40%—40%—20%. (1) At the moment of the beep I am wondering why the beep hasn't come already; I'm thinking that the beeper is supposed to beep at least twice an hour. I clearly experience this content at the moment of the beep. At the same time I feel a tingling in the muscles in the inside of my cheeks at the sides of my mouth as if I am speaking aloud. This is an imaginary sensation (I am not in fact speaking and as far as I know the muscles are not in fact moving) but it is clear in my experience. At the same time I experience my voice as somehow speaking—my normal voice normally inflected. However, I do not directly experience words. The words themselves either do not exist in my experience or exist so faintly as to be unrecognizable. Thus I have a sense of speaking; I have a muscular sensation of speaking; I know the content that I am speaking; I have sense of my voice as speaking. But the words that I seem to be speaking are experientially nonexistent or at most nearly nonexistent.

(2) I experience myself as running out of time, which I feel as a physical sensation in my chest as if I am beginning to run out of breath. This physical sensation has an emotional component—like a modifier or coloring or tingeing of the running-out-of-breath sensation—I don't feel exactly like I am running out of breath, but I *anxiously* feel that I'm running out of breath. That is, the anxiousness colors or suffuses the sensation of running out of breath and somehow subtly transforms it into an emotional-physical feeling of running out of breath rather than merely a physical feeling of running out of breath.

(3) I feel the mouse where it contacts my fingers—not just the finger tips but most of the fingers. I feel the mouse itself, not the pressure in my fingers caused by the mouse. Separately but simultaneously, I feel my hand moving left to right. I experience my whole hand moving, not merely the fingers. Thus experience (3) could be called two separate experiences—of the mouse and of the movement.

NOTE: For the record, the beep comes at least once an hour, on average once every 30 minutes.

Sample 6.3. I'm reading the phrase "we tested this possibility" on my computer screen. There are two or three simultaneous aspects of my experience: (1) the contour of the words; (2) innerly speaking the words; and maybe (3) experiencing the meaning of the words. The first two are about equally salient; it's hard to know whether the third should be counted as a separate aspect or as a portion of (2).

(1) I see the shape, contour, or edge of the words "we tested this possibility." The letters of each word are seen to comprise a black mass, so that each word is solid black, or maybe black with occasional white

holes where openings of the letters would be. Russ used the following metaphor, which seems pretty good: it was as if the words were made out of black chocolate that had melted together so that the letters themselves were no longer clearly discernible. My metaphor was that it was as if the words were printed in a hyper-bold font, so bold that the shape of the letters nearly disappeared. I think an external observer might have been able to make out the words. Here is Russ's rendering:

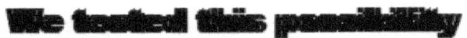

I am attending particularly to the outside edges of these words. I see this display clearly on the screen that I am looking at, even though the words themselves are not particularly clearly readable, and even though the words do not look like the actual words that fall on the retina. That is, I clearly see a distortion of or modification of the actual words, but I don't immediately feel them to be distorted words—I am merely looking at the outline of black words. Furthermore, I see a white rectangular area around these words, extending a millimeter or two beyond them in all directions, with straight edges and rounded corners.

(2) I am innerly speaking these words to myself in my own voice with a relatively flat affect. I do not feel any sensations (that is, I don't feel any kind of tingling in my mouth as I did in sample 6.2).

(3) At the same time I have a direct experience of the semantic meaning and also of the significance of the words, which I experience as being somehow attached to the words so that if I were to say these words aloud I would somehow stress (italicize) them, even though they are not being stressed or italicized in my inner speaking.

Q: Marco, from your perspective, do these descriptions capture your experience?

MARCO: Two months after the samples (and after discussing them with Russ), I reread these descriptions and had a mixed feeling of familiarity and foreignness. I know that these are my experiences, and I remember that Russ and I put a great deal of effort into capturing them. Yet I am also surprised by the speed with which I have forgotten most or all of these instants. It is as if the experiences that we tried to faithfully describe here had left no trace in me: seen on the page, they seem distant, they could almost belong to someone else. Perhaps this sense of remoteness of my own experiences evidences *the fact that the DES method has been successful in bracketing my presuppositions about myself: these are Marco's experiences, to be sure, but not experiences that I emphatically recognize as mine; they do not reflect my entrenched presuppositions about who I am.*

On the other hand, the feeling of "not-mineness" that I get when I read these descriptions is, I think, related to the distancing power of language, and how it can preserve an instant that would otherwise be lost in the flow of my interactions with the world. This is part of what I find poetic about Russ's DES (see my email of June 3 in the next chapter): it achieves something akin to what literary theorist Shklovsky (1991) called "defamiliarization." By stripping away my presuppositions it makes my own experience look (almost) like somebody else's.

XIX

A VERY SMALL QUIBBLE ON WORDING

May 27
Dear Russ,
I've now finished reviewing your descriptions of my sampled experiences [those of the previous chapter], and there is no doubt that these are high-fidelity descriptions. We are in a *very* high level of agreement about the descriptions of the 4 + 4 + 4 + 6 + 3+ 3 = 24 beeped experiences, with the slight exception of sample 6.2 described below.

I have some more general points to make about DES, but I thought that it would be best to stick to the descriptions and what's in there for this round.
Thanks again and all the best,
Marco

NOTE: The following is Marco's main change to Russ's descriptions.

RE [202] Sample 6.2.
 Here is how I would edit sample 6.2:

Sample 6.2. I'm at the computer. I have three simultaneous experiences: (1) wondering why the beeper hasn't beeped; (2) feeling myself running out of time; and (3) feeling the mouse beneath my fingers and my hand moving; approximately 40%—40%—20%. (1) At the moment of the beep I am wondering why the beep hasn't come already; I'm thinking that the beeper is supposed to beep at least twice an hour. I clearly experience this content at the moment of the beep. At the same time I feel a tingling in the muscles in the inside of my cheeks at the sides of my mouth as if I am speaking aloud. This is an imaginary sensation (I am not in fact speaking and as far as I know the muscles are not in fact moving)

[203] but it is clear in my experience. At the same time I experience my voice as somehow speaking—my normal voice normally inflected. ~~However~~ I have the impression that words are implied in this experience, but I do not directly experience words. The words themselves ~~either do not exist in my experience or~~ seem to exist so faintly as to be unrecognizable. Thus I have a sense of speaking; I have a muscular sensation of speaking; I know the content that I am speaking; I have sense of my voice as speak-

[204] ing. But the words that I seem to be speaking ~~are experientially nonexistent or at most nearly nonexistent~~ present themselves in a raw, inarticulate, prelinguistic form (however paradoxical this may sound).

(2) I experience myself as running out of time, which I feel as a physical sensation ~~in~~ on my chest (in the recording I mention a sensation of pressure on my chest—this refers to a previous experience, probably sample 3.4, but I think this experience was fundamentally similar) as if I am beginning to run out of breath. This physical sensation has an emotional component—like a modifier or coloring or tingeing of the running-out-of-breath sensation—I don't feel exactly like I am running out of breath, but I *anxiously* feel that I'm running out of breath. That is, the anxiousness colors or suffuses the sensation of running out of breath and somehow subtly transforms it into an emotional-physical feeling of running out of breath rather than merely a physical feeling of running out of breath.

(3) I feel the mouse where it contacts my fingers—not just the finger tips but most of the fingers. I feel the mouse itself, not the pressure in my fingers caused by the mouse. Separately but simultaneously, I feel my hand moving left to right. I experience my whole hand moving, not merely the fingers. Thus experience (3) could be ~~called~~ seen as two separate experiences—of the mouse and of the movement, but these two sensations were tightly integrated.

June 1
Hi Marco—
Below please see my very slight comments about your comments about the sample descriptions.

RE [203] "The words themselves seem to exist so faintly as to be unrecognizable."

I think your edit removes perhaps too completely the possibility that there were no words present in experience at the moment of the beep. It seems to me that no-words-present remains a possibility.

I think your alteration of sample 6.2(1) gives words an experientially certain reality that they perhaps did not deserve at the moment of beep 6.2. When you say that "the words themselves seem to exist so faintly as to be unrecognizable," you imply (as I read it) the unquestioning existence of the words. I understand the phrase "seem to exist" as modifying the faintness, not the words, so your sentence to my ear reads: "The words themselves unquestionably exist; however, their manner of (unquestionable) existence seems to be so faint as to make the (unquestionably existing) words unrecognizable." (I understand that to a large degree you are adopting my own writing of this beep description, which I think also regrettably gives a reality to the words that they do not necessarily deserve. But I think my infelicity was worsened when you stripped out the explicit acknowledgment that words might not have existed in experience at the moment of the beep.)

[205]

RE [204] "But the words that I seem to be speaking present themselves in a raw, inarticulate, prelinguistic form (however paradoxical this may sound)."

I have the same observation about this sentence as you modified it. Your grammar (again, adapted from mine) seems to imply that one can remove the relative clause "that I seem to be speaking" (I'm no grammarian, so if my usage is not correct, please let me know), leaving your sentence to read: "But the words present themselves in a raw, inarticulate, prelinguistic form (however paradoxical this may sound)." In that sentence there is no equivocation about the existence of the words, so your sentence to my ear reads: "But the words, which themselves unquestioningly exist, present themselves as unquestioningly existing in a raw, inarticulate, prelinguistic form (however paradoxical this may sound)."

I think that words may not deserve such unquestioned existence in your pristine experience at sample 6.2. You yourself seem to say this when you write "I have the impression that words are implied in this experience, but I do not directly experience words." To say that "words are *implied in* this experience" is to say that the words do not exist in experience.

The bottom line: I think we should keep the possibility of no words present to experience in the sample description of 6.2.

I note that the "size" of the quibble here is experientially very small. I say *little or no* experience of words, whereas you say *a little* experience of words. That is, what is at stake here is the possibility there were *no* words in experience 6.2, or whether there were *ever-*

so-faint-but-raw-inarticulate-prelinguistic words. From the standpoint of experience, that is a microscopic distinction, probably smaller than is possible for either of us to make on the grounds of experiential evidence. That's the point of Hurlburt and Schwitzgebel (2011), where I tried to show that experientially we are not in a position to discriminate reliably between "no" and "little or no."

If our task is to judge the fidelity of descriptions of pristine experience, it doesn't much matter. It's rather like saying about András Schiff's recording of *The Well-tempered Clavier*: "There may be some noise in the background, but if there is noise it's so faint that I can't hear it." Perfection? No. Very high fidelity? Yes. This is the largest quibble we have about the 24 samples, and this quibble is microscopic. Therefore I conclude that we agree that these descriptions of experience are of very high fidelity.

I emphasize that our task is to create descriptions that rest lightly and faithfully on your pristine experience, and that I am not infallible, nor am I the ultimate authority about experience in general or yours in particular. However, I also think that you are not infallible or the ultimate authority about your own experience, even though the pristine experience is yours. I think we both come to this descriptive task as flawed human beings, trying to do our best with the limitations we have.

Q: Russ, if I've been following you correctly, that paragraph seems to be about as good a description of DES as there is.
RUSS: I agree!

June 2
Dear Russ,
Below please find my response to your comment on sample 6.2.
Thanks and all the best,
Marco

RE [205] "Your alteration of sample 6.2(1) gives words an experientially certain reality that they perhaps did not deserve."
I think you're right that in the rewritten text I'm implying too strongly the existence of words in my experience. What I wish to convey is this: I had a sense of words in my experience, but the words themselves may

(or may not) have existed. You may compare this to tasting a dessert without knowing the ingredients and sensing a hint of chocolate. However, you can't remember anything that looked like chocolate in your spoon. The chocolate-y sensation may come from chocolate or cocoa, but it may also result from an exotic ingredient that tastes almost like chocolate (carob?) or from some unexpected combination of other ingredients. Or you may just have made up the chocolate-y taste. Outside of the allegory, I think there are three different possibilities here: (1) my reporting a sense of words reflects a presupposition; thus, neither the sense of words nor the words themselves were experienced; (2) I really had a sense of words but no words were experienced; (3) I really had a sense of words and could faintly experience some words. I can't rule out any of these possibilities, but (2) and (3) look more plausible than (1) for several reasons, including the fact that this was the last sampling day and that the experience occurred very close to our conversation.

All in all, I'd suggest rewriting the paragraph in the following way:

At the same time I experience my voice as somehow speaking—my normal voice normally inflected. I have the impression that words are implied in this experience, but I do not directly experience words (and indeed no words may be experientially present). If words are experientially present (which they seem to me to be), the words themselves seem to exist so faintly as to be unrecognizable: <u>they present themselves in a raw, inarticulate, prelinguistic form (however paradoxical this may sound)</u>. Thus I have a sense of speaking; I have a muscular sensation of speaking; I know the content that I am speaking; I have sense of my voice as speaking. <u>However, the sense of words that I have may not correspond to any actual words in my experience.</u>

Does this look okay?

June 2
Hi Marco—
Yes, I agree with your edit.
—Russ

June 3
Dear Russ,

Below please find a few general remarks about my sampling experiences. My commentary on the sampling is hardly exhaustive, but I thought it would be good to set the ball rolling.
Thanks and all the best,
Marco

Personal reactions to the sampling

Here I distinguish between my personal reactions to the sampling and some more general remarks (below).

[206]

[207]

[208]

1) On Day 2 during or shortly after our conversation I thought: the whole DES method strives for clarity and distinctness, but what if (some aspects of) experience are inherently, and irreducibly, vague? You make room for this possibility by stressing that the questions you ask may not have an answer, but I still saw a danger that DES questioning may encourage people to be more specific than their experience actually was. I believe I was thinking this in relation to beep 2.2, when you asked me if my experience contained words or not, and I had the sense that it both contained words (in the implied form that we've already discussed) and did not contain words (because I couldn't remember any).

[209]

2) Throughout the sampling (I don't know when exactly) I was surprised by the salience of sensory and bodily awareness in the samples. At some point I related this with recent trends in cognitive science and the philosophy of mind, which hold that perception and bodily patterns of interaction with the world are much more pervasive and cognitively central than posited by traditional, computational cognitivism (see Lakoff and Johnson, 1999; Gibbs, 2005).

General remarks about my sampling experiences

I start with practical limitations of the method that I'm sure you're well aware of, but I'm bringing them up here in case you have something to add beside the argument that "every method has limitations, and for all its limitations DES is still the best way we've found for studying pristine experience"—to which I would have nothing to object, of course. I've grouped my comments under three different headings: practical

A VERY SMALL QUIBBLE ON WORDING • 239

limitations, broad vs. pristine experience (again!), and metaphor and creativity.

PRACTICAL LIMITATIONS OF DES AND INTERSUBJECTIVITY

I found that sampling in intersubjective contexts was complicated by both social and pragmatic factors. First, one always has to explain why one is wearing an earphone, often by describing the purposes and framework of the study—which inevitably ends up increasing the participant's awareness that he or she is wearing a beeper.

Second, interrupting one's activity in order to take notes can be difficult or even impossible, since it requires both time and concentration. Once I was speaking on the phone when I heard the beep and I couldn't do anything, so I had to skip the beep entirely. This makes some kinds of experiences difficult or impossible to capture—again, because of practical limitations—through DES. It is likely that some meaningful areas of human experience (think of intimacy and sexuality, or any activity that requires complete absorption such as intense physical exercise) will always remain beyond the reach of DES. This alone is, in my view, a strong argument for the importance of studying broad experience along with pristine experience.

Further, my hunch is that there might be a link between these practical limitations of the method and your claim that experience is inner, private, and difficult to genuinely share with others. I wonder if it wouldn't be possible to study intersubjectivity *through* DES, and if this wouldn't teach us something about the issues we've been discussing for some time now. Wouldn't it be interesting, for example, to ask two participants to wear the beeper while they spend time together, and find a way to beep them at the same time? Have you already tried doing something along these lines? Julian Hanich, a colleague of mine here in Groningen, is studying how people can share experiences while watching movies (he's a film scholar; see Hanich, 2014), and I think it would be extremely productive to put his claims to the test through DES.

ON THE PRISTINE EXPERIENCE VS. BROAD EXPERIENCE DISTINCTION

I have two related points to make here. First, in the interviews you often stress that the questions you ask may not have an answer, but I have

[212] the sense that the DES set-up may still place demands on participants to provide more experiential detail than was actually available in pristine experience. The detail may come from memories of the context in which the experience took place, or of previous or subsequent experiences, or from the imaginary reenactment of the experience itself. All this is to some extent inevitable: experience has a temporal structure (Husserl's retention/protention), so that previous and future experiences seem to extend into the present moment. You're the first to acknowledge this, I think, when you argue (Hurlburt, 2011b) that DES reports are referential,

[213] not molecular. What I wonder is if this does not inject into descriptions of pristine experience at least a tiny fraction of broad experience (i.e., context-based and generalizing reports).

Second, many of the background feelings that I described (irritation in 2.1, anxiety in 2.2, sadness in 4.3, anxiety again in 6.2) were vague and resistant to high-fidelity description. In most cases they were not particularly salient in pristine experience. These background sensations seem to be at the outer edge of pristine experience; they straddle the divide between pristine experience (what is experienced at a given moment)

[214] and broad experience (generalizations). But can't a sensation that has relatively little weight in pristine experience take on importance because it is present for a long time? And is DES fully equipped to deal with this ongoingness of background feelings, or doesn't this again point to the need for broad experiential descriptions as a more efficient way of capturing patterns in experience?

METAPHOR AND ARTISTIC CREATIVITY

In our conversations we've made use of several metaphors or similes: imaginary forces or objects pressing down my body (sample 2.2; handkerchief in 5.1), spring (2.3), running out of breath (6.2), melted chocolate and hyper-bold font (6.3). Doesn't this point to a deep connection between metaphor as a linguistic/conceptual tool and experience? I have made a case for this view in a recent article (Caracciolo, 2013b). The article deals with fictional characters' pristine experiences—as conveyed by literary texts—but I believe there is still a lot of work to be done on this topic, and extending the investigation to nonliterary experiential reports is crucial. This could take the form of a linguistic analysis of a set of DES

[215] transcripts, for example. Could it be that there is a correlation between people's use of metaphor and their skill at DES? In other words, could it

be that the more experienced participants become, the more they tend to employ metaphors and similes in order to describe their pristine experiences? This is only a hypothesis, of course, but it may be worth examining in more detail.

Moreover, since metaphors are one of the trademarks of creative (and artistic) language, their use in the DES context also ties in with what is, for me, one of the most fascinating aspects of this method. I find that [216] there is something deeply *poetic* about experience sampling and the way in which you practice it. Virginia Woolf remarked that art seeks to capture what she called "moments of being" (see, e.g., Banfield, 2003), and while sampling I couldn't help thinking that these carefully and laboriously described instants had a value that goes even beyond the scientific project of studying pristine experience. They reminded me of the many passages in literature that attempt to convey experience with the same degree of clarity, texture, and attention to detail that characterizes the DES method. By saying this I don't mean to diminish the scientific merits and value of DES. As we've already agreed, literature does not make any claims as to the real-world fidelity of the (mostly fictional) experiences it describes. Yet I think that learning to appreciate consciousness-focused narrative might [217] actually be a good preparation for (or complement to) DES training.

NOTE: Here Marco sends Russ a copy of his paper on metaphor: Caracciolo (2013b).

June 4
Hi Marco—
I'll have more to say later when I have more time. In the meantime, let me respond to one comment:

RE [207] "I still saw a danger that DES questioning may encourage people to be more specific than their experience actually was."

It seems to me that you have yourself provided a potential response when you said "I was surprised by the salience of sensory and bodily awareness in the samples." Do you think it possible that your (Marco's) sensory and bodily awareness was the result of my (Russ's) encouraging you to be more specific about your experience than your experience actually was?
—Russ

June 5
Dear Russ,

[218] There is no doubt that the salience of sensory and bodily awareness in my samples was *not* the result of your questioning, or of an implicit demand for specificity. When and if it operates, that demand must exist at the level of experiential details. Take, for instance, beep 3.1, when you asked me what my seeing of the actor was like, and I answered that I was attending to the color and shape of his body. I responded to the best of my ability and in all sincerity, but I can't rule out the possibility that my answer overspecifies my seeing by drawing on memories of the moments before or (especially) after the beep. In other words: I'm confident about the big picture of each beep (including the salience of sensory and bodily awareness), but I can't be sure—not always, anyway—about the details. [Cf. RE 235 in chapter XXIII.]

All the best,
Marco

XX

SALIENT CHARACTERISTICS OF MARCO'S EXPERIENCE AS CHARACTERIZED BY RUSS

June 6
Hi Marco—

Here is a draft of a description of the salient characteristics that I think emerge from your samples. Except in a few places where I thought it necessary to clarify, these descriptions are (I think) tightly constrained by the individual-sample descriptions of your pristine experiences [as described in chapter XVIII].

So please have a look and provide whatever commentary/criticism seems appropriate. My object is to craft characteristic descriptions that rest lightly on the pristine experiences, and if you think I've fallen short or have alternative ideas, I'd like to hear about it.

Once we finish whatever discussion we might have about this description, I'll return to the several rounds of general discussion that are in my court.

—Russ

SENSORY AWARENESS

Sensory awareness is a construct defined by DES (Hurlburt, Heavey, and Bensaheb, 2009; reprinted as chap. 16 in Hurlburt, 2011a) where a person is "immersed in the experience of a particular sensory aspect of his or her external or internal environment without particular regard for the instrumental aim or perceptually complete objectness" (Hurlburt, Heavey, and Bensaheb, 2009, 232). Hurlburt, Heavey, and Bensaheb (2009) provided many examples of sensory awareness, including this one:

> Andrew is dialing his cell phone. At the moment, he has just "zeroed in" on the shiny blueness of the brushed aluminum phone case. He is not, at that moment, paying attention to the number he is dialing; his experience has momentarily left that task (which continues as if on autopilot) to be absorbed in the shiny blueness. . . . Andrew's momentary interest is not instrumental: he's dialing but he's attending to the shiny-blueness, not the dialing. And his momentary interest is not in the complete object: he is drawn not to the phone, which happens to be shiny-blue, but to the shiny-blueness, which happens to be of the phone. (231–32)

Such sensory awareness appeared in 18 of Marco's 20 samples: 90%; or 22 of 24 (92%) if we count the first sampling day; or 24/24 if we count the rectangle in Scanning (see below) as sensory awareness. Furthermore, at most of Marco's samples, there were multiple separate sensory awareness occurring simultaneously, so there were about 35 separable sensory awareness in his 20 samples. Thus, no matter how one counts, sensory awareness was a highly frequent characteristic of Marco's experience.

Marco's sensory awarenesses were frequently bodily (10/20) including imaginary bodily, frequently visual (7/20) including imaginary visual, frequently tactile (6/20) including imaginary tactile, and frequently auditory (3/20). Here are some examples. *Bodily*: sample 4.1 (muscular tension in arm). *Imaginary bodily*: sample 6.2 (imagined cheek muscles tingling while innerly speaking). *Visual*: sample 4.4 (noticing the obliqueness and red-brownness of the tiles). *Tactile*: sample 4.3 (feeling the edges of the bottle cap). *Auditory*: sample 5.1 (hearing the aural qualities of a voice). Marco's sensory experiences were apparently very differentiated; for example, he confidently and convincingly differentiated between bodily sensory awarenesses (where the focus was on a bodily sensation per se) and tactile sensory awareness (where the focus was on the feel or sensation of an object that Marco was touching). For example, at sample 4.2, Marco was drinking from a glass and felt the pressure of the glass against his lips. This was primarily a sensation of pressure in his lips rather than a sensing of the glass itself, and therefore is an example of bodily, *not* tactile, sensory awareness. By contrast, at sample 4.3 Marco was holding a bottle cap, and the sensation was of the bottle cap itself, *not* the pressure that the cap exerted in his fingertips.

READING/SCANNING

Marco was reading text on his computer screen on 5 of 20 occasions (6 of 24 counting the first day). Half of those involved what Marco called "scanning"; half involved sensory awareness of the words; half involved innerly speaking while reading (but none of those involved innerly speaking as the main experiential feature).

Scanning: Marco's "scanning" involved the seeing of a white rectangle moving left to right along a line of text. This rectangle was seen to have straight edges but somewhat rounded corners, to be a half a centimeter or a centimeter high (extending roughly half way between the lines of printed text), and 3 to 6–8 centimeters wide. There may or may not have been a border at the edge of this rectangle—if there was a border, it was very faint. The white rectangle existed on a white computer screen; nonetheless, the white rectangle was clearly seen differentiated from the white screen. (How that is optically possible is not the issue here.) This rectangle enclosed words, and the words were sometimes blurred or indistinct; sometimes clearly seen but not attended to; sometimes distorted and clearly seen but attended to for their sensory qualities. That is, the experience of scanning involved primarily seeing a moving rectangle, *not* experiencing the words that the rectangle enclosed. For example, at sample 5.2 Marco was reading an article on his computer screen and saw the "scanning" rectangular area moving from left to right as he read "criticism voiced by readers." He was both scanning and innerly speaking (in his own natural voice) those words. The text within the scanning rectangle was *not* sharper or more salient than the surrounding text—that is, it was the rectangle itself that drew his attention, not the text within it. Sample 3.4 included the experience of a scanning movement but without the visually seen rectangle. [219]

(Marco's use of the term "scanning" is very different from most DES subjects' use of that term. DES subjects frequently report themselves to be scanning, by which they mean that they are quickly looking through or down an article, trying to find something in particular. Marco himself had one instance of this kind of experience: In sample 6.1, Marco was scanning through—using the typical definition of "scanning," *not* Marco's idiosyncratic use—an email looking for the names that would be listed farther down in the email. He knew that he was expecting to find names, and when his eyes would come upon the names, he would stop the scanning-down. This typical-DES-subject use of "scanning" does *not* involve a white rectangle; does *not* involve any sensory experience at all. The typical scanning experience is of being on hold, waiting for what is being searched for to appear.)

None of Marco's reading samples included a simple semantic apprehension of what he was reading. He read with comprehension, but the comprehension for the most part seemed to happen entirely outside of experience. The closest Marco came to the experience of comprehension was the innerly speaking of the words being read on two of the six reading occasions (5.2 and 6.3), and both of those experiences included an equally salient sensory awareness of the features of the words (6.3) or the seen scanning rectangle (5.2).

WORDS

Words were somehow important in 17 of the 20 experiences (19 of 24 counting the first day). Most often, words were important *by their experiential absence* when it would be reasonable to expect the experience of words to be present. For example, when Marco heard someone speaking (including himself speaking), his experience was not of meaningful utterances but instead of aural characteristics. When Marco saw printed words, he often attended to the color, shape, or outline of the letters rather than to the semantic meaning being conveyed. This by no means implies that words had no semantic nature for Marco; on the contrary, he skillfully processed the meaning of the words. However, this processing was for the most part entirely outside of his direct experience.

On two occasions (5.2, 6.3), Marco experienced inner speech while reading; sample 5.2 ("criticism voiced by readers") was described above. But on two occasions (3.3, 6.1) Marco was reading without speaking the words. On one occasion, Marco experienced inner speech while typing. At sample 4.6 Marco was typing "Because of the cognitive basicness" on his laptop. As he typed, he innerly said "Because of the cognitive basicness" in his own voice. On one occasion (2.3) he was typing without speaking the words.

On one occasion (6.2), Marco experienced himself to be speaking, and to be speaking in words, but did not experience the words themselves. At the moment of beep 6.2 Marco was wondering why the beep hasn't come already, thinking that the beeper is supposed to beep at least twice an hour. He clearly experienced this content at the moment of the beep. At the same time, he felt a tingling in the muscles in the inside of his cheeks at the sides of his mouth as if he were speaking aloud. This was an imaginary sensation (he was not in fact speaking and as far as he knew the muscles were not in fact moving) but it was clear in his experience. At the same time he experienced his voice as somehow speaking—his normal voice normally inflected. Marco had the impression that words were implied in this experience, but he did not directly experience words (and indeed no words may have been experientially present). If words were experientially present (which they seemed to Marco to be), the words themselves seemed to exist so faintly as to be unrecognizable: they presented themselves in a raw, inarticulate, prelinguistic form (however paradoxical this may sound). Thus Marco had a sense of speaking; he had a muscular sensation of speaking; he knew the content that he was speaking; he had the sense of his voice as speaking. However, the sense of words that he had may not correspond to any actual words in his experience.

MOVEMENT

Marco frequently experienced movement (11 or 12 out of 20; or 13 or 14 out of 24 counting Day 1). The Scanning samples described above count as movement, as does the experience of the eye movements that occasionally accompanied scanning. Marco experienced movement in many parts of his body. For example, at sample 4.4 he was walking into a store and had a bodily sense of moving—his whole body moving. This movement was in the direction of into-the-store, but the into-the-storeness direction was not in his experience. It was his whole body that was moving all in the same direction, even though in reality parts of his body were swinging in the opposite direction, etc.

Marco's experience separated the experience of the translation of motion and the kinesthetics of motion. For example, at sample 5.1 Marco was stirring tea and feeling the circular motion, *not* the kinesthetics or tactile sensations of making the motion. But in sample 4.1, where he was moving his arm from the bottle to his face, he felt the muscular tension but not the movement.

On two occasions (2.1 and 6.1) Marco was specifically noticing the quickness of his movement, which seemed to be part of the experience of apprehension or anxiety.

Against the potential criticism that Marco's way of performing the DES task is, after the beep, to survey his environment and report any ongoing movement as having been experienced at the moment of the beep, I note that at sample 5.3 Marco was walking and reported neither the movement nor the kinesthetics thereof.

FEELING

On seven (of 20) occasions, Marco experienced a subtle tinge of emotional feeling. Usually, this feeling seemed to pervade all aspects of his experience, like a drop of food coloring in a bathtub, rather than be distinctly felt as a directly apprehended emotion.

Marco's clearest feelings were at samples 3.4, where he felt apprehension on the surface of his chest, but with no particular characteristics (not pressure, not tension, not tingling or tickling, etc.); and sample 5.3, where he felt (on the surface of his chest, a slight pressure on the skin) a slight apprehension that he couldn't find the place he was looking for.

The other samples that Marco experienced as including feeling had only this tinge or suffusion of feeling. For example, at sample 2.1 Marco was walking somewhat too fast and talking somewhat fast, and Marco apprehended the fastness as tinged with irritation.

(Marco did not experience in any of his samples the kinds of emotion sensations that some DES samplers report as conveying, or being, feelings: heaviness in the heart, lightness in the chest, clenching of the fists, dryness of mouth, hotness of skin, and so on.)

INNER SPEAKING

Marco experienced himself as innerly speaking on four occasions (of 20 or 24): Samples 4.6, 5.2, 6.2, and 6.3. Inner speaking occurred only while reading or writing—that is, there was no occasion of inner speech that was not directly driven by simultaneously present external words.

As we saw in the Words section above, at one of these samples (6.2), Marco experienced himself as speaking without the experience of words themselves.

XXI

TWO MORE QUIBBLES ON WORDING

June 7
Dear Russ,
Many thanks for your work on this! The description looks both extremely interesting and accurate. See below for my only two concerns. Let me know what you think.
All the best,
Marco

RE [219] "Scanning."
    Here and throughout, I think you're making too much of my use of the phrase "visually scanning a text" at beep 5.2.   [221]
    By "scanning" I meant "reading at a quicker pace than usual," although I now realize that this isn't standard English usage. I'm not sure if the computer metaphor ("scanning" as in digitizing a text by taking pictures) played a role in my choice of this word, but it seems likely.
    I would agree that "scanning" (in my sense) is indeed different from "scanning-through" (which occurs at 3.3, 3.4, 6.1): in "scanning," the movement through the text is mainly along a horizontal axis; it is quicker than in reading, but it is still a word—word—word movement. By contrast, "scanning-through" is (or so I perceive it) more vertical than horizontal. Further, in "scanning-through" there is a sense of being on the lookout for something.
    However, when I first used the word "scanning" I didn't mean to associate it with the rectangle experience. Thus, I think it's too strong to say that "Marco's 'scanning' involved the seeing of a white rectangle moving left to right along a line of text."
    At beep 6.3, for example, I saw the rectangle but I wasn't "scanning" (in the sense that I was reading at my normal pace, or so I think). At beep 6.1 I saw the rectangle around the word "Utrecht" while scanning-

through. Thus, I have qualms about linking too closely the rectangle experience with what I called "scanning" at 5.2. At the very least, I'd indicate that the terminological choice is yours, although it's inspired by my nonstandard use of the term. Or I'd distinguish more carefully in the text between the rectangle experience while reading and "scanning" per se.

Let me know if you want me to suggest some changes, or if you'd prefer to take care of that yourself.

RE [220] "On one occasion (6.2), Marco experienced himself to be speaking, and to be speaking in words, but did not experience the words themselves."

[222] What about 2.2, where "I'm thinking that I should find that file. It somehow seems like there are or should be words present in this thinking, but I can't say what the words were, whether they were voiced, or even what language they were in (I could speculate that they were in English, but that would come from my knowledge of the task, not recollection of the phenomenon)." Wouldn't this also count as possible inner speech?

June 8
Hi Marco—
All things considered, I'd say your quibbles about my sample descriptions are pretty darn small, and I take that as evidence that these are pretty darn high-fidelity descriptions of your pristine experiences during these samples. That is not to say that the quibbles are not important—I'll respond to each below. But if the big-picture question is, "Can we create high-fidelity descriptions of Marco's experience?" I think the answer is Yes.

This is a small number of samples (20 or 24) during a small period of time (a few weeks in May), and therefore may or may not be representative of Marco during those weeks at times other than while wearing the beeper, or at other periods. Were we worried about that, we might be able largely to solve those problems by sampling more often, or at more varied times, and over a longer haul. The DES method improves with use, unlike most psychological methods (questionnaires, structured interviews, etc.) that deteriorate with use, so there is no theoretical limit to the potential size of a data pool.

And no matter how long we sampled, we will never (or at least may never) get to the essence of Marco. The method has limitations.

I will respond to your June 7 comments now. When we are (more or less) finished with this discussion of the collected samples and their description, then I will return to respond to your general concerns from May 11 and later.

RE [221] "I think you're making too much of my use of the phrase 'visually scanning a text' at beep 5.2. By 'scanning' I meant 'reading at a quicker pace than usual.'"

The discussion of "scanning" takes place at 21:30 into the audio of day 5 [the audio is on the Companion Website]. To my ear, there is nothing in the interview that implies, or could be taken as implying even vaguely, that "By 'scanning' I meant 'reading at a quicker pace than usual.'" Perhaps it is implied elsewhere in the series of interviews; I'd be happy to know where. In fact, I think there is evidence (implied, not explicit) that the pace is *not* quicker than usual: I asked (just ahead of 22:46) "You've used the term 'scanning' and you've used the term 'reading.' What do you mean by that?" Here's your answer:

> M: Um, I guess that the. . . . So I was in the process of reading this text. And, um, just before the beep interrupted me I was moving my gaze along the text. And in particular I was . . . well my gaze was aimed at the words "criticism voiced by readers."
> R: So you don't mean *scanning* as if . . . , as . . . , as in a *quick* take-in of this page and then the next page. You mean *scanning*: your eyes are moving across the line."
> M: Yeah. Exactly. Yeah, yeah.

By the structure of the question and the answer, your phrase "moving my gaze along the text . . . my gaze was aimed at the words 'criticism voiced by readers'" could be taken as your definition of "scanning." That is a description of movement tied to reading, and in particular tied to reading in inner speech, and the inner speech is not described as fast paced. (I emphasize that that is mild evidence.)

There are at least three possible understandings of the discrepancy between the interview's *not-quicker* and the retrospective account's *quicker-pace-than-usual*: (1) unskilled apprehension of the pristine experience; (2) inadequate interview; and (3) unfaithful retrospection of the pristine experience.

With respect to (1) and (2), I think your skill and my interviewing technique were adequate, so that if the rectangle were indeed moving fast, we would have said that unambiguously. I can't be certain of that, of course, but you frequently reported the quick pace of events in other samples.

Also as before, if I had to bet, I would (with all the same caveats as before) bet on (3). I think it possible or likely that in retrospection you are captured by your own word "scanning." That is, I think it possible or likely that your thought process was something like, "If I said 'scanning' I must have meant 'rapid' like Webster." I accept that Webster's "scanning" implies a rapid pace, and I accept that you are a highly skilled language user, but from that it does *not* follow that your use of "scanning" when applied to your own inner experience follows Webster. I think the words people use to describe their own inner experience come from early childhood and are not shaped by the external verbal community. (Recall my discussion of the word [223] "thinking" above [at marginal 190 in chapter XVI].) I think it possible or likely that when you learned to read, at age 3 or 8 or whenever, you used this (rather unusual) seen-rectangle technique, and naturally assumed (without thinking a bit about it) that everyone else did so too (which is not true, but you would not have known that then), and that therefore when people happened to use the word "scanning" in external conversation, you came (organically, fundamentally) to associate it with the moving rectangle. (You weren't consulting Webster in that process.) That is, in your puerile idiographic lexicon, "scanning" meant "moving rectangle." Eventually you learned that in the external world, "scanning" means fast pace, but that does *not* erase the inner experiential significance—scanning [inner] and scanning [external] exist as homophones, one highly differentiated [external] and one idiosyncratically intimate [internal].

[224] All that is *highly* speculative, and if you can show me anywhere in the interview where "scanning" has the connotation of rapid, I'd be happy to trash the whole idea. But in the meantime, I would bet (not a large amount) that this is an exemplar of Sherlock Holmes's observation that "Insensibly one begins to twist facts to suit theories, instead of theories to suit facts" (A. C. Doyle, *A Scandal in Bohemia*, 1891/2015, 3).

I re-re-emphasize that I am no mind reader; I'm just trying to make sense of the evidence. And I re-emphasize that if I'm right about this (that you misremember things and that you distort your own evidence to align with your self-theories), I don't hold it against you, nor should others. Everyone that I know (including me) is susceptible to distorting facts. The difference here is that the DES situation is such that such misrememberings can be exposed: we have a specific moment, a skilled interviewer, videotaped interview, energy to explore and transcribe the videotapes, and so on. That is a very rare nexus; as a result, people are rarely so directly confronted with their own distortions of facts. I re-emphasize that I recognize that *I* am just susceptible to Sherlock's insensible twistings as you are. I go to the trouble of videotaping, transcribing, trying to be as explicit as I can about what I think and why, and so on, as my way of practicing trying to keep my own insensible twistings at bay.

And as above, we should keep in mind what is at stake here: we agree about the existence of rectangles; we agree that they move left to right; we agree that they have straight edges and rounded corners; we agree that there are no borders; we agree that they are white. We may disagree about, or leave unresolved, the speed at which they move. That strikes me as a fairly minor detail.

Q: *What's wrong with Marco's memory?*
RUSS: *Nearly everyone is susceptible of distorting facts, and this is why pristine experience has to be documented very close to the moment it occurs, and why retrospective generalizations are not to be trusted. Here's one more example.*

Sample 5.3 concerns Marco's apprehension that he is not finding the place he's looking for. That apprehension was experienced as being on the surface of his chest. During the interview about that sample (at 52:15), Marco said about his chest experience, "I think it's um, I mean, [pause] I think it's on the surface this time. I remember at other times it was more inside, whereas this time it's almost on the skin, Yeah, more superficial anyway."

Actually, at Marco's previous samples he had never experienced feelings as being inside his chest. The one previous chest experience (sample 3.4) involved apprehension on the surface of his chest, very much like sample 5.3. During the 5.3 interview, Marco misremembered his sample 3.4 experience despite the fact that we had discussed it in explicit and extended detail.

Marco is not an unusually bad recaller; quite the contrary. But I think he has a presuppositional theory that feelings are down deep, and as Sherlock says, theories are more powerful than facts.

The moral for the study of pristine experience is clear: pristine experience must be documented with minimal delay.

RE [222] "What about 2.2, where 'I'm thinking that I should find that file.' . . . Wouldn't this also count as possible inner speech?"

Preliminarily, we must distinguish clearly between (1) Marco's pristine experience at the moment of beep 2.2, (2) our interview about beep 2.2, (3) my contemporaneously written description of Marco's pristine experience at beep 2.2, and (4) my written description of Marco's salient characteristics. From my perspective, the phenomenon of interest is (1), Marco's pristine experience. Everything else is a tool that points, more or less adequately, toward Marco's pristine experience.

The quotation you cite here is of type (3); that is, you seem to be making more of my contemporaneous description than it deserves. The interesting question is about Marco's pristine experience, not my contemporaneous description of it. Just as you wouldn't judge the painting on the ceiling of the Sistine Chapel by the quality of Michelangelo's brushes or the scaffolding he built to lie on (although those are somewhat interesting in their own right), you shouldn't make too much of my contemporaneously written descriptions. Those descriptions are tools, useful only (or at least primarily) as facilitators, pointers, ways of accessing the thing of interest, Marco's pristine experience.

So I will understand your question as reading, "Doesn't Marco's pristine experience at sample 2.2 count as possible inner speech?"

The best evidence we have about Marco's pristine experience at beep 2.2 is the videotape of the interview [the audio is on the Companion Website]. Here's the relevant excerpt:

Sample 2.2, 25:39 in the audio file

R: Let's start with the thinking [M: OK.] "I should find that file." How does that thinking present itself to you?
M: Hmm. [long pause] I think it has a slight um sensory element, I mean, of hearing myself ah saying "I should find that file" or something similar. Um. But that's very, very slight, um especially in this case, and it's [pause] yeah.
R: So, are the words quote "I should find that file," seems like you're not sure of the exact words, or if there are words or, what are the words . . .

M: Well, I guess, like, uh I mean I don't want to, um, but, yeah, like, last time, uh, I think, um, I have the sense that the words are there but I'm [pause] I'm not sure, I mean, but I, but at the same time I have the sense that this is only a paraphrase, so these are not the words that actually occurred to me um in that moment. So I have a sense that there is . . . that there are some words involved in that thinking process, but I wouldn't be able to say which words, and these words are clearly y'know a summary of what was going on but not the words that I had in mind.

First, let's note that your responses in this passage are *highly* subjunctified. I've written at length about subjunctification (all of chapter 8, most of chapter 5, *passim* elsewhere) in my 2011 book, but in brief, a subjunctifier (my coinage) is any word, vocalization, or action that undermines the simple declarative flow of speech. I'll reprint your 26:30 utterance with the subjunctifiers underlined; I'll alternate single and double underlining to indicate the separate subjunctifiers:

M: Well, I guess, like, uh I mean I don't want to, um, but, yeah, like, last time, uh, I think, um, I have the sense that the words are there but I'm [pause] I'm not sure, I mean, but, but at the same time I have the sense that this is only a paraphrase, so these are not the words that actually occurred to me um in that moment. So I have a sense that there is . . . that there are some words involved in that thinking process, but I wouldn't be able to say which words, and these words are clearly y'know a summary of what was going on but not the words that I had in mind.

We might quibble about whether one or another of these actually count as subjunctifiers (or that some not marked should be counted), but there are about 27 subjunctifiers in a 120 word paragraph. No matter how you slice it, that's a lot!

Subjunctification is Marco's grammar producer's (or heart's, or body/mind/complex's, or whatever's) way of saying that what he is saying is not to be understood literally, or at least not to be understood as simply literal (the rationale for that understanding is in Hurlburt, 2011a, but here I will say that subjunctification is more important in DES interviews than in most non-DES situations because DES is aimed at specific, circumscribed experiences). Marco's subjunctification is (or at least probably is) Marco's way of saying that he doesn't know what he is talking about, or that he himself doesn't believe what he is saying.

However, this is only the second sampling day, and I accept that your ability to apprehend your experience likely improved over time, and had you been more skilled at the moment of beep 2.2, you might have been better able to apprehend the nature of the experience and to transmit it to me.

So did Marco's inner experience at the moment of beep 2.2 include inner speech, or possibly include inner speech? I think probably not. If one is actually engaging in inner speech, and one experiences oneself as engaging in inner speech, one must have the experience of speaking, and I can see little evidence of that. I accept that I am not sure.

Could his pristine experience at 2.2 be of wordless inner speaking, similar to 6.2? Perhaps so, but that presumes that we have apprehended with fidelity Marco's experience at 6.2, and I think there is reason to be somewhat skeptical about that. It is possible that at 6.2, (a) Marco was innerly speaking without experiencing words; I have encountered that phenomenon in other subjects (rarely), so I don't rule that out. But it is also possible that (b) Marco is not innerly speaking but instead is encumbered by a presupposition that the kind of thought he is having *must* take place in inner speech. I don't think we have a way of sorting this out with the data at hand. It is likely that if we sampled longer (perhaps a lot longer), we could sort this out.

But we should keep in mind the size of the quibble: I wrote (and you quibbled) "there were no occasions of inner speech that were not directly driven by simultaneously present external words." You might be right, and if you are, then I should change that sentence to read: "there were no occasions of *innerly spoken words* that were not directly driven by simultaneously present external words." I agree that those two characterizations are different, but the size of the difference is pretty small. I said you had four inner speech occasions. Maybe it should have been five (including 2.2). Maybe it should have been three (excluding 6.2). Either way, less than a quarter of your sample included inner speech, far less if you exclude inner speech while reading or typing. That we can't discriminate confidently between 20% or 15% or 25% is inconsequential by comparison to the widespread view that inner speaking in words occurs continuously throughout the waking day.

So we may come to agree about, disagree about, or leave unresolved these details, but the big picture, as it seems to me, is that we have a pretty darn high-fidelity view of Marco's experiences during a few weeks in May, and we could refine and extend that view if we wished to spend the effort. If you agree with that, then it is about time to return to the general discussion, informed by this effort.

June 9
Dear Russ,
Please find below a few brief responses to your June 8 comments. I think our disagreements are indeed very small, so I look forward to your reactions to the more general points I raised over the last weeks.
All the best,
Marco

RE [224] "If you can show me anywhere in the interview where 'scanning' has the connotation of rapid, I'd be happy to trash the whole idea."
   For example, about 44:00 minutes into the recording of day 3 (beep 3.4) I said "I'm scanning through the email visually," but maybe you're distinguishing between scanning and scanning-through here. In any case I agree that the interview does not suggest that I was reading at a quicker-than-usual pace at beep 5.2 (but it doesn't rule that out either). So the slightly increased reading speed that I tend to associate with my use of the term "scan" (both in general and in my recollection of that particular beep) will have to remain a broad experience for now.

RE [223] "I think it possible or likely that when you learned to read, at age 3 or 8 or whenever, you used this (rather unusual) seen-rectangle technique, and naturally assumed (without thinking a bit about it) that everyone else did so too (which is not true, but you would not have known that then), and that therefore when people happened to use the word 'scanning' in external conversation, you came (organically, fundamentally) to associate it with the moving rectangle."
   It's entirely possible that I used and still use the seen-rectangle technique to read, but it's unlikely that I connected it with the word "scanning" when I was a child, because that word just doesn't exist in Italian (nor is there a similar-sounding word for a similar concept). Moreover, the evidence for the association between the rectangle experience and the term "scanning" is, in my view, flimsy. As far as I can tell I used the verb "scan" without "through" only at beep 5.2. I'm quite sure that this was a creative, nonidiomatic use of an English expression that is

[226]

258 • CHAPTER XXI

normally accompanied by "through" in this context. And I can also add—again, in broad experience—that the meaning I was trying to express was that of the Italian verb "scorrere" (skim or scan through a text).

Anyway, the point I am raising here is more terminological than content-related, so I agree that the quibble is very small. The important thing is that we've discovered this peculiarity of my reading method, of which I was unaware until now.

[227] RE [225] "The big picture, as it seems to me, is that we have a pretty darn high-fidelity view of Marco's experiences during a few weeks in May, and we could refine and extend that view if we wished to spend the effort. If you agree with that, then it is about time to return to the general discussion, informed by this effort."

Yes, I agree with that, and I think it's time to go back to the general discussion.

June 10
Hi Marco—
OK, I will go back to the general discussion. It might take me a while. Before I do that, let me respond to a few particulars here.
—Russ

RE [226] "The evidence for the association between the rectangle experience and the term 'scanning' is, in my view, flimsy."

I agree. I would note in passing something about which I have never written in general terms, although I have (as my own broad experience reveals to me) encountered it frequently in DES interviews, namely: Very often subjects who have a fairly unusual feature of experience (more or less of the moving-rectangle-while-reading ilk) (a) don't have any broad experience of such a feature; but (b) have a word for that feature that they have idiosyncratically defined; but (c) don't have any broad experience of having such a word; and (d) don't know the word's idiosyncratic definition; but (e) use the word consistently anyway; and (f) don't know where the word came from. It is possible that your use of "scan" follows that pattern. I'm not asserting that with confidence, but I would bet a small amount.

I have written about one such word in chapter 20 of my 2011 book, where 14-year-old RD referred to some of his thoughts as being "solid." He used "solid" in a matter of fact way, with the same natural familiarity as he might use "blue" in the sentence "My father's car is blue." However, when we asked him what he meant by a "solid" thought, he couldn't say, even though he used the term or its apparent antonym "light" in a consistent way. Eventually we could piece together what "solid" meant: a solid thought was one in which he was deeply engrossed, totally occupied. He said that if you wanted his attention when he was having a solid thought, you'd have to shake him by his shoulders. By contrast, if he was having a light thought, then he was easily permeable to external stimuli.

I think it possible that you use "scan" in approximately the same way that RD used "solid": skillfully, unknowingly, idiosyncratically, consistently, ignorant of its origin. I don't know whether that is true of you. I don't know how common such use is. Neither does anyone else, I think, because one needs something like DES to discover such phenomena. But knowing the answers to such questions seems very near to the heart of linguistics. [228]

June 11
Dear Russ,
You'll find one brief comment below.
All the best,
Marco

RE [228] "I think it possible that you use 'scan' in approximately the same way that RD used 'solid': skillfully, unknowingly, idiosyncratically, consistently, ignorant of its origin."

It is possible, but it doesn't seem very plausible (to me) because unlike RD I used the term "scan" without "through" only once. But I agree that RD's "solid" and my "scan" (if we accept your interpretation) are fascinating cases of idiolect for inner experience. It would indeed be interesting to ask a linguist's opinion about all this.

FOURTH PART
CLARIFICATIONS

XXII

WHERE RUSS TRANSITIONS BACK TO THE GENERAL

June 12
Hi Marco—
It might be useful for you to document, now that we are transitioning from the specific back to the general, how what you found in your (specific) sampling did or did not agree with your (broad) opinion prior to sampling. For example, you have said, I think, that you hadn't known that you frequently engaged in the kinds of sensory awarenesses we found; and that you hadn't known about the moving rectangle while you read. I'm suggesting that you collect such observations in one place, as a sort of reference point: this is what I expected to find and actually did find; this is what I was surprised to find; this is what I was surprised not to find; and so on. [229]

In doing so, I think you should be explicit about the source of your "prior" opinions, distinguishing among what I might call *documented prospection* ("Prior to sampling, I explicitly wrote down X about my experience; now I note Y"); *contemporaneous noting* ("On sampling day N, I explicitly noted my surprise about Z, which would not have occurred to me to write about prior to sampling"); *retrospective prospection* ("When I look back, I think that prior to sampling I expected to find W"); and whatever other categories seem natural. That is, I think we should accept that memory (or any kind of retrospection) is (or at least may be) a construction of the present that looks backwards, and therefore that what is "remembered" is (or at least may be) affected, created, or otherwise colored by present circumstances. That is, I think, the human condition, so we should be as explicit as possible about the data sources.

So if that seems like a good idea, go for it, and I will return to May 11.
—Russ

June 13
Dear Russ,

[230] Yes, that sounds like a very good idea. Unfortunately I don't think I will have many documented prospections (since I should have started keeping track of them before the sampling, which I didn't). However, comparing retrospective prospections and what we actually found in the experience samples should be an interesting exercise in itself.
All the best,
Marco

June 14
Hi Marco—
I've had a lot of catching up to do, going back to May 11, so the installment below is pretty long.

Furthermore, trying to respond to this has left me pretty far behind in my other demands, so I feel like I have not been quite as careful in this turn as I would like. If you discover mistakes or infelicities, please let me know and I will try to fix them.
—Russ

RE [227] Russ: "The big picture, as it seems to me, is that we have a pretty darn high-fidelity view of Marco's experiences during a few weeks in May." Marco: "I agree."

As we transition back toward the general, it might be worthwhile to review the characteristics of our description of your experience, what that description is and is not:

- The description is not perfect—we could wordsmith it.
- The description does not guarantee that Marco's pristine experience is stable. We have a relatively few samples (24) in a relatively short window (a few weeks in May) and in only a handful of situations. Were we concerned about any of those limitations, we could sample in more varied situations and across a longer time frame. A mature science of experience would work out how long and in how many situations. That said, I don't see any reason to believe that your samples during this period were not more or less representative of Marco on a larger scale. For example, I think it likely that you have frequent sensory awarenesses

in almost every situation and in almost every time frame. That is a speculation, verifiable by additional sampling.
- The description is about Marco's pristine experience as discovered by the DES method. There may be kinds of pristine experience that DES systematically overlooks, masks, or exaggerates (experience that is disturbed by an audible beep, for example). A mature science of experience would work out what kinds of experiences are overlooked or exaggerated, and whether other methods can discover them with higher fidelity, and so on.
- The description is entirely about Marco. The particularities of the situations in which Marco happened to find himself when beeped (eating with his friend, talking with his wife, working at his computer, walking to an appointment, etc.) fall away.
- The description is entirely about Marco, not about Marco and some specific externality. For example, "Marco has frequent sensory awareness" is not, for example, about *Marco's experience of traveling through India,* which would confound Marco with India travel.
- The description is about Marco himself, *not* Marco relative to some group. Marco has frequent sensory awareness regardless of whether anyone else or everyone else in the universe does or does not have frequent sensory awareness.
- The description is of Marco's pristine experience, *not* a score on a questionnaire. It is *not* the case that Marco has a high score on some sensory awareness questionnaire; it is that Marco has a lot of sensory awareness. Those are two very different things, one fundamentally idiographic, the other fundamentally comparative to some norm group; one about phenomena, the other about responses to specific probes.
- The description is idiographically about Marco. When we say "Marco has frequent sensory awareness," we do *not* mean that sensory awareness is a thing that exists independently of Marco, which Marco then "takes off the shelf" and engages in. Marco engages in his own idiographically unique experience, which we call sensory awareness. We can subsequently observe that what we call Marco's sensory awareness is similar to quite a few other people's experience that we called sensory awareness, and that may (probably does) indicate that sensory awareness is a frequently occurring way of experiencing. But that is downstream

from the idiographic observations of Marco's experience. "Idiographic" does not mean "different from everyone else"; it means relating specifically to Marco. Marco's idiographic experience may or may not be similar to some or many other people's idiographic experience. His sensory awareness is similar to many others'. On the other hand, the moving rectangles that he saw when he read may be highly unusual (I have not encountered them before). From the standpoint of an idiographic description, it doesn't matter.

- This description is not about Marco's *reports*; it is about his *pristine experience*. It is Russ's responsibility to help Russ and Marco filter out the merely reported from the actually apprehended (by noting subjunctifications, etc.).

[231]
- The description is not about Russ—any investigator with adequate skill would, I think, arrive at a similar description of Marco's experience. The fact is that there are not too many investigators with the requisite skill, because bracketing presuppositions is not easy and is not widely appreciated. That is unfortunate, but it does not change the fact that there *might sometime be* many skilled investigators, and if there were, they would find largely the same things about Marco's experience. At least that's what I think; a mature science of experience would verify that or debunk it.

RE [230] "Unfortunately I don't think I will have many documented prospections."

As in most things human, there are advantages and disadvantages to documenting prospections prior to sampling. *Now* it would have been nice to have documented prospections. *During sampling itself,* however, such documentation might have had an interfering effect—entering into the operation of presuppositions in some unknowable way. Early in my sampling career, influenced by the Duquesne school of phenomenology, I required subjects to document prospections, but I have abandoned that practice as being usually a waste of time and sometimes making things more difficult.

As you may recall, in the introductory interview [25:05 in the audio on the Companion Website] I did weakly and ambiguously raise the possibility of your writing a prospective account. You didn't jot down what you thought we would find, probably because you wanted to engage in sampling as similar to a regular DES subject as possible, and

I think that was probably a good strategy. The downside is that now we don't have documented prospections, but as is often the case, one can't have things both ways.

Now I respond to comments you made in your May 11 turn

RE [192] "All this seems to presuppose that the question that we're trying to address in this conversation is: how can Marco learn to skillfully and effectively apprehend pristine experience?"

That's not the central question from my point of view. I think the central question is: How can Marco learn to appreciate the differences between pristine experience and broad experience? To answer that question, I think Marco has to know something about how pristine experience is skillfully and effectively apprehended and described, and how that is different from the way broad experience is described. In particular, I think that Marco (and everyone else) should not apply to broad experience the methods that are appropriate to pristine experience (or vice versa), nor should he (they) presume that characteristics that are appropriate to pristine experience are also characteristics of broad experience.

RE [193] "When you write that 'you [have] sincerely to act *as if you know nothing about* similarities between people' . . . , I wonder what exactly the scope of application of this principle is."

I meant specifically that *on those occasions when you wish to apprehend pristine experience* you have sincerely to act as if you know nothing about similarities between people's pristine experience.

RE [194] "But apprehending pristine experience is not everything."

I agree and think that I have said so consistently. My harp is not that pristine experience is everything; it is that pristine experience is *something,* and that that something is different from broad experience (and from most other things), and that those differences should be appreciated and respected. My harp is that pristine experience is usually overlooked completely, usually on the (mistaken) assumption that everyone already knows about it.

RE [196] "Phenomenologists from Husserl onwards have offered some pretty interesting insights into experience. What's the relationship between your science of experience and the work of these philosophers? Can one really afford to ignore them?"

[232] If you would care to specify concretely and exactly the specific "pretty interesting insights" about which you'd like to know the relationship to my work, I'd be happy to try to respond. But I think you need to be specifically concrete about the insights. Modern references to Husserlian insights are often insufficiently specified, on the assumption that everyone knows what the important Husserlian insights are. But I don't think that's true—even the later Husserl didn't agree with the earlier Husserl about some important things—so it is very difficult for me to be confident I know what people are referring to when they refer to Husserl. So if you would like to point be to a specific passage in Husserl (or someone else) and ask how my work aligns or doesn't align with that passage, I'd be happy to try to respond.

RE [195] "Can a mature science of experience be a purely empirical, inductivist endeavor, in the sense that you would approach not only the sampling activity (where presuppositionlessness is essential) but your *analysis* of the samples without 'a theoretical perspective'?"

I have not presumed to know what a mature science of experience would look like, except for this one detail: it would know what pristine experience is, how it must be investigated, and how it is similar to and different from other things (including broad experience). I have no quarrel with theoretical perspectives per se, and I think I have never held myself up as an example of someone without a theoretical perspective. What I have consistently said (I think) is that theoretical perspectives can wreak substantial havoc on the attempt to apprehend pristine experience, and that if one is interested in pristine experience, one has to figure out some way to deal with that havoc. DES is one set of structures that (I think) constructively deal with the potential havoc of theoretical perspectives. A mature science of experience will doubtless advance other ways, parallel to or better than DES, and a way of integrating them.

My *analysis* of your samples has discussed sensory awareness, and I happily accept that that reflects some sort of theoretical perspective. For example, I could have discussed your frequency of using the word "the," or the occasions that you looked leftward or upward during the interview, or any of a myriad of other things. I choose to discuss sensory awareness because of a theoretical perspective (largely unreflected upon) that suggests that sensory awareness is more interesting than the frequency of "the." And I happily acknowledge that there may be important aspects of your experience that I am (or we are) blind to, based on my (our) presuppositions or theoretical perspectives. We need others with differing blindnesses to engage in pristine experiential work. But none of that changes the fact that your pristine experience is frequently populated by sensory awareness, and whereas a few details might be corrupted by my (our) theoretical perspectives, the big picture is starkly clear.

RE [197] "After years spent on sampling and studying experiences, can you still claim that 'you know nothing about similarities between people'?"

I don't believe I have claimed anywhere in my correspondence with you that I know nothing about similarities between people. I have claimed that *it is desirable to act as if* I know nothing about similarities between people. Those are two very different things. It is desirable for the actor Daniel Day-Lewis to *act as if* he were Abraham Lincoln, but that does not require him to believe that *he is* Lincoln.

RE [198] "I'm saying that his experience sounds familiar after reading an elaborate description of his faithfully apprehended experience of hunger."

I find "experience sounds familiar" particularly problematic: people often mistakenly take what sounds familiar as being unequivocally known, and those are very different things. "That sounds familiar" lulls one into complacency, leads one unwarrantedly to believe that one understands. That is anathema for science. (Also see next).

RE [200] "I accept that words and concepts referring to internal events may be less precise—and precisely employed—than words and concepts referring to the public world. I wonder why that is the case, however. Is that because we don't spend enough time talking about inner events? . . . Further, don't philosophers and in part also literary texts—at least those that focus on the representation of (fictional) consciousnesses—give us a vocabulary to talk about inner lives?"

I agree that philosophers, novelists, and poets (and others) do give us a vocabulary to talk about inner lives, but sometimes the philosophers' use of that vocabulary is dead wrong (see the discussion on Bernard Baars (2003) below, at RE 201), and sometimes that vocabulary is not adequate for describing pristine experience. For example,

[233] philosophic and literary texts have been describing consciousness for centuries (or millennia), but have largely ignored "unsymbolized thinking" (Hurlburt and Akhter, 2008a, b), "sensory awareness," and, for that matter, "pristine experience" itself, terms that I have had to invent.

The problem is *not* a lack of time talking about inner events. The problem is primarily a failure to appreciate the fact (or at least the likelihood) that we often talk past each other when we talk about inner events. When people say "I'm saying that his experience sounds familiar," they often (usually, I think) assume that "sounds familiar" means "is pretty much the same as mine."

Failing to recognize that referents are different is a far more difficult problem about inner experience than about the external world. If I assert about the external world that "my car is blue," it is easy for you to clarify my assertion with as much precision as you wish: You can ask, "What do you mean by blue—dark blue like the New York Yankees logo? Robins egg blue? Turquoise blue?" I can answer with a publicly observable gesture (that is, I could in principle display a particular New York Yankee's logo and say, "Like this!"). I grant that those concepts like NY Yankees blue, robin egg blue, and turquoise blue may differ somewhat from one person to another (recall our Winawer Russian discussion from March 22 onward), but in external conversation we can to a very great (albeit not perfect) extent overcome those differences (by for example inspecting swatches of colors or specifying wavelength).

But such refinement/validation/verification is not nearly so easy (and is probably impossible) with mentalisms. If I assert about my inner world that "I feel blue," it is not at all easy (and is probably impossible) for you to clarify my assertion with anything that remotely approaches precision. You can ask, "What do you mean by blue—sad like having lost your girlfriend? Unhappy like having gotten a C on a test? Crying frequently?" However, those questions do *not* refer to publicly observable *experiences*. They refer to publicly observable *events* (e.g., losing a girlfriend), but the blueness that innerly ensues from those events is both not publicly observable and doubtless differs greatly from one person to the next: losing a girlfriend differs, or at least may differ, greatly from one person (it's the end of my world) to another (actually, in a way I'm relieved). Crying frequently is a publicly observable event, but tears are *not* experience—at best the tears are a *correlate of* an experience of blueness, not the blueness itself.

Therefore it is at best very difficult, and probably not possible despite philosophers,' poets,' and novelists' efforts, to refine with confidence mentalistic terms like blueness (or hunger, etc.).

I have claimed that pristine experiences are not mentalisms; that is, whereas pristine experiences are private, they are refinable with substantial precision and confidence. For example, in your sample 3.4 you were, at the moment of the beep, apprehensively questioning whether you have done the right thing in signing a contract to rent a house. I asked a series of refining questions, all aimed at your experience at the moment of the beep, something like:

> Did you innerly see the house? *No.* Were you innerly speaking something at the moment of the beep? *No.* Were you apprehensive? *Yes.* Did your experience include anything bodily? *Yes.* Where in your body? *In my chest.* Down deep or on the surface? *On the surface, or maybe not exactly on the surface but within a few millimeters of the surface.* Pressure? Tingling? Heat? *None of that. Somehow my chest, particularly the surface of it, made itself present to me.*

That chesty-surface-experience description is pretty darn, but not perfectly, precise, not probably as precise as the blue of my car, but much more precise than "feeling blue."

We have agreed that all language use is metaphorical to a greater or lesser degree. Pristine experience is at the not-very-metaphorical end of that range. That is, I am not claiming that pristine experience (e.g., chesty-surface experience) is *perfectly* nonmentalistic, only that it is pretty darn nonmentalistic.

Thus, I think we have a series of pretty darn well described bits of Marco's pristine experience, and in chapter XX, on June 6, I have formed some real generalizations about them. We could quibble about the exact words I have used in that chapter to describe the general characteristics of your experiences, and doubtless improve what I have written. But such quibbles will not produce, for example, frequent inner speakings and inner seeings in Marco's experience—you just didn't have many of those, regardless of my descriptive infelicity.

I think that statement about Marco's pristine experience (with whatever refinements we care to make) is a pretty darn objective characterization of Marco's experience, objective in the sense that it does not depend much on the subjective states of the characterizer (Russ, in this instance). That Marco has frequent sensory awarenesses but not

272 • CHAPTER XXII

frequent inner speakings are facts independent of Russ, independent of Marco's use of language. It's just the way it *is*, not the way Russ or Marco *wants it to be*.

Pristine experiences are by definition private, but they are experientially specifiable in a way that mentalisms like blueness and hunger are not.

ROAD MAP: *Russ's comments wrap up our discussions of mentalism and pristine experience (theme g) and the relationship between concepts and experience (theme j).*

RE [199] "Despite your claims to the contrary, you seem—at times—to consider DES a one-size-fits-all solution to the questions raised by experience."

From my side of the chasm, I do not consider DES a one-size-fits-all solution to anything, and as far as I know I have never said that. I accept my own potential for distortion/delusion, so if you can point me to where I have indeed said that I would sincerely appreciate it.

The situation, metaphorically, is this. Imagine that a guy named Russ lives on a planet where jewelry is greatly valued, and jewelers set shiny bits that the natives call "diamonds" in valuable metals like gold and platinum. Now suppose that Russ discovers that some of these so-called diamonds are metastable allotropes of carbon with extremely high hardness and remarkable optical properties, whereas some are a crystalline form of zirconium dioxide (ZrO_2), which, like the metastable carbon allotrope, is also very hard and optically flawless. So this guy Russ says to the jewelers, "You have two kinds of things here, both of which you call diamonds, but one is carbon and the other is zirconium dioxide." The jewelers say: "We have diamonds, we sell diamonds, we make lots of money, and the world is good." Russ says, "No, you have carbon and you have zirconium, and those things have different properties." The jewelers say, "We have beautiful rings that are made out of diamonds." Russ says, "No, you have beautiful rings, some of which are made out of carbon and some out of zirconium." The jewelers say, "We have beautiful necklaces that are *very* made out of diamonds." Russ says, "No, you have beautiful necklaces, some of which are made out of carbon and some out of zirconium." At which time the jewelers say, smugly, "We talk about diamonds and gold and platinum and rings and necklaces—we talk about all manner of interesting things. By contrast, all you ever talk about is carbon and zirconium. The distinction between carbon and zirconium is not everything. Despite your claims to the contrary, you seem to consider this distinction between carbon and zirconium a one-size-fits-all solution to all important jewel questions. It seems unreasonable to assume that the tool for determining whether something is carbon or zirconium should be the only standard for how jewelry is judged, described, referenced, or even studied." Russ says, "No, the distinction is not the Ultimate Distinction, but it is an important distinction. In a mature science of jewelry, jewelers would know the difference between carbon and zirconium, the properties of each, and when each is useful."

RE [201] Russ said [at marginal 191]: "If subsequent sampling days do not produce any sayings-to-herself, then I think we can be confident that there were not sayings-to-herself on the first day either—that her first-day *report* of saying was driven by presupposition, not phenomena." Marco replied [at marginal 201]: "This line of reasoning is based on the assumption that people's experiences are always somewhat similar to themselves."

That characterizes my position as being more extreme than it is. I have written (in my 1993 book) about people whose experiences are dramatically *not* consistent across time. See also chapter 2 of my 2006 book with Chris Heavey. So I do not blindly assume similarity across occasions.

The case of inner speaking as reported on the first sampling day is a rather special situation. Very many people hold the deep and unquestioned presupposition that all people always (or at least always when thinking) talk to themselves. For example, this is from Bernard Baars:

> Human beings talk to themselves every moment of the waking day. Most readers of this sentence are doing it now.... Overt speech takes up perhaps a tenth of the waking day; but inner speech goes on all the time. (Baars, 2003, p. 106)

Baars is a highly regarded consciousness scientist, and that statement appeared in *Journal of Consciousness Studies*, a highly regarded journal. I think Baars's statement is entirely false, but (a) Baars stated it with boundless confidence; (b) there was, as far as I know, no editorial resistance; and (c) there has been no readership complaint. I am not especially critical of Baars—he is by no means unusual. There are powerful forces that lead people (including very smart people) to make and accept false statements about the appearance of inner speech in inner experience. As a result, any method that seeks to explore inner experience in high fidelity cannot merely ignore those forces—they must be actively countered somehow.

So I don't think it is right to say that "This line of reasoning is based on the assumption that people's experiences are always somewhat similar to themselves." The line of reasoning is this: I have seen hundreds of people report inner speaking in their experience on the first day who do not report inner speaking on their later days. There are three possibilities that I can see: (1) I badger them out of reporting inner speech; (2) experience is variable across occasions and almost always varies in the direction *away from* inner speech; or (3) their first-day reports are based more on their presuppositions about inner speech than on their direct experience thereof.

About (1), you yourself get to be one judge of the severity of my badgering: your own sampling included some speculation on the first and second sampling days that inner speech was present in your experience. [Here Russ sends Marco an annotated transcript of a portion of his first DES interview, wherein he shows that, far from badgering, Russ *supported* Marco's tentative reports about inner speech. For space considerations, we have excised that from this account, but you can see these comments on the Companion Website]. Did you feel pressure from me to abandon talk about inner speech?

About (2), I accept that as a possibility, but it seems highly unlikely that inner speech would always happen to recede just after sampling begins. I think I can document that I'm happy to discuss inner speech in experience if there be inner speech in experience—across all my sampling, I discover inner speech in approximately 25% of samples. So I'm pretty sure I have no wholesale prejudice against inner speech. Furthermore, when inner speech is present, sampling interviews are generally easy, so it's to my selfish advantage to find inner speech.

About (3), lots of people (think Baars and his editors and readers) have strong presuppositions about the ubiquity of inner speech, so it shouldn't be surprising that such presuppositions seep into early sampling reports.

So my line of reasoning is that of those possibilities that might lead to inner speech disappearing across sampling interviews, (3) seems by far the most likely. However, I'm acutely sensitive to the other potentials, and I strive to make the playing field level for all of them.

You may wish to consult Hurlburt (2009a), which is largely reprinted as chapter 10 of Hurlburt (2011a).

Now I respond to comments you made in your June 2 turn

RE [210] "Practical limitations of DES and intersubjectivity."

I largely agree with what you say about practical limitations, although I think you may be somewhat overly broad. For example, I think DES could provide some useful insight into sexuality. Some sexual dysfunction is said to be related to performance anxiety, or to assuming a spectator role while engaged in sexual activity. I think it would be possible to structure investigations that could shed light on such theories. There are some procedural hurdles to overcome, but I think those are not necessarily insurmountable. However, such studies have not been done.

RE [211] "Wouldn't it be interesting, for example, to ask two participants to wear the beeper while they spend time together, and find a way to beep them at the same time? Have you already tried doing something along these lines?"

I have performed one such investigation but never written about it. The couple who engaged in this task found it very enlightening and useful, but they were not or at least may not have been a typical couple. There are very many details that might arise in such sampling that can be very problematic, and the couple needs to be able to withstand that or accept the consequences of it: Suppose A and B are the couple, and the beep happens when A is feeling sexually aroused by C; or B is thinking that A is fat; or A is not listening to what B is saying; and so on. Not everyone happily wants to know such details or could handle them if they knew them. Furthermore, people customarily are quite dishonest about such details, and that may make honest reporting in DES difficult. But if you could overcome those things, then yes, I think it would be fascinating.

What people actually experience while simultaneously watching a movie is, quite amazingly from my point of view, largely unknown. Exploring it has some of the same risks/difficulties as described in the previous paragraph, in addition to the problematic expectation that the experience *must be* about the movie. But I think those things are overcomable as well.

ROAD MAP: *Russ and Marco now have set aside discussion of whether experiences can be shared (theme b).*

RE [212] "I have the sense that the DES set-up may still place demands on participants to provide more experiential detail than was actually available in pristine experience. The detail may come from memories of the context in which the experience took place, or of previous or subsequent experiences, or from the imaginary reenactment of the experience itself."

I agree that DES doubtless distorts/overspecifies/underspecifies details. That's why I prefer to say that DES can produce "high-fidelity" descriptions, rather than that DES can produce "accurate" descriptions. DES descriptions can be faulty in the details (and thus *not accurate*) and yet be faithful to the main aspects of the experience (and be thus *of high fidelity*). And because of the specificity of the moment, the contemporaneity of the jottings, the iterativeness of the training, and the open-beginningedness of the interview, I might argue that that distortion/overspecification/underspecification is likely to be less in DES than in other methods.

[235]

Some maintain the point of view that DES is *not good enough* in its apprehension of detail, and therefore that all DES descriptions should be scrapped. I happily accept that point of view as being logically unassailable. But if one adopts that view, then I think one must scrap all reports of experience, and that, while logical, may not be productive.

RE [218] "When and if it operates, that demand must exist at the level of experiential details. Take, for instance, beep 3.1, when you asked me what my seeing of the actor was like, and I answered that I was attending to the color and shape of his body. . . . I can't rule out the possibility that my answer overspecifies my seeing."

As I just said, I accept that DES may distort details. However, I am not at all sure that the black/whiteness of Sample 3.1 is an experiential *detail*. I think it likely (or at least possible) that the black/whiteness was *the central or dominant experiential feature* of your experience at that moment, not a mere experiential detail. I'm not sure about that, but most subjects who experience a lot of sensory awareness take a few sampling days to realize (or admit!) the centrality of the sensory, so you may have just been coming into your own (so to speak) in the reporting of sensory awareness. In a photo (or a video), the black/whiteness would in fact be a detail, one among many hundreds or thousands of other details one could point to in the photo ("Look here at the black and whiteness!"). But in *experience,* the pointing-to has already taken place, and I think it likely that you had already zeroed in, for whatever reason, on the black/whiteness of the TV person. I'm not sure of that, and don't wish to defend it too strongly, but it turns out that in *most* of your samples you had zeroed in on a sensory aspect.

RE [213] "I wonder . . . if this does not inject into descriptions of pristine experience at least a tiny fraction of broad experience (i.e., context-based and generalizing reports)."

I fully accept that apprehensions of pristine experience are shaped to some degree by context and generalizing, and that that shaping is created by events that take place distant or far distant from the moment of the beep. I'm agnostic about whether it makes sense to say about those factors that broad experience has been injected into pristine experience. *Something* has been injected into apprehensions of pristine experience; what that something is, I'm not sure.

RE [214] "Can't a sensation that has relatively little weight in pristine experience take on importance because it is present for a long time?"

I presume it can, but I have neither affirmed nor denied that position. I can say that some people never experience feelings. Some of those people are even-keeled, unemotional types, but some have obviously massive ongoing emotions and yet feel nothing, such as the guy who slams the door but honestly and apparently correctly denies feeling anger: Emotion ongoing? Yes! Feeling ongoing? No. Ongoing emotion and the experience of feeling are not necessarily connected (Heavey, Hurlburt, and Lefforge, 2012). Is ongoing emotion without the sense of feeling important? Yes: the guy beats his wife. Would he be healthier if he experienced the feeling while the emotion is ongoing? Probably so—as it is, the emotion "takes him by surprise"; his anger builds and builds but he doesn't notice it until he erupts, and then it is too late.

The bottom line is that I have never claimed that pristine experience is the most important aspect of human nature. I have claimed that it is or may be an important aspect, perhaps even claimed that it is or may be a *very* important aspect, but that is substantially short of asserting that it is the most important aspect.

RE [215] "Could it be that there is a correlation between people's use of metaphor and their skill at DES? In other words, could it be that the more experienced participants become, the more they tend to employ metaphors and similes in order to describe their pristine experiences?"

I have thought a lot about metaphor (which I will not distinguish from simile here) over my career, and written some stuff about it but never written anything coherent about it. Here's what I think.

I like metaphors. I use metaphors. I think metaphors are important features of communication. I think metaphors are or can be beautiful, forceful, and effective. I'm a fan of metaphors.

[236] As I have said, I think all or most communication has at least a hint of metaphoricity.

[237] I have not collected the relevant data, but my sense is *not* that DES participants (interviewer and subject) use *more* metaphors, but rather that they are clearer about the metaphoricity of their metaphors when they use them. For example, when I used the melting-chocolate-letters metaphor, I was 100% aware of the metaphoricity of that statement. It would never have occurred to me, for example, to try to investigate the melting point of inner words, or to investigate the taste of inner words, and so on. You might be thinking "Of course not!" but I think much of psychological science is caught up (wittingly or unwittingly) in reifying metaphors and then investigating the real properties suggested by the metaphor. For example, one can say the mind is like a computer, and I have no problem with that metaphor. But we have a generation of scientists who are investigating inputs and outputs and control functions and executive systems and programs and so on, which are real properties of real computers but not necessarily properties of minds. Those investigations follow from the reification of the metaphor rather than from the direct observation of phenomena, and I think that is a very bad thing for science.

So I think being unclear about the extent to which one's communication is metaphorical is highly problematic. And I think being unclear about the ambiguity that can be inherent in metaphor is highly problematic. I felt comfortable in advancing the melting-chocolate metaphor because we had already largely nailed down the phenomenon of interest, and I thought the metaphor might add something in the realm of details.

Elsewhere (e.g., Hurlburt and Schwitzgebel, 2007, 72, 160; Hurlburt, 2011a, 253) I have argued that when some people say "I was thinking in the back of my head," "I was green with envy," "I see the world through rose colored glasses," "I feel blue," "I'm so angry I see red," and so on, they mean to be taken literally. I'll use "I see red" as an example, but everything I will say for the rest of this response should be understood as also applying to the other phrases.

When some people say "I see red," "red" has an entirely literal referent—they are indeed visually seeing the color red infusing their visual field. When others say "I see red," "red" has an entirely metaphorical referent—"seeing red" for them is a linguistic device that has been shaped by the verbal community and that has, for them, no direct relationship to the color red.

Many people (perhaps most, but I don't really know) who use "I see red" with the literal referent are surprised or even shocked to discover that their utterance does indeed have a literal referent. A typical exchange in a DES interview might be something like this:

SUBJECT: My wife had taken money out of the account again and I was angry. She pisses me off when she does that! I was seeing red.
INTERVIEWER: How does this anger or pissed-off-ness present itself to you?
SUBJECT: I was yelling at her, and I was seeing an image of the bank statement. [They discuss the image.]
INTERVIEWER: You said you were seeing red. Does that . . . ?
SUBJECT: Nah! That's just a figure of speech. I was yelling . . . Wait a minute! That's not right! My image of the bank statement *was* red! It was like I was seeing the statement in red light. Oh my god! I *was actually* seeing red. That's really weird!

I've seen enough such interviews, and iteratively examined several occasions from the same person, and conducted my explorations on an adequately level playing field, to be convinced that the redness was experientially visually present at the moment of the beep, and was *not created* to be consistent with having said "I was seeing red" in the interview. That is, I'm confident that "I was seeing red" referred to a pristine experience at the moment of the beep, and that the person did not know prior to sampling that the color red was actually a characteristic of his pristine anger experience. I'm just as confident of that as I am that you were seeing blueness with white above it in your pristine experience at sample 5.3.

I happily accept that I might be mistaken, both about the redness and about your blue/white experience (but I think the probability of both is low). I happily accept that the in-the-world frequency of literally seeing red might be smaller than I take it to be (that I have, by luck, interviewed more than my share of such people, or inflated my recollections thereabout). But there is, I think, a good enough chance that I'm largely right about this literal seeing of red that a science of experience should take it seriously. In particular, I might notice:

1) This is another example of where people's broad experience of their own pristine experience does not comport with their actual pristine experience.
2) It demonstrates that one cannot (or cannot always) judge the metaphoricity of an expression from the expression itself. There is nothing about the words "I see red" that determines the metaphoricity of that expression.
3) It demonstrates the skill required in a DES interview—neither to assume that "I see red" is metaphorical, nor to pressure the subject into claiming it to be sensory.
4) It demonstrates that people do not necessarily know the metaphoricity of their own speech.
5) It seems reasonable at least to speculate that it provides some insight into the development of language. "I see red" may well be retained by the linguistic community not as arbitrary metaphor but because *some people* (probably many but not all) *actually see red*. (Maybe the linguists know all about this, and I'm just ignorant about what they know.)
6) Following from (2) and (4), I think in real life and literature we have to be cognizant that what seems like metaphor might be declarative description. Let's take an example from your paper on the use of metaphor Ian McEwan's *Saturday* (thanks for sending this paper!): "These diaphanous films of sleep are still slowing him down—he imagines them resembling the arachnoid, that gossamer covering of the brain through which he routinely cuts" (Caracciolo, 2013b, 65). You provide two alternative

understandings of that metaphor: that Henry himself creates the metaphor, and that the narrator creates the metaphor for Henry. But there is a third alternative, which you don't mention, namely, [238] that Henry *actually sees* (imaginarily, of course) gossamer arachnoid. Under that interpretation, the passage includes no metaphor at all, but rather is merely a literal description of Henry's experience. I am not arguing that the third alternative is most likely the author's intent—I have no idea about that. Instead, I am suggesting that . . .

7) . . . There probably is not a clear dividing line between literal [239] expression and metaphor. (Here again, the linguists may know all about this, and I'm just ignorant about what they know.) Our above subject who says "I see red" may well be uttering some amalgam of literal and metaphorical expression, and it is not at all necessary (and may well be counterproductive in general) for him to be explicitly cognizant of the relative contribution of each. However . . .

8) . . . DES, at least in some situations, can disentangle metaphorical from literal expression, and sometimes that can be quite enlightening.

RE [216] "I find that there is something deeply *poetic* about experience sampling and the way in which you practice it. . . . I couldn't help thinking that these carefully and laboriously described instants had a value that goes even beyond the scientific project of studying pristine experience."

I agree. I think every genuine human endeavor, whether it be in science, poetry, music, religion, athletics, or whatever, is the same at its heart: the object of each is to cultivate human skill, to push the limits as constrained by the real world. However, much of what passes as science, poetry, music, religion, athletics, or whatever is not very genuine in this sense, instead being corrupted by greed or insecurity or whatever.

The bottom line: I think when you get down deep enough into genuineness, everything looks pretty much the same. You practice your art, trying to make it conform to reality, not asking too much of it, not asking too little of it, not lying about it, not hiding it, learning to communicate about it, trying to figure out which way to push it and then doing so. All that is genuine humanism, pretty much independent of the discipline.

ROAD MAP: *Russ's remark concludes the discussion of the difference between the humanistic and the scientific approach to experience (theme d).*

RE [217] "I think that learning to appreciate consciousness-focused narrative might actually be a good preparation for (or complement to) DES training."

If by "appreciate" you mean, or at least include, learning to recognize the advantages, disadvantages, ranges of convenience, traps, vantage points, pitfalls, temptations, beauties, and so on, for what they are and not more nor less (that is, being genuinely humanistic as I described in the previous paragraph), then I agree with you. [Marco later replies: All this surely is part of what I mean by "appreciate."]

Now I respond to comments you made in your June 3 turn

RE [206] "The whole DES method strives for clarity and distinctness, but what if (some aspects of) experience are inherently, and irreducibly, vague?"

I think that misrepresents DES. The striving is for fidelity, not (necessarily) clarity. If experience is clear and distinct, then fidelity urges clarity and distinctness. But if experience is vague or blurry, then fidelity urges vagueness or blurriness. To resist the temptation of exaggerating clarity is high art, and I am not in a position to claim that I do that well. But I'm pretty sure (a) that I explicitly work at such resistance; (b) that I resist that temptation better than do most of my co-interviewers, with whom I have had many conversations and watched many videotapes aimed at exactly this issue. That said, I imagine that there are many who might be more skilled at this than I.

RE [208] "I had the sense that it [beep 2.2] both contained words (in the implied form that we've already discussed) and did not contain words (because I couldn't remember any)."

I thought we came very close to such a conclusion about sample 6.2 [see RE 202–205 on May 27, and later], so I think I do not blindly rush toward clarity when clarity does not exist. Sample 2.2, as I have discussed above [see RE 222 on June 8], is a different story, because I think there were lots of reason to be skeptical about your description of that experience. However, "skeptical" as I (and Webster) use the term does not mean "disbelieving"; it means that I don't know what to make of it and so will have to keep an open mind. You may wish to look at chapter 2 of my 2006 book with Chris Heavey; that chapter was a case study about unclarity.

RE [209] "I was surprised by the salience of sensory and bodily awareness in the samples. At some point I related this with recent trends in cognitive science and the philosophy of mind, which hold that perception and bodily patterns of interaction with the world are much more pervasive and cognitively central than posited by traditional, computational cognitivism."

If your implication is that philosophers'/psychologists' understanding of sensory awareness is behind the embodied cognition movement, I think you are grossly mistaken. I think philosophers and psychologists know little or nothing about sensory awareness as you and others experience it.

Some people, like you, have ubiquitous salient sensory and bodily awareness in their pristine experience. You probably engage in sensory awareness roughly 20,000 times a day (20 times a minute [that's a new sensory awareness every three seconds, which is a very rough estimate but probably in the ballpark] × 60 minutes × 16 hours), which works out to about 70,000,000 sensory awarenesses over the past 10 years. Other people (more than half, I think is safe to say, but there may well be cultural differences that I have not investigated, sorry to say) have approximately zero percent sensory or bodily awareness. As I believe you have seen for yourself, having or not having sensory awareness is not a mere linguistic distinction, as if everyone's experiences are the same but some include the word "sensory awareness" in their descriptions but some don't. There is, I think you would agree, a huge phenomenological difference between sensory awareness and other forms of pristine experience. That difference is huger than the difference between black and white, roughly as huge as the difference between black and 17, roughly as huge as the difference between white and "perhaps."

Just as you were surprised that your own experience included so many sensory awarenesses, cognitive science and the philosophy of mind are ignorant of the fact that many people (like you) engage in roughly 20,000 sensory awareness experiences a day, whereas many others engage in none or a few. I don't think it is possible to paper over that ignorance with a notion such as embodied cognition.

Cognitive science (including embodied cognitive science) is a universalist doctrine: it presumes (without much thought and no investigations thereabout) that people who engage in 20,000 sensory awarenesses a day are cognitively no different from those who engage in no sensory awarenesses. There are two possibilities here: (a) Cognitive science is right: sensory awareness has no functional significance. Sensory awareness is merely epiphenomenal and has no role in cognition, embodied or otherwise; or (b) Cognitive science is wrong: sensory awareness does have functional significance—your 20,000 sensory awarenesses a day do impact (or are impacted by) your way of being in the world, including your cognition, in a way that is different from someone who has no sensory awarenesses. If that is the case, then cognitive science (including embodied cognitive science) *should be* taking sensory awareness into consideration *but isn't*.

[240]   Either way, it is a gross mistake to think that sensory awareness is behind or somehow drives the embodied cognition movement. If sensory awareness is epiphenomenal, then cognitive science has been right to ignore it. If sensory awareness does matter, then cognitive science should investigate it, but so far it hasn't. I suspect that people who have 20,000 sensory awarenesses a day are indeed different in some important ways (including, probably, cognitive ways) from people who have 0 sensory awarenesses a day. That is a guess; neither I nor anyone else has conducted such studies.

We should be clear about the implications of your own surprise at the frequency of your sensory awarenesses. You are very typical in this regard. That implies that no retrospective interview, armchair introspection, or questionnaire prior to sampling is likely to discover who does and who does not engage in 20,000 sensory awarenesses a day. So if cognitive scientists or anyone else is to investigate the implications of having frequent sensory awareness, they will likely have to eschew their most commonly used investigative methods and engage in something like DES as a starting point.

XXIII

FEELING HOOKS INSIDE ONE'S CHEST; METAPHOR AND EXPERIENCE

June 17
Dear Russ,
Thank you so much for your illuminating comments and responses. You'll find below my further thoughts on these issues.
All the best,
Marco

RE [231] "The description is not about Russ—any investigator with adequate skill would, I think, arrive at a similar description of Marco's experience."

　I agree with you here (and indeed with the whole list of "characteristics of our description of [my] experience" [see RE 227 in chapter XXII]). Thus, I think we can return to one of our earlier points of discussion—whether DES reports are influenced by the interlocutor; I can safely conclude that you were (and are) right about the relative interlocutor-independence of DES.

ROAD MAP: Marco had been convinced that even pristine experience is interlocutor-dependent (see RE 113 in chapter XI), but he changed his mind after his personal encounter with DES: Russ was right, there is indeed a sharp difference between broad experience and pristine experience with respect to their degree of interlocutor-dependence.

　This concludes the discussion of the difference between DES reports and what people say about their experience (theme c).

RE [232] "If you would care to specify concretely and exactly the specific 'pretty interesting insights' [into experience offered by phenomenologists]

285

about which you'd like to know the relationship to my work, I'd be happy to try to respond."

You've indirectly answered my question here. What I was asking is not your opinion on some specific insight offered by Husserl or someone else, but your general attitude toward phenomenology as a philosophical school focusing on experience. I think your response implies: I don't believe in any insight into experience unless it aligns with what one can (or cannot) find by practicing DES. That may be a slightly exaggerated way of describing your stance toward phenomenology, but it is not too off-target in my view. Further, I have the sense that—while your analysis of experience samples does indeed "reflect some sort of theoretical perspective"—you've built that perspective yourself through years of DES. This does look like an inductivist method, but I'm neither a scientist nor a philosopher of science, so I may be wrong, and in any case I cannot criticize you for this. But I wanted to better understand how DES relates to phenomenological philosophy.

RE [233] "Philosophic and literary texts have been describing consciousness for centuries (or millennia), but have largely ignored 'unsymbolized thinking,' 'sensory awareness,' and, for that matter, 'pristine experience' itself."

[242] This does sound a little overstated, at least as far as sensory awareness is concerned. Take, for example, this description from Joyce's *A Portrait of the Artist* (appearing a few lines after the passage quoted above [see chapter X]): "There were two cocks that you turned and water came out: cold and hot. [Stephen] felt cold and then a little hot: and he could see the names printed on the cocks. That was a very queer thing" (Joyce, 2000, 8). Wouldn't you say that these sentences focus on the character's sensory awareness?

RE [234] "Did you feel pressure from me to abandon talk about inner speech?"

Not at all, and your analysis of our exchanges proves that beyond doubt.

Q: Why do you ask about abandoning inner speech?
RUSS: Many people, including many if not most consciousness scientists, believe that people talk to themselves all the time (recall the discussion of Baars at RE 201 in chapter XXII). DES finds that inner speech

occurs about a quarter of the time. That's a big difference! The 100% folks think I must in some way discourage people from reporting inner speech. This question was a small exploration of that issue.

RE [235] "DES descriptions can be faulty in the details (and thus *not accurate*) and yet be faithful to the main aspects of the experience (and be thus *of high fidelity*)."

Yes, that is a helpful distinction, and I would agree with you that the black-and-whiteness of the man I saw in sample 3.1 may be more than an experiential detail. I think the reason why I was tempted to see it as a detail is that I remember having some difficulties answering your questions about what in particular was in my visual experience. I went back to the video of the interview [4:48 into sample 3.1 in the audio on the Companion Website] and found that my description is highly subjunctified, and it is possible that your questions may have led me to describe more than I could possibly report about this visual experience. I remember—but again I don't have any contemporaneous note to prove—that I was still a bit unsure about the distinction between shape and black-and-whiteness after our conversation: the shape and color were fused into a single blob, and I couldn't confidently say whether I was attending to the one or the other.

RE [236] "I think all or most communication has at least a hint of metaphoricity"; and

RE [239] "There probably is not a clear dividing line between literal expression and metaphor."

I think any cognitive linguist working in the wake of Lakoff and Johnson's *Metaphors We Live By* (1980) would agree with you that metaphors are everywhere and that they underlie many linguistic constructions that we tend to consider "literal" (through so-called "conceptual metaphors" such as GOOD IS UP or BAD IS DOWN, LIFE IS A JOURNEY, etc.).

RE [237] "I have not collected the relevant data, but my sense is *not* that DES participants (interviewer and subject) use *more* metaphors, but rather that they are clearer about the metaphoricity of their metaphors when they use them."

Yes, that is quite possible. But I was thinking about a more linguistic analysis of the metaphors; it seems to me that it can be difficult to disentangle "unintentional" from "intentional" metaphor on the basis of language alone.

I was at a conference last Friday where psychologist Katalin Bálint was illustrating a series of qualitative interviews aimed at investigating the experience of "absorption" in narrative texts. [This study was later published as Bálint and Tan, 2015.] Needless to say, the participants used a number of metaphors to describe their experiential states; after all, "absorption" itself is a metaphor, and so are most terms used to capture this phenomenon in literary studies, media psychology, and even in everyday language: immersion, transportation, captivation, etc. While looking at the speaker's slides (which showed the transcripts of the interviews) I was struck by some patterns in the metaphors employed by the participants: some of the interviewees used more or less conventional metaphors (those I have just listed); others offered creative

[243] variations on these conventional metaphors (for instance, a participant said that she felt "hooks inside [her] chest," which I take to build on the idiom "being hooked"); others, finally, used completely novel metaphorical language (e.g., someone declared that the novel was "swelling up in her head"). In this set-up, where the participants are instructed to freely describe an experience of absorption in a novel, the risk of fauxity and confabulation is obviously very high (as in the reviews of *The Road*). The speaker was arguing that these metaphors demonstrate the readers' bodily involvement while reading (i.e., in pristine experience), but this is—of course—questionable. What I wonder, however, is if creative or novel metaphors are not *more likely* to reflect the readers' pristine expe-

[244] rience in high fidelity than are conventional metaphors. I think it would be interesting to examine DES reports in this light, trying to establish whether the novelty (rather than the frequency) of the metaphors used by the participants increases with their skill at observing and reporting pristine experience.

RE [238] "There is a third alternative, which you don't mention, namely, that Henry *actually sees* (imaginarily, of course) gossamer arachnoid. Under that interpretation, the passage includes no metaphor at all, but rather is merely a literal description of Henry's experience."

[245] I think a lot depends on how we define metaphor. If metaphor is seen as a mapping between two or more semantic-conceptual domains, as in recent, cognitive-linguistic theories of metaphor (see, e.g., Fauconnier

and Turner, 2002), then the passage *does* contain a number of metaphors. The character imaginarily blends his sleepiness with some "diaphanous films," which are compared to the "arachnoid," which in turn resembles a "gossamer." All this may well correspond to the character's experience. So Henry—and people more generally—may *actually* experience a metaphorical construct through mental imagery. To put this point otherwise: metaphorical is not, for me, the opposite of "real" or "actual." Metaphorical only implies a particular cognitive mechanism—the blending of different semantic-conceptual domains—which may indeed lead to imaginary experiences.

There have been some, mostly speculative, claims that metaphors are processed by way of mental simulation, i.e., by literally blending together concrete images and sensations. Compare Gibbs and Matlock: [246] "People understand metaphors by creating an imaginative simulation of their bodies in action that mimics the events alluded to by the metaphor. . . . We claim in this chapter that the recruitment of embodied metaphors in some aspects of verbal metaphor understanding is done imaginatively as people recreate what it must be like to engage in similar actions" (Gibbs and Matlock, 2008, 162). If this could be demonstrated at the level of pristine experience, it would show that at least *some* metaphors are not purely linguistic constructs but, on the contrary, ride piggyback on somatosensory experience. (I say *some* because conventional metaphors are more likely to be processed through category extension, which I would characterize as a cognitive-level, unconscious process. See Bowdle and Gentner's (2005) "career of metaphor" theory. Glucksberg (2008) provides psycholinguistic evidence for metaphor processing through category extension.)

RE [240] "It is a gross mistake to think that sensory awareness is behind or somehow drives the embodied cognition movement."

I would agree with you that the embodied cognition movement has not (so far) engaged in a careful investigation of pristine experience, and that only methods such as DES can support that project. However, experience seems to have a far more central role in embodied and situated cognitive science than in AI-inspired cognitivism, and I am reasonably optimistic that scientists will undertake such an investigation going forward. After all, isn't the rise of interest in consciousness studies—and in the DES method itself—a sign of this turn toward experience?

June 19
Hi Marco—
Thanks very much. Here are my comments.
—Russ

RE [241] "I think your response implies: I don't believe in any insight into experience unless it aligns with what one can (or cannot) find by practicing DES."

That is an extreme position that I think fairly represents my views if we narrow it a bit. I'll italicize my additions: I don't believe in any insight into *pristine* experience unless it aligns with what one can (or cannot) find by practicing DES *or some other method as good or better*.

I think it is a mistake to make claims about pristine experience unless one examines pristine experience in a way dictated by the phenomena (that's the point of my 2011 book). Many people, including many phenomenologists, have tried to skip that step, but not with success, as it seems to me.

(By the way, believing that it is necessary first to examine pristine experience if one wishes to make claims about pristine experience does not imply that pristine experience is of ultimate importance or even that it is important.)

RE [242] Russ said [at marginal 233]: "Philosophic and literary texts have been describing consciousness for centuries (or millennia), but have largely ignored 'unsymbolized thinking,' 'sensory awareness,' and, for that matter, 'pristine experience' itself." Marco replied [at marginal 242]: "This does sound a little overstated, at least as far as sensory awareness is concerned."

I accept that literary texts have frequently described *examples of* sensory awareness, such as the one you cite. However, the point I was trying to make was that texts have largely ignored discussing sensory awareness as a feature of human pristine experience. Here is a litmus test: If a text is discussing *sensory awareness as a feature of human pristine experience* (rather than merely providing an example of sensory awareness), then that text should state that some people have lots of sensory awareness whereas others have none. That is a basic, (I think) obvious fact about sensory awareness as a phenomenon of human pristine experience. I know of no philosophic or literary texts that discuss that fact, and therefore I conclude that philosophic and literary texts have largely ignored sensory awareness as a phenomenon of human pristine experience.

RE [243] "A participant said that she felt 'hooks inside [her] chest,' which I take to build on the idiom 'being hooked.'"

I recommend not discounting the possibility that the participant intended her chest-hooks expression as a literal description of a sensation inside her chest. Your "which I take to build on the idiom" is typical (to my ear) of the way many or most philosophers and psychologists would understand the participant's locution, an understanding that presumes that words are primary and that many other things including descriptions of experience are derivatives of (or buildings on) some presumed network of words. Certainly words are sometimes or to some degree influential, as Winawer's Russian language study shows (see near marginal 121 in chapter XI). However, I find it problematic that when such claims are made, little space is typically left for the oppositely directed causality—that the experiential hooks *create* rather than build on the idiom. [247] [248]

In your own pristine experience, of which we have two dozen samples, to what degree did your network of words/idioms affect your pristine experience? For example, I chose a sample at random and found this:

> Sample 5.1. I'm feeling the motion on the skin or surface of my thumb and forefinger and to a lesser extent the rest of my hand. This is a circular motion; I feel the motion, not the kinesthetics of making the motion. This is felt as a slight pressure on the skin or surface of my hand, as if a handkerchief rests lightly on my hand and weighs it down slightly. I feel my hand and this pressure make a circular motion. Note that I do *not* feel the spoon in my thumb and forefinger, even though I am in reality holding the spoon there and stirring with it.

To what degree do you think your network of words/idioms created, distorted, shaped, or otherwise built the motion-feeling on the surface of your thumb and forefinger? I think not very much. I think to a very great degree your finger sensations were what they were, regardless of whatever words/idioms might exist in your personal lexicon. [249]

RE [244] "I think it would be interesting to examine DES reports . . . to establish whether the novelty (rather than the frequency) of the metaphors used by the participants increases with the skill at observing and reporting pristine experience."

I agree that this might be interesting. Acknowledging that my suspicions about what I might find in a DES study are often substantially wrong, I suspect that there might be large individual differences in metaphor use. There may be some people, as perhaps you would predict, who start out their DES participation being not particularly skilled in metaphor, but as they become more involved in trying to describe their experience, they become more creative in their metaphor. But there might be others who start out their DES participation being highly metaphorical, perhaps as a way of defending against or being estranged from their own real experience; increasing DES skill for them may result in a decrease in metaphor in general and in novel metaphor as well. And there might be others who don't use much metaphor prior to sampling and still don't use much metaphor during or after sampling. Three bottom lines: First, as my mother often instructed me, don't judge others by yourself. Second, I don't really know the answer to your question—that's why the study might be interesting. Third, perhaps even more interesting than your question would be these: What are the characteristics of people's inner experience that lead one to use metaphor frequently? Infrequently? In novel ways?

In passing, I note that your question (like almost all those posed by philosophers and psychologists) is a universalist question, presuming that all people are the same and therefore would be similarly influenced by DES participation (anything else would be error). My "perhaps more interesting" questions are individual-difference questions, presuming (or at least acknowledging) that people are importantly different and therefore might be affected by DES in importantly different ways. The distinction between universalist and individual-difference perspectives is, I think, of fundamental importance if science is to advance. I think it plausible that some or much of the resistance to DES stems from unwillingness or inability of many scientists to abandon their universalist perspectives.

RE [245] "If metaphor is seen as a mapping between two or more semantic-conceptual domains, as in recent, cognitive-linguistic theories of metaphor, then the passage *does* contain a number of metaphors."

I would be the last person to argue that the passage does not contain a number of metaphors, because I think almost all communication is metaphorical. The question, as it seems to me, is not about metaphors in general but about metaphors as Marco-the-metaphor-paper-author meant the term when he wrote the paper. For example, when you cited "he imagines them resembling the arachnoid, that gossamer covering of the brain through which he routinely cuts" (Caracciolo, 2013b, 65), did you have in mind a literal reading, in which Henry was actually literally innerly seeing the arachnoid? If so, the metaphoricity you had in mind was, for example, in the word "gossamer," extending its literal meaning (cobwebs floating in the air) to the actually heavier and more substantial real arachnoid. Or did you have in mind a completely metaphorical arachnoid reference? If so, the metaphoricity was in the entire mention of arachnoid. My speculation, about which you may correct me, is that Marco-the-metaphor-paper-author meant the latter, that you saw the sentence as metaphorical through and through. [250]

I don't know whether McEwan (2005) meant a literal inner seeing or an entire metaphor, or whether it would be desirable for him to know the difference between the two.

RE [246] "Compare Gibbs and Matlock: 'People understand metaphors by creating an imaginative simulation of their bodies in action that mimics the events alluded to by the metaphor. . . . We claim in this chapter that the recruitment of embodied metaphors in some aspects of verbal metaphor understanding is done imaginatively as people recreate what it must be like to engage in similar actions.'"

I agree with your characterization of this claim as "mostly speculative," made in substantial ignorance about pristine experience, even though pristine experience should lie close to the center of the discussion.

XXIV

METAPHOR TABLES

June 21
Dear Russ,
Please find my comments below.
All the best,
Marco

RE [247] "I recommend not discounting the possibility that the participant intended her chest-hooks expression as a literal description of a sensation inside her chest."

That's not what I was suggesting. I was arguing that the (possible) influence of the idiom "being hooked" would make the expression slightly more suspect of *not* accurately reflecting a pristine experience. But I don't think that the superficial similarity between the idiom and the participant's locution conclusively proves anything. So I agree with you that the possibility that the participant really felt hooks in her chest shouldn't be discarded (but see also my next comment).

RE [248] "However, I find it problematic that when such claims are made, little space is typically left for the oppositely directed causality—that the experiential hooks *create* rather than build on the idiom."

As I said in the previous paragraph, I think you're right. Consider, however, that in Bálint's study of absorption in reading (Bálint and Tan, 2015), the participants were invited to describe "what it was like for them to be immersed/absorbed in a book." Although all efforts were made to anchor the description to a particular reading experience of a particular book, I'd say that the study is very far from the methodological rigor of DES. In other words, it is a study of broad experience, not of pristine experience. And in broad experience (I would say) a locution that builds on a conventional metaphor is more likely to be influenced by presuppositions about what a particular experience feels like than is a novel metaphor. But that's pure speculation, of course. In any case I fully agree with you that if the expression "I felt hooks in my chest" appeared in DES, it would be a presupposition to discard or take it "metaphorically" because it is reminiscent of the idiom. (Cf. my discussion of the term "metaphorical" in RE 250 below.)

RE [249] "To what degree do you think your network of words/idioms created, distorted, shaped, or otherwise built the motion-feeling on the surface of your thumb and forefinger? I think not very much."

I also think not very much. But, again, you've convinced me that pristine experience and broad experiential descriptions are radically different in this respect.

RE [250] "For example, when you cited 'he imagines them resembling the arachnoid, that gossamer covering of the brain through which he routinely cuts' (Caracciolo, 2013b, 65), did you have in mind a literal reading, in which Henry was actually literally innerly seeing the arachnoid?"

Your suspect may be right; perhaps I was taking the whole sentence as metaphorical in the sense that Henry wasn't innerly seeing the arachnoid. In any case I think we should be careful with the adjective "metaphorical," because it can mean many things: one can say that something is "metaphorical" because it contains linguistic metaphors, or because it doesn't have any basis in reality (it is imaginary, even though it may be experienced), or because it doesn't have any basis in pristine experience. I'd rather use other terms or phrases for "doesn't have any basis in reality" and "doesn't have any basis in pristine experience." I think part of the problem is that when we say that something is "metaphorical" we typically don't specify whether the frame of reference is "external" reality or pristine experience.

Consider table 7. I think the first two rows are uncontroversial. In the first, someone says "I felt hooks in my chest" and refers to a situation in which he really *had* hooks in his chest. No metaphor here (or at least not much—I agree with what you said at RE 245, that all communication is metaphorical at least to some degree). In the second row, someone says "I felt hooks in my chest" but refers to a situation in which he had no hooks in his chest; what is more, his expression has no pristine-experiential correlates: he just felt captivated or "hooked" by a book. This (I think you would agree) is a linguistic metaphor. However, we might disagree about the metaphoricity of the expression in the last row. Suppose that someone says "I felt hooks in my chest" as a way of capturing his pristine experience: does his phrase contain a metaphor? You may say: "No, because his experience is real and apprehended in high fidelity." I don't deny that. Yet I would argue that the participant arrives at that description because he compares his pristine experience with the way he imagines it would feel like to have hooks in his chest. That comparison, in my view, is at the heart of metaphor—so as far as I'm concerned it still makes sense to say that the participant's expression contains a metaphor.

[251] Table 7. Meanings of "metaphorical"

EXPRESSION	TYPE	IS THE COMMUNICATION ABOUT A REAL OBJECT? (Does it occur in the world?)	IS IT REAL SUBJECTIVELY SPEAKING? (Does it occur in pristine experience?)	DOES IT CONTAIN A METAPHOR? (Is it metaphorical in the linguistic sense?)
I felt hooks in my chest	Real occurrence	Yes	Yes	No (or not much)
	Linguistic metaphor	No	No	Yes
	Describing experience	No	Yes	Yes/No?

Also, consider my beep 6.3. I used the hyperbold font metaphor, while you suggested the melted-chocolate metaphor. These images are not identical (in terms of the roundedness of the borders, for example), but they were for me (almost) equally valid ways of capturing a prelinguistic, premetaphorical experiential content. Which is also why they are still metaphors even though they are not "metaphorical" in the sense of "purely imaginary" (that is, they correspond to a *real* experiential content).

June 23
Hi Marco—
Here are my latest comments.
—Russ

RE [251] Table 7
I think this table is very helpful in advancing our understanding of metaphor, and I agree that the controversy arises from the Yes/No?

cell. But I think the answer in that cell is not either/or but *both* Yes *and* No. Yes, that row is a metaphor because (nearly) everything is a metaphor. However, No, that row is *not* metaphorical in the purely linguistic sense of the second row of your table. As a result, that ambiguity suggests that the either/or question of metaphoricity needs to be divided in some way.

A metaphor is a way of calling attention to some aspect of one concept (which Julian Jaynes (1986) called the *metaphrand*) by referencing another concept (which Jaynes called the *metaphier*). When I say "Love is a rose," the statement is about "love" (the metaphrand), and I call attention to love's qualities by invoking the notion of the rose (the metaphier). Now which characteristics of the rose do I actually wish to invoke? Its beauty? its stateliness? its unfoldingness? its scent? its transience? its thorniness? its need for water? its expense? All of the above? Jaynes called such things *paraphiers*, and paraphiers are not specified by the metaphor, which makes the metaphor an ambiguous communication. Ambiguity is not inherently bad—ambiguity can give lilt, energy, beauty, interest to a communication (think of the *Mona Lisa*).

When I say, "That stop sign is red," I believe that statement, properly understood, is to some degree a metaphor. I am calling attention to some aspect of the metaphrand (the stop sign) by referencing the metaphier (red). "Red" does not mean "light with a wavelength of 700 millimicrons." "Red" is something with a variety of meanings: the color of an apple; the color of an old fire engine; the color when you blush; the color of fresh blood; the color of dried blood; and so on. Now, which of those characteristics of "red" (which paraphier) do I actually wish to invoke? That is not specified, which makes "That stop sign is red" an ambiguous communication. I think you will grant that "That stop sign is red" is a tighter metaphor (has a smaller range of paraphiers) than does "Love is a rose." But it is always a matter of degree, so all communication is metaphorical, and I therefore endorse the "(or not much)" in your "real occurrence" row.

The statement "All communication is metaphorical" is of course itself metaphorical. I wish to call attention to communication (the metaphrand) by invoking the concept of the metaphor (the metaphier). Now which aspect of the metaphor am I invoking? Its poeticness? its imprecision? its ubiquity? its vitality? its association with Mrs. King's 9th grade English class? The specifically intended paraphier or set of paraphiers is not specified (as usual).

All communication is ambiguous. The object of DES is therefore not to eliminate metaphor, as that would be impossible. The DES object is to get our understanding to "rest lightly on" (that, of course, is a metaphier) pristine experience, rather like chocolate syrup on ice cream. Does the syrup take the shape of the ice cream? Largely, yes. Does it distort the ice cream shape in so doing? To some degree, yes. Can you find out something useful about the shape of the ice cream by examining the shape of the syrup? Probably, yes.

When a DES participant invokes a metaphor (which, of course, participants do all the time), we have to evaluate the tightness of the expression, narrow down the paraphier possibilities, ask additional questions until we can be pretty darn confident that we know what he's talking about.

So, back to the Yes/No? cell of your table. It seems to me that the confusion in that cell arises because of confusion about the metaphrand. Table 8 tries to clear that up. In this revised table your "Does it contain a metaphor?" column becomes useless—everything is metaphorical to some degree.

Your beep 6.3 is a good example of the "describing experience" row of table 8. The metaphrand is your experience (you saw "We tested this possibility"). In our interview, you used hyperbold font as a metaphier, I used melted chocolate as a metaphier. When you say these were "(almost) equally valid ways of capturing a prelinguistic, premetaphorical experiential content," I think you are saying that the interview made the range of the paraphiers relatively small, so that the characteristics of your visual experience of "we tested this possibility" can emerge with relatively little ambiguity (the degree of roundness of the edges remained ambiguous). Said another way, the metaphrand at the moment of 6.3 was a pretty-darn-present-to-your-experience inner seeing. There was little struggle over the metaphrand itself—at the moment of the beep you were seeing "we tested this possibility." The struggle was in *conveying* the metaphrand, that is, in describing something that you could see but I could not. So you invoked an ambiguous metaphier ("hyperbold"); I, in trying to grasp what was and was not the intended paraphier, advanced another (also ambiguous, as they all are) metaphier (melted chocolate), which has an overlapping but different batch of paraphiers.

"Hooked on reading" is a good example of the "linguistic metaphor" row of the table. The broad experience of being interested in, or involved in, or absorbed in, or valuing reading is the metaphrand, and

Table 8. Meanings of "metaphorical," Russ's revision

EXPRESSION	TYPE	IS THE COMMUNICATION ABOUT A REAL OBJECT? (Does it occur in the world?)	IS IT REAL SUBJECTIVELY SPEAKING? (Does it occur in pristine experience?)	METAPHRAND	METAPHIER	SIZE OF THE PARAPHIERS (degree of metaphoricity of the expression)
I felt hooks in my chest	Real occurrence	Yes	Yes	Reality	The term "hooks" as a classification of real objects	Can be close to zero with proper definition
	Linguistic metaphor	No	No	Broad experience	The term "hooks" as existing in a network of conventional metaphors	Large, and resists being made small
	Describing experience	No	Yes	Pristine experience	The term "hooks" as a characterization of past pristine experiences of being stabbed, cut, punctured, pulled, etc.	Can be made small by proper method

being hooked is the metaphier. I don't think it is possible to reduce the ambiguity of this metaphor. It is important to be interested in, or involved in, or absorbed in, or valuing reading (reading is arguably the most important skill to modern success), but I don't think there is any way to disambiguate the metaphrand—there are simply too many different people with too many different ways of being interested in, or involved in, or absorbed in, or valuing reading. We can advance the metaphier "hooked on" reading, and that may well have important political and social ramifications. But it does not disambiguate the metaphrand. In fact, there is now a double struggle: a struggle over what is the metaphrand, and a struggle over how literally to take the metaphier.

ROAD MAP: *Our discussion of metaphor and experience (theme h) ends here.*

XXV

RETROSPECTIVE PROSPECTIONS

June 26
Dear Russ,
Here's table 9, which I will refer to below.

Table 9. Comparing Marco's retrospective prospections with what we found

RETROSPECTIVE PROSPECTIONS	WHAT WE FOUND
Sensory and bodily awareness plays an important role in experience.	Marco's experience almost always includes sensory and bodily awareness, although (Russ explains) this is not the case for all DES subjects.
Inner speech (verbal thinking) is common, although by no means always present.	Inner speech is not common at all in Marco's experience; apart from one borderline case (beep 6.2), in which a sense of words is present even if no distinct words were involved in the experience, inner speech appears only while Marco is reading or typing.
Visual imagery is common, especially while reading narrative.	Marco experiences only two visual images (3.2, 4.5), both of them not particularly rich. There is no trace of visual imagery while reading (although Marco's reading was exclusively nonfiction in the samples). Marco experiences comparatively more imaginary bodily sensations (1.2, 2.2., 3.2, 4.5, 4.6, 6.2) than visual imagery.
Judgments, evaluations, and interpretations are an important component of experience.	None of the samples contains anything that resembles a judgment, an evaluation, or an interpretation.
Emotion is pervasive.	A minority of samples (7 out of 20) contains emotional feelings.
Meaning is pervasive.	Only on one occasion (beep 4.5) is meaning directly experienced.

Table 9. (*Continued*)

RETROSPECTIVE PROSPECTIONS	WHAT WE FOUND
People's experiential engagement with the world is guided by a background of cognitive predispositions and memories of past events.	Memory plays virtually no role in the samples. Predispositions may be present, but they are never directly experienced.

Russ, we've been discussing some general issues. Now I return to the specifically personal thread about my own sampling.
All the best,
Marco

RE [229] "How what you found in your (specific) sampling did or did not agree with your (broad) opinion prior to sampling."

In table 9 I compare my retrospective prospections with what we've actually found.

June 27
Hi Marco—
Here is one comment on your table.
Russ

RE [252] Your "Retrospective prospections" table.

I found one noteworthy aspect of your table 9. As an exercise for Marco, I'd ask you to look at it again and see if you can spot what I might think would be noteworthy. Then I will tell you.

I might suggest jotting down some notes about your reactions to this exercise-for-Marco, as they occur.

Later, Russ sends this:

Hint: What I found remarkable occurs in the first row of the table:

RETROSPECTIVE PROSPECTIONS	WHAT WE FOUND
Sensory and bodily awareness plays an important role in experience.	Marco's experience almost always includes sensory and bodily awareness, although (Russ explains) this is not the case for all DES subjects.

Does that help you spot what I might think would be noteworthy?

Later, Russ sends this:

Before I answer this, let me reiterate that I am no mind reader; I don't have access to the Truth about Marco or anything else. I will describe something that I found remarkable, but that may be more a characteristic of me than of you.

I think that an objective reader of that row in the table would conclude that, prior to sampling, Marco viewed himself as having frequent sensory and bodily awareness, and that such sensory and bodily awareness is common and has some important role in experience. The objective reader would conclude (I think) that if, as a result of sampling, Marco was surprised about anything sensory-awareness-wise, it would be that Russ says that not everyone has the same high level of sensory/bodily awareness that Marco himself has.

That is, bluntly abbreviated, I think that row of the table says:

(JUNE 26, BLUNTLY ABBREVIATED)

RETROSPECTIVE PROSPECTIONS	WHAT WE FOUND
Sensory/bodily awareness is key.	Marco found in himself the sensory/bodily awareness he expected.
	The surprise: Russ says not everyone has salient sensory/bodily sensory awareness.

However, on June 3 (chapter XIX, marginal 209; and discussed frequently thereafter), you said: "Throughout the sampling (I don't know when exactly) I was surprised by the salience of sensory and bodily awareness in the samples." That seems quite different from the June 26 (original or blunt) table, as if the row in the table had read:

304 • CHAPTER XXV

(JUNE 3, BLUNTLY ABBREVIATED)

RETROSPECTIVE PROSPECTIONS	WHAT WE FOUND
Sensory/bodily awareness is **not** key.	The surprise: Marco has salient sensory/bodily sensory awareness.
	Marco found what he expected about people other than himself—Russ says some people do not have salient sensory and bodily awareness.

The June 3 and June 26 views of sensory awareness seem very different—almost opposite. There are at least three alternative explanations: (1) Russ has made a mistake in his understanding/analysis here; (2) the June 3 and June 26 writings refer to different things or different situations; or (3) Marco's June 26 view is inconsistent with his June 3 view. I accept possibilities (1) and (2), and would be happy to have them demonstrated to me; that they seem less likely than (3) may well be due to my own biases.

[253] The exercise-for-Marco was designed with possibility (3) in mind: that Marco has presuppositions/biases about sensory awareness that operate prior to his rational analysis, with the result that inconsistencies can exist but not be recognized. I reemphasize that I am not an authoritative judge about such things, that there is no way that I can know for sure whether I'm right about this, and that I would be just as happy to be wrong as right.

I have structured the exercise-for-Marco so that you would have a chance to explore this for yourself. If I am wrong about (3), that is, that you had no important presuppositions/biases active here, then when I originally directed your attention back to the table, you might have jotted a reaction in the vicinity of: *I bet Russ thinks that my sensory awareness row is inconsistent with what I said on June 3*. If you did jot something like that, then (3) is *not* correct—you do *not* have important presuppositions/biases. Possibility (3) is correct only if you are blind to an important distinction. If (3) is correct, that is, if you do have important presuppositions/biases active here, then when I directed your attention to the table, everything should have looked OK, even when I zeroed you in on the sensory awareness row of the table. That is, if (3) is correct, it would be difficult or impossible for you to have seen a discrepancy between the June 26 and the June 3 tables.

I say again: I don't know whether (3) is correct. But if (3) is correct, it serves as an example of why contemporaneous apprehensions of pristine experience and of broad experience are vitally important.

That is, if (3) is correct, you had on June 3 one broad experience of your own relationship to sensory awareness, and on June 26 you had a quite opposite broad experience of your own relationship to sensory awareness.

It seems to me that the evidence suggests that your June 3 broad experience fairly accurately characterizes your pristine-experience sensory awareness, and if so, then your June 26 broad experience is misleading. I recognize that there is nothing *false* in your June 26 view of sensory awareness—everything you said in that row is correct except that the retrospectivity of your retrospective prospection does not go back to your prior-to-sampling view, as the context of the table requires. That is, it seems to be a true statement about your *current* broad experience that "Sensory and bodily awareness plays an important role in experience; Marco's experience almost always includes sensory and bodily awareness, although (Russ explains) this is not the case for all DES subjects." The question is whether that was a true statement about your broad experience *prior to sampling*.

I re-reiterate that I am not the Judge nor the omniscient being. I may be off the track as far as my explication of (3) is concerned. I have tried to set up an exercise that is specifically designed for you, but whether that has been successful I don't know. If I have misrepresented you, I apologize.

June 28
Dear Russ,
Please find my response to your latest comment below.
All the best,
Marco

RE [253] "The exercise-for-Marco was designed with possibility (3) in mind: that Marco has presuppositions/biases about sensory awareness that operate prior to his rational analysis, with the result that inconsistencies can exist but not be recognized."

There are two ways in which I can explain what you characterize as the inconsistency between the retrospective prospection and my surprise of June 3.

- a) It is not experientially impossible to be surprised about something that one expects. Maybe one didn't expect one's predictions to be confirmed as clearly and indisputably as they turned out to be. Maybe what I meant on June 3 is that I was *pleasantly* surprised by the degree to which our findings match my theoretical presuppositions about sensory awareness. It's a "hah, I knew it!" kind of response.

b) Thinking that sensory/bodily awareness is key does not necessarily involve thinking that sensory/bodily awareness is always present. Logically, something can be very important without being always present. Hence, even if I did think that "sensory/bodily awareness is key," there was still room for being surprised (on June 3) by the fact that almost every single sample contains experiences of sensory/bodily awareness.

[254]

I believe (b) is probably a better explanation for the apparent inconsistency. Perhaps the problem here is that "Sensory and bodily awareness plays an important role in experience" has the form of a theoretical statement, not of a hypothesis or prospection that can (or cannot) be confirmed. But the fact is that prior to the sampling I didn't write down or even mentally form any specific hypotheses about what we would find, so all I can report is (what I think were) my presuppositions about experience. Thus, in my view saying on June 26 that prior to the sampling I thought "Sensory and bodily awareness plays an important role in experience" is *not* a (completely) faux generalization. What is true, however, is that the *language* I used to phrase this sentence is probably the language of Marco after discussing the samples with Russ. What (I think) I would have written before we started analyzing the samples is: "Embodiment and perception play an important role in experience." And the difference (I now realize) is significant: embodiment and perception are cognitive-level phenomena that may not have any repercussion on pristine experience.

[255]

June 29
Hi Marco—
Thanks for your comments. Please see below.
—Russ

RE [255] "The fact is that prior to the sampling I didn't write down or even mentally form any specific hypotheses about what we would find."

If, prior to sampling, I had set you (or you had set yourself) the task of explicitly recording what you expected to find in sampling, I suspect it would not have been very informative, because people in general (including you) are not in a position to know the remarkable features of their experience. Prior to sampling it would not any more have occurred to you, I think, to predict ubiquitous sensory/bodily awareness than it would have been to predict "If I see people walking, they will be walking on their feet" or "If I have a stomach ache it will be above my knees and below my shoulders." Of course!

But I'm pretty confident that the ubiquity of sensory/bodily awareness was pretty darn surprising to you as it unfolded across your sampling. You referred to it explicitly in your writing on June 3, but I think if we watched the videos we would see ample and repeated expressions of surprise (verbal and behavioral) early in sampling and resignation later in sampling as the repetitive sensory/bodily awareness examples accumulated. That is, throughout sampling I heard you repeatedly saying (explicitly or between the lines) that you were surprised at your own amount of sensory/bodily awareness.

Therefore I found it striking when your what-I-found description didn't mention the surprise over sensory/bodily awareness.

RE [254] "Hence, even if I did think that 'sensory/bodily awareness is key,' there was still room for being surprised (on June 3) by the fact that almost every single sample contains experiences of sensory/bodily awareness."

I entirely agree with that. However, that doesn't get at what I find remarkable: that you were surprised on June 3, and on many other sampling days, but that you didn't recall any of that surprise on June 26. [256]

I have no direct access to anything, and no omniscience, but I'd suggest a third explanation (c), and would bet on that:

> c) Marco has, and probably always has had, ubiquitous sensory/bodily awareness. Prior to sampling, he was ignorant of his ubiquitous sensory/bodily awarenesses, and so was surprised when they repeatedly arose during sampling, and said (or otherwise indicated) so repeatedly during sampling including on June 3. But between June 3 and June 26, Marco came to accept about himself that he has, and probably always has had, ubiquitous sensory/bodily awarenesses, and now notices them as they

frequently occur in everyday (nonbeeped) life. But now that he naturally accepts his ubiquitous sensory/bodily awarenesses, it is much harder (nearly impossible) to recall ever having been surprised by them, and therefore much harder to recall saying or otherwise indicating that he was surprised by them.

Explanation (c) is an instantiation of a natural part of the human condition, it seems to me, in line with Sherlock's "Insensibly one begins to twist facts to suit theories, instead of theories to suit facts" (Doyle, 1891/2015, 3). Your current (correct) theory is that you have ubiquitous sensory/bodily awarenesses, and one of the facts that gets twisted (forgotten) is that at one point (mostly throughout your life, actually) you didn't know that about yourself.

This is *not* an idiosyncratic Marco failing, as if anyone else in the same situation would have a clearer recollection. It is an example of Marco's participation in the human condition, where retrospection, which seems like a recalling of past events, is actually a construction *in the present* of events that are understood as taking place in the past. We do not recall events as they were experienced when they originally occurred; we construct experiences *as it seems to us now that* they originally occurred. And we are exquisitely blind to the alteration, because the results of our alterations are absolutely perfectly in synch with our idiosyncratic manner of alteration. That is, not only do we twist things, but part of the twisting skill is that we systematically overlook the twisting process (whatever that is).

The "we" in the preceding paragraph includes you, me, and (I think) everyone else that I know. My twistings are just as real-seeming to me as yours are to you.

I think we now have a fairly well documented laboratory example of broad experience, simpler than but parallel to Marco's broad experience of traveling through India: we have Marco's broad experience of traveling through (or, slightly less metaphorically, participating in) DES. I think Marco's broad experience of DES participation is not merely a characterization of experiences that happened during his DES participation. It is a present-tense creation of experiences that plausibly-from-his-present-perspective might have happened during his DES participation. Some of those plausible constructions are in accord with the actual experiences; some are not; and Marco cannot be expected to know the difference, because he is doing his best to recall actual experiences, and whatever might warp that "recalling" (I put the term in scare quotes because I think it is not actually a recalling) also in exquisite parallel warps his sense of plausibility/actuality.

DES is the result of taking all of that seriously: If it is the human condition to twist recollections, and that applies as much to me as to any of the participants in research I might conduct, how should one proceed if one wants to investigate experience? My answer is to minimize retrospection, to focus on concrete instances, to insist on contemporaneous commitment to details, and so on, all simply honest ways of accepting the failings of the human condition (including my own).

I wish to re-emphasize that I am *not* saying that broad experience is worthless—as I have often said above, broad experience is important, and often it is the only experiential avenue we have. But, as I think we have agreed, broad experience should be understood as a past-looking construction of the present, partially informed by what actually happened in the past, partially informed by what actually was experienced in the past, partially infused by some present experience, partially shaped by the present context, and so on. (All of that is true of DES pristine experience as well, but I think far less, for the reasons I have harped about.)

Q: Russ, you put scare quotes around "recalling" when applied to broad experience. Shouldn't you also put scare quotes around DES reports? After all, they are recollections, too.

RUSS: Yes, I agree that "recalling" without scare quotes doesn't exist, so the "recollection" of a pristine experience is indeed a fabrication and thus deserves scare quotes. However, I also think the "size" of the scare varies substantially across situations. Consider these "recollections": your "recollection" of a specific moment that occurred a few seconds ago and which you were trained to apprehend; your "recollection" of where you were when the Challenger space shuttle exploded; your "recollection" of your experience of traveling through India. A science of experience has to keep these things distinct even though we use the term "recollection" for each.

June 30
Dear Russ,
Please find a comment below.
All the best,
Marco

RE [256] "That doesn't get at what I find remarkable: that you were surprised on June 3, and on many other sampling days, but that you didn't recall any of that surprise on June 26."

Your explanation (c) for why I didn't mention my surprise of June 3 on June 26 sounds plausible to me. I am happy to accept that as a possibility, and I am happy to acknowledge that my broad experience could have distorted my reactions to DES.

[257] It is true that neither when I wrote down the prospections nor later on, when I looked at your exercise-for-Marco, I could see the inconsistency between my surprise of June 3, my broad experience of June 26, and what we've found in DES. Yet I think the distortion is less clear-cut than you make it sound. If you had asked me: "tell me what surprised you during the sampling," I am reasonably confident that I would have remembered my surprise on June 3 and answered "the pervasiveness of sensory awareness." However, the task involved making some retrospective prospections and comparing them to what we've actually found. As I said above, I couldn't recall any specific prospections, so I resorted to listing what were, for me before the sampling, the characteristics of experience *in general*. The reason why I didn't see the inconsistency is that my surprise, my broad experience, and what we've found are not precisely equivalent or at the same level. Maybe this discrepancy does not by itself explain my forgetfulness, but it does seem to complicate the picture you paint.

Your reasoning works along these lines: I (Marco) was surprised by the pervasiveness of sensory awareness on June 3; hence there must be a presupposition in me that says (A) "(my) sensory awareness is not very pervasive"; on June 26 I wrote that prior to the sampling I thought (B) "sensory/bodily awareness is key (in general, for everyone)," and that this was to some extent confirmed by (C), the pervasiveness of sensory awareness in my samples. According to you, my judgment that (B) is supported by (C) is incongruous because there was no reference to (A), which clashes with (C). I agree that there is a clash, and that my omission of (A) seems to hint at a distortion, but in my view such distortion is partly mitigated by the fact that (B) is a judgment of importance, not of pervasiveness in pristine experience; and that (B) applies to everyone, not just to Marco, so it is not strictly comparable to (A) and (B).

July 1
Hi Marco—
Here is my response to your last comment.
—Russ

RE [257] "If you had asked me: 'tell me what surprised you during the sampling,' I am reasonably confident that I would have remembered my surprise on June 3 and answered 'the pervasiveness of sensory awareness.'"

As I have said, I'm no mind reader, and what you say in these paragraphs might be right.

However, your response prompts me to clarify my explanation (c). Preliminarily, because I will refer to it frequently, let's abbreviate "sensory awareness/bodily awareness" by "SABA," and put a subscript on it so that 1 indicates before sampling and 2 indicates during or after sampling. Then prior to sampling, you thought, as a general principle, that $SABA_1$ was key. And as a result of sampling, you discovered very frequent $SABA_2$ in your own experience. In one manner of speaking, as you say, the high frequency of $SABA_2$ corroborates (or at least appears to corroborate) your understanding of the importance of $SABA_1$.

However, $SABA_1$ and $SABA_2$ are not at all the same thing. $SABA_1$ is a sensation that gets incorporated into a perceptual process. $SABA_1$ is an ingredient, or a constitutive entity, which, along with many other ingredients, somehow becomes a perception of reality. $SABA_1$ is the kind of thing that leads the embodied perception people to notice that distances are distorted when walking uphill. By definition, and by practice, $SABA_1$ is mostly or entirely unnoticed; its effect is to contribute to that which is noticed (which is other than $SABA_1$ itself).

By diametric contrast, $SABA_2$ is the perceptual entity itself, the main focus of consciousness. It is *not* constitutive of something else. When, at sample 3.1, you were attending to the sweetness and crunchiness of the cereal, that sweetness/crunchiness was not a building block incorporated into the perception of the cereal (in which case it would be a $SABA_1$); the sweetness/crunchiness was the ($SABA_2$) perception itself.

Said another way: $SABA_2$ is a directly apprehended phenomenon of pristine experience, whereas the existence of $SABA_1$ is an inference about cognitive process. $SABA_1$ and $SABA_2$ exist in two entirely different realms.

My guess is that you knew little or nothing about your (or anyone else's) $SABA_2$ prior to sampling, even though you yourself have engaged, across your lifetime, in some millions of $SABA_2$ experiences. $SABA_2$ was a (pretty close to total) surprise to you.

By diametric contrast, your belief in $SABA_1$ has remained pretty stable across sampling: you thought $SABA_1$ was key before sampling, and you still think it is key.

So when you write "on June 26 I wrote that prior to the sampling I thought (B) 'sensory/bodily awareness is key (in general, for everyone),' and that this was to some extent confirmed by (C), the pervasiveness of sensory awareness in my samples," I think that is not correct. $SABA_1$ has nothing to do with whether $SABA_2$ is frequent for some people, and therefore your high-frequency $SABA_2$ does not confirm (nor disconfirm) anything about $SABA_1$. Similarly, when you write "(B) is a judgment of importance, not of pervasiveness in pristine experience; and that (B) applies to everyone, not just to Marco, so it is not strictly comparable to (A) and (C)," I think you are on the wrong track. $SABA_1$ and $SABA_2$ are not comparable because they are not the same thing, not because one applies to Marco and the other doesn't.

Returning to why you might have forgotten being surprised: $SABA_2$ as a concept did not exist for you prior to sampling. Now it exists as a differentiated, florid, rock solid, clearly demarcated, unambiguous concept. In general, it is almost impossible (or perhaps entirely impossible) to imagine not having a concept that one currently has, so one "remembers" as if one always had the concept. Therefore it is difficult (or perhaps impossible) to recall being surprised by the arising of a concept, because once the concept has arisen, surprise is no longer possible. Applied here: Once your conceptual scheme includes $SABA_2$, it is difficult to recall being surprised by $SABA_2$. The talk about $SABA_1$ is a red herring, but it is difficult to disentangle because the words used are the same.

July 2
Dear Russ,

I agree with your explanation. I have said this myself, I believe, when I wrote (in my June 28 email) that "the difference (I now realize) is significant: embodiment and perception [your $SABA_1$] are cognitive-level phenomena that may not have any repercussion on pristine experience [your $SABA_2$]."
All the best,
Marco

ROAD MAP: *These are our closing remarks on the role of presuppositions and delusions (theme e) and the personal dimension of our conversation (theme i).*

XXVI

IN LIEU OF A CONCLUSION

July 3
Hi Marco—
It seems to me that the conversation we have been having could be of interest far beyond simply you and me. That is, the issues we have been grappling with are important not only for Marco and Russ but for anyone who is interested in experience of any kind, and that's a lot of people. And I think we have something important to say. We've undertaken these conversations in (I think) an original and constructive manner, combining real human confrontation, thoughtful consideration, knowledge, and writing skill.

If you agree with all or most or even part of that, then it might be time to start thinking about how to make this conversation public. I think conversations like ours never really end, but I think that we are close to reaching the end of an episode, a place where it makes sense to pause and consider what we have done.

I think that the conversation from beginning to end, with some very light pruning to remove redundancy, mistakes, irrelevance, and the like, would make a valuable book.

If we do edit like that, I think it important to keep enough of the flavor of the discussion, even though (or especially because) the conversation is sometimes redundant. When such redundancy is an integral part of the conversation, as I think it is when presuppositions are involved, then I think it should stay.

There is a human tension in this project that I think we should preserve. That is, at just about every turn I was nervous about offending or being otherwise out of line, and relieved when I received the reply from you that indicated that you understood what I was saying and the motives for it. I think readers will grasp that, and so that tension should not be edited out.

There are lots of possibilities: you're not interested; you're not interested *now* because there is more to be done first; you are interested if we do it in X manner; and so on. I'd like you to feel yourself as a free agent in the discussion of what if anything we should do about this.

So please give it some thought and let me know.

July 4
Dear Russ,
I completely agree that we should try to make this conversation public somehow. On both sides there is (I think) a sense of urgency, a willingness to invest ourselves in what is not just a research interest but a matter of personal relevance and resonance. Our conversation could be read almost as a manifesto for a creative way of doing interdisciplinarity across the sciences/humanities divide, one that is based on your view that "science is an entirely human endeavor, embodying the highest values of humanism" (at chapter IX, RE 88), and that "when you get down deep enough into genuineness, [every human endeavor] looks pretty much the same" (at chapter XXII, RE 216). I think the value of personal involvement and commitment has to be reasserted as a humanistic path to the "consilience" of knowledge. I also think that if we succeed in framing our project that way, it would make a fascinating read.
All the best,
Marco

July 5
Hi Marco—
I'm delighted that you're delighted with the prospect of making these conversations public in some way. It's difficult for me to be objective about the originality or creativity of our interactions. From my view, our interactions have been quite simple: You have said things that, by their implication or denotation, moved me to clarify, question, challenge, generalize, particularize, or whatever, and I have done so. Likewise for you. From my view, there have been no particular general principles that drove that discussion, other than (a) each of us trying to disambiguate what we both said; (b) trying to apply our discussion to concrete, directly accessible specifics; and (c) accepting the

confrontational nature of the discussion and trying to rise above the petty personal aspects of it.
—Russ

Q: *That's it? You're just stopping?*

RUSS AND MARCO: *Here, as in most important relationships, there is no real end. We have opened ourselves to dialogue, paid uncompromising attention to phenomena, and tried to let go of our presuppositions, and now have paused to share what has happened. It is up to you, dear reader, to determine the extent to which our struggles resonate with your experience.*

WORKS CITED

5TOORMTROOPER. (August 14, 2011). Excellent book, difficult style. *Amazon.com customer reviews*. Retrieved from www.amazon-associate.com/gp/customer-reviews/R1NUTHCC915IYA

Abbott, H. P. (2011). Reading intended meaning where none is intended: A cognitivist reappraisal of the implied author. *Poetics Today* 32(3): 461–87.

Akhenatonio. (November 12, 2009). Poetic justice. *Amazon.com customer reviews*. Retrieved from www.amazon.com/review/R2QXK17GJ7V4J9

Angry Warrior. (August 21, 2008). Simple, heartfelt and brilliant. *Amazon.com customer reviews*. Retrieved from www.amazon.com/review/R4HSL48Y49C2N

Aristotle. (335 AD/1967). *Poetics*. Trans. Gerald F. Else. Ann Arbor: University of Michigan Press.

Baars, B. J. (2003). How brain reveals mind: Neural studies support the fundamental role of conscious experience. *Journal of Consciousness Studies* 10: 100–14.

Bálint, K., and Tan, E. (2015). "It feels like there are hooks inside my chest." The construction of narrative absorption experiences using image schemata. *Projections: The Journal for Movies and Minds* 9(2): 63–88.

Banfield, A. (2003). Time passes: Virginia Woolf, post-impressionism, and Cambridge time. *Poetics Today* 24(3): 471–516.

Black Brain. (October 1, 2001). Slightly confused on what to think of this book. *Amazon.com customer reviews*. Retrieved from http://www.amazon.com/review/RPRQ9AKX73315

Borges, J. L. (1964). Funes the memorious. In J. E. Irby, trans. *Labyrinths*. New York: New Directions. 59–66.

Bortolussi, M., and Dixon, P. (2002). *Psychonarratology*. Cambridge: Cambridge University Press.

Bowdle, B. F., and Gentner, D. (2005). The career of metaphor. *Psychological Review* 112(1): 193–216.

Caracciolo, M. (2012). On the experientiality of stories: A follow-up on David Herman's "Narrative theory and the intentional stance." *Partial Answers* 10(2): 197–221.

———. (2013a). Narrative space and readers' responses to stories: A phenomenological account. *Style* 47(4): 425–44.

———. (2013b). Phenomenological metaphors in readers' engagement with characters: The case of Ian McEwan's *Saturday*. *Language and Literature* 22(1): 60–76.

———. (2014a). Beyond other minds: Fictional characters, mental simulation, and "unnatural" experiences. *Journal of Narrative Theory* 44(1): 29–53.

———. (2014b). *The experientiality of narrative: An enactivist approach*. Berlin and New York: Walter de Gruyter.

Cohn, D. (1978). *Transparent minds: Narrative modes for presenting consciousness in fiction*. Princeton: Princeton University Press.

Craig, A. (December 21, 2006). An unsettling, profound tale of love and survival. *Amazon.com customer reviews*. Retrieved from www.amazon.com/review/R2PQMEUVDX1SCZ

Doyle, A. C. (1891/October 10, 2015). *A scandal in Bohemia*. Retrieved from www.pagebypagebooks.com/Arthur_Conan_Doyle/The_Adventures_of_Sherlock_Holmes/ADVENTURE_I_A_SCANDAL_IN_BOHEMIA_p3.html.

Eco, U. (1979). *The role of the reader: Explorations in the semiotics of texts*. Bloomington: Indiana University Press.

Epictetus. (108AD/1865). *The works of Epictetus*. Trans. E. Carter and T. W. Higginson. New York: Little, Brown and Co.

Esrock, E. J. (2005). Visualisation. In D. Herman, M. Jahn, and M.-L. Ryan, eds., *Routledge encyclopedia of narrative theory*. New York: Routledge.

Fauconnier, G., and Turner, M. (2002). *The way we think: Conceptual blending and the mind's hidden complexities*. New York: Basic Books.

Fludernik, M. (1996). *Towards a "natural" narratology*. London: Routledge.

Gibbs, R. W. (2005). *Embodiment and cognitive science*. Cambridge: Cambridge University Press.

Gibbs, R. W., and Matlock, T. (2008). Metaphor, imagination, and simulation: Psycholinguistic evidence. In R. W. Gibbs, ed., *The Cambridge handbook of metaphor and thought*. Cambridge: Cambridge University Press. 161–76.

Glucksberg, S. (2008). How metaphors create categories—quickly. In R. W. Gibbs, ed., *The Cambridge handbook of metaphor and thought*. Cambridge: Cambridge University Press. 67–83.

Hanich, J. (2014). Watching a film with others: Towards a theory of collective spectatorship. *Screen* 55(3): 338–59.

Heavey, C. L., Hurlburt, R. T., & Lefforge, N. (2012). Toward a phenomenology of feelings. *Emotion* 12(4): 763–77.

Heidegger, M. (2001). *The fundamental concepts of metaphysics: World, finitude, solitude*. Trans. W. McNeill and N. Walker. Bloomington: Indiana University Press.

Herman, D. (2003). Stories as a tool for thinking. In *Narrative theory and the cognitive sciences*. Stanford: CSLI Publications. 163–92.

———. (2008). Narrative theory and the intentional stance. *Partial Answers*, 6(2), 233–60.

Herman, D., ed. (2011). *The emergence of mind: Representations of consciousness in narrative discourse in English.* Lincoln and London: University of Nebraska Press.

Hogan, P. C. (2003). *Cognitive science, literature, and the arts: A guide for humanists.* London: Routledge.

Holland, N. N. (1975). *5 readers reading.* New Haven and London: Yale University Press.

Hurlburt, R. T. (1993). *Sampling inner experience in disturbed affect.* New York: Plenum Press.

———. (2009a). Iteratively apprehending pristine experience. *Journal of Consciousness Studies* 16(10–12): 156–88.

———. (2009b). Descriptive experience sampling. In T. Baynes, A. Cleermans, and P. Wilken, eds., *Oxford Companion to Consciousness.* Oxford, UK: Oxford University Press. 225–27.

———. (2011a). *Investigating pristine inner experience: Moments of truth.* Cambridge: Cambridge University Press.

———. (2011b). Nine clarifications of descriptive experience sampling. *Journal of Consciousness Studies* 18(1): 274–87.

Hurlburt, R. T., and Akhter, S. A. (2008a). Unsymbolized thinking. *Consciousness and Cognition* 17(4): 1364–74.

———. (2008b). Unsymbolized thinking is a clearly defined phenomenon: A reply to Persaud. *Consciousness and Cognition* 17(4): 1376–77.

Hurlburt, R. T., and Heavey, C. L. (2001). Telling what we know: Describing inner experience. *Trends in Cognitive Sciences* 5(9): 400–403.

———. (2006). *Exploring inner experience: The descriptive experience sampling method.* Philadelphia and Amsterdam: John Benjamins.

———. (2015). Investigating pristine inner experience: Implications for experience sampling and questionnaires. *Consciousness and Cognition* 31: 148–59.

Hurlburt, R. T., Heavey, C. L., and Bensaheb, A. (2009). Sensory awareness. *Journal of Consciousness Studies* 16(10–12): 231–51.

Hurlburt, R. T., and Kane, M. J. (2011). Experience in Tourette's Syndrome. In R. T. Hurlburt, *Investigating pristine inner experience: Moments of truth.* Cambridge: Cambridge University Press, 94–103.

Hurlburt, R. T., and Schwitzgebel, E. (2007). *Describing inner experience? Proponent meets skeptic.* Cambridge, MA: MIT Press.

———. (2011). Little or no experience outside of attention? *Journal of Consciousness Studies* 18(1): 234–52.

Hurlburt, R. T., and Sipprelle, C. N. (1978). Random sampling of cognitions in alleviating anxiety attacks. *Cognitive Therapy and Research* 2: 165–69.

Hutto, D. D. (2000). *Beyond physicalism.* Philadelphia and Amsterdam: John Benjamins.

Iser, W. (1978). *The act of reading: A theory of aesthetic response.* Baltimore and London: Johns Hopkins University Press.

Jaynes, J. (1986). Consciousness and the voices of the mind. *Canadian Psychology/Psychologie canadienne* 27(2): 128–48.

Joyce, J. (1916/2000). *A portrait of the artist as a young man.* London: Penguin.

Kuiken, D., Miall, D. S., and Sikora, S. (2004). Forms of self-implication in literary reading. *Poetics Today* 25(2): 171–203.

Kuzmičová, A. (2014). Literary narrative and mental imagery: A view from embodied cognition. *Style* 48(3): 275–93.

Lakoff, G., and Johnson, M. (1980). *Metaphors we live by.* Chicago and London: University of Chicago Press.

———. (1999). *Philosophy in the flesh: The embodied mind and its challenge to Western thought.* New York: Basic Books.

Lutz, S. L. (May 13, 2007). The road. *Amazon.com customer reviews.* Retrieved from www.amazon.com/review/RL547GVFFFXI6

maya j. (July 3, 2007). Hope road. *Amazon.com customer reviews.* Retrieved from www.amazon.com/review/R1G4XLIPJFLG3G

McCarthy, C. (2006). *The road.* New York: Knopf.

McCarthy-Jones, S., and Fernyhough, C. (2011). The varieties of inner speech: Links between quality of inner speech and psychopathological variables in a sample of young adults. *Consciousness and Cognition* 20(4): 1586–93.

McEwan, I. (2005). *Saturday.* Toronto: Vintage.

McHugh, P. R. (2008). *Try to remember: Psychiatry's clash over meaning, memory and mind.* New York: Dana Press.

Miall, D. S. (2006). *Literary reading: Empirical and theoretical studies.* New York: Peter Lang.

Miall, D. S., and Kuiken, D. (1995). Aspects of literary response: A new questionnaire. *Research in the Teaching of English* 29(1): 37–58.

Mitchell, W. J. T. (1994). *Picture theory.* Chicago and London: University of Chicago Press.

Moore, A. T., and Schwitzgebel, E. (August 28, 2013). The experience of reading: Imagery, inner speech, and seeing the words on the page. *The Splintered mind.* Retrieved from schwitzsplinters.blogspot.com/2013/08/the-experience-of-reading-imagery-inner.html

Nabokov, V. (1980). *Lectures on literature.* Ed. F. Bowers. London: Weidenfeld and Nicolson.

Nell, V. (1988). *Lost in a book: The psychology of reading for pleasure.* New Haven and London: Yale University Press.

Noë, A. (2004). *Action in perception.* Cambridge, MA: MIT Press.

O'Regan, J. K., Myin, E., and Noë, A. (2005). Sensory consciousness explained (better) in terms of "corporality" and "alerting capacity." *Phenomenology and the Cognitive Sciences* 4: 369–87.

O'Regan, J. K., and Noë, A. (2001). A sensorimotor account of vision and visual consciousness. *Behavioral and Brain Sciences* 24(5): 939–1031.

Peter G. (2007, May 17). Wow! Incredible writing. *Amazon.com customer reviews.* Retrieved from www.amazon.com/review/RO9AV1FVC09GI

Phelan, J. (2007). *Experiencing fiction: Judgments, progressions, and the rhetorical theory of narrative.* Columbus: The Ohio State University Press.

Phelps, E. A., Cannistraci, C. J., and Cunningham, W. A. (2003). Intact performance on an indirect measure of race bias following amygdala damage. *Neuropsychologia* 41(2): 203–8.

Pollio, H. R., Henley, T. B., and Thompson, C. J. (1997). *The phenomenology of everyday life: Empirical investigations of human experience.* Cambridge: Cambridge University Press.

Richardson, A. (2004). Studies in literature and cognition: A field map. In A. Richardson and E. Spolsky, eds., *The work of fiction: Cognition, culture, and complexity.* Aldershot, UK: Ashgate Publishing. 1–29.

Roxane. (March 22, 2009). Difficult book to rate; loved it and hated it. *Amazon.com customer reviews.* Retrieved from www.amazon-associate.com/gp/customer-reviews/R32RVJDDU4YBZU

Ryan, M.-L. (2001). *Narrative as virtual reality: Immersion and interactivity in literature and electronic media.* Baltimore and London: Johns Hopkins University Press.

Scarry, E. (2001). *Dreaming by the book.* Princeton: Princeton University Press.

Schmid, W. (2005). Defamiliarisation. In D. Herman, M. Jahn, and M.-L. Ryan, eds., *Routledge encyclopedia of narrative theory.* London and New York: Routledge.

Seemann, A. (Ed.). (2011). *Joint attention: New developments in psychology, philosophy of mind, and social neuroscience.* Cambridge, MA: MIT Press.

Shklovsky, V. (1991). Art as device. In B. Sher, trans. *Theory of prose.* Champaign and London: Dalkey Archive Press. 1–14.

Skinner, B. F. (1953). *Science and human behavior.* New York: Macmillan.

———. (1971). *Beyond freedom and dignity.* New York: Knopf.

———. (1974). *About behaviorism.* New York: Knopf.

———. (1977). Why I am not a cognitive psychologist. *Behaviorism* 5: 1–10.

Troscianko, E. (2010). Kafkaesque worlds in real time. *Language and Literature* 19(2): 151–71.

———. (2014). *Kafka's cognitive realism.* New York and London: Routledge.

Van Peer, W., Hakemulder, J., and Zyngier, S. (2007). *Muses and measures: Empirical research methods for the humanities.* Cambridge: Cambridge Scholars.

Winawer, J., Witthoft, N., Frank, M. C., et al. (2007). Russian blues reveal effects of language on color discrimination. *Proceedings of the National Academy of Sciences of the United States of America,* 104(19): 7780–85.

Zachary Breakstone. (January 2, 2008). I highly recommend. *Amazon.com customer reviews*. Retrieved from www.amazon-associate.com/gp/customer-reviews/R20Q3FPZO2HPM

Zemeckis, Robert. (November 29, 2012). Interview with Dave Davies. *Fresh Air*. NPR

Zwaan, R. A., and Radvansky, G. A. (1998). Situation models in language comprehension and memory. *Psychological Bulletin* 123(2): 162–85.

INDEX

5 Readers Reading (Holland), 52

Abbott, H. Porter, xi, 65
About Behaviorism (Skinner), 154
Aiken, Conrad, 43
Akhter, Sarah A., 270
ambivalence in linguistic meaning, 79, 100, 204–5, 297–98
arachnoid, 280–81, 289, 293, 295
Aristotle, 155

Baars, Bernard J., 269, 273–74, 286
Bálint, Katalin, 288, 294
Beyond Freedom and Dignity (Skinner), 154
blue, as emotion vs. as color, 270–71; in Russian, 133, 139–41
Bortolussi, Marisa, 30
Bowdle, Brian F., 289
bracketing presuppositions, and defamiliarization, 232; definition of, 18, 121; difficulty of, 38, 202–3, 208, 266; importance of, 13–22, 35, 76–77, 98, 207, 210; role of repetition in, 7–8
braided conversation, 7–8, 17
bulimia nervosa, 176–77

Cohn, Dorrit, 113

Coleridge, Samuel Taylor, 121
concepts and experience. *See* experience

Davies, Dave, 93
Day-Lewis, Daniel, 269
delusion, awareness of, 128, 135, 272; and intersubjectivity, 5, 7, 97, 192; and presuppositions, 18–20; standards for, 96, 100, 102; ubiquity of, 86, 105, 114–15
Dennis (DES subject), 189–90, 199–200, 206, 213–14
Descriptive Experience Sampling (DES), and adulteration, 113, 123–25, 133, 135, 138–39, 149; basic description of, 9, 28, 194–97; and experiential details, 239–40, 242, 276–77; and language, 84, 90–92; poetic aspect of, 241, 281. *See also* bracketing presuppositions; experience; fidelity in experiential descriptions
diamond, 272–73
Dickens, Charles, 103–4, 111
Dixon, Peter, 30
Donald (DES subject), 161–64, 168
Doyle, A. C., 252, 308

Eco, Umberto, 30
embodied cognition, 283–84, 289
emotion, as a feature of broad experience, 59, 68, 184; vs. feeling, 277; in

pristine experience, 205, 229–30, 248, 301; in reader response, 11, 29, 40, 51, 69–70

enactivism, 60, 95

engagement with, vs. experience of, 56–57, 59, 62; offline, 65–66

Epictetus, 15

escape velocity, 202–3

Esrock, Ellen J., 71

experience, and cognitive science, 283–84, 289; and concepts, 95, 97, 100–101, 185–86, 188–91, 199–200, 204–5, 215, 269–72, 312; humanistic (historical) vs. scientific approaches to, 98, 104, 107–9, 114–15, 281; and language, 133, 139–41, 204–5, 271, 280, 288 (see also inner speaking); is not an object, 84, 89, 101, 105, 148; of vs. while reading, 35–36, 55–56; pristine vs. broad, 58–59, 77–78, 88–90, 92–94, 106–9, 125–27, 134–37, 144–46, 148–69, 176–78, 183–85, 239–40; and significance, 137, 149, 154. See also Descriptive Experience Sampling; science of experience

Experiencing Fiction (Phelan), 30

Farm Basket turkey (DES case). See Michaels, John

Fauconnier, Gilles, 288

faux generalizations, 157, 163, 166, 176, 198, 209; degrees of fauxity, 187–88

fidelity in experiential descriptions, 50–51, 89, 107–8, 134–35, 144–45, 151, 236; vs. accuracy, 276; vs. clarity, 282

Fludernik, Monika, 31

Forrest Gump (Zemeckis), 93–94

Freud, Sigmund, 88, 158

Gentner, Dedre, 289

Gibbs, Raymond W., 238, 289, 293

Glucksberg, Sam, 289

Great Expectations (Dickens), 103–4

Hakemulder, Jèmeljan, 31

Hanich, Julian, xi, 239

Heavey, Christopher L., xi, 18, 154, 179, 197, 204, 209, 215, 243, 273, 277, 283

Heidegger, Martin, 113

Henley, Tracy B., 77

Herman, David, 65, 113, 185

Hogan, Patrick Colm, 31

Holland, Norman, 30, 52

human condition, and delusions, 87, 96–97, 99, 105, 188, 214, 263; and messiness, 114; and pristine experience, 146; and retrospection, 307–9

hunger, 154–55, 165, 171–73, 175, 185–87, 189–91, 199–200, 206, 213–14

Husserl, Edmund, 213, 240, 268, 286

Hutto, Daniel D., 95, 111

immersion, in engaging with art, ix, 11, 28, 32, 39, 48, 69, 288, 294; in pristine experience, 185, 243

individual differences in experience, 15, 58, 140–41, 292

inner speaking, 118–19, 205, 208–9, 273–74, 286–87; in Marco's experience samples, 220–21, 228, 231, 234–36, 246–48, 250–51, 254, 256, 301

inner speech. *See* inner speaking

intentions in literary writing, 65–66, 68

interdisciplinarity, 71, 315

intersubjectivity, 83, 87–88, 133–34, 149–50, 214, 239, 275. *See also* sharing experiences

Iser, Wolfgang, 30

James, William, 9, 158
Jaynes, Julian, 297
John (DES subject). *See* Michaels, John
Johnson, Mark, 238, 287
Joyce, James, 112, 119–23, 130, 132–33, 142, 286
Juanita (DES subject), 156–57
judgments, 11, 51, 53, 69, 137, 153–54, 165, 169–71, 183, 187–88, 198, 301, 310, 312. *See also* faux generalizations

Kafka, Franz, ix, 3, 22, 51, 59, 61, 63, 65, 68, 97, 167
Kane, Michael (Mike) J., 115–19, 123, 125–27, 131, 139–40
"Kubla Khan" (Coleridge), 121
Kuiken, Don, 31, 41
Kuzmičová, Anežka, xi, 31

Lakoff, George, 238, 287
language and experience. *See* experience
Lincoln, Abraham, 269
literary representations of consciousness, 112–13, 119–20, 122, 132, 215, 241, 269, 286
literary theory, 51–52, 70, 113, 130, 232
Lovecraft, H. P., 43

Matlock, Teenie, 289, 293
McCarthy, Cormac, 68–71, 73–76, 97
McEwan, Ian, 280, 293
Melanie (DES subject), 115–16, 123, 139, 141–42, 150
memory, 47, 90, 194, 263, 302, 309; false memory syndrome, 169, 176, 184; Marco's memory, 253–54
mental imagery. *See* visual imagery

mentalism (Skinner), 154–59, 164–66, 171, 173, 176, 194, 270–72
mental state, 154–57, 159, 165–66, 171, 174–75. *See also* mentalism
The Metamorphosis (Kafka), ix, 3, 4, 22–26, 29, 31, 35, 38, 40, 43–47, 49, 51, 54–66, 85, 156, 219
metaphier, 297–300
metaphor, and artistic creativity, 69, 240–41, 281; in Marco's experience samples, 221, 231, 249; and psychological processes, 5, 154–55, 158, 160, 166, 175, 271, 278–80, 287–89, 292–93, 293–300; as used in this book, 37, 88, 137, 170, 175, 185, 202, 209, 272
Metaphors We Live By (Lakoff and Johnson), 287
metaphrand, 297–300
Miall, David, 30–31, 41
Michaels, John (DES subject), 143–46, 148, 151–54, 159–60, 165, 169, 183, 187–88
Michelangelo, 254
Mike (DES subject). *See* Kane, Michael (Mike) J.
misunderstanding, 83, 86–87, 97
Mitchell, W. J. Thomas, 70
molecular vs. referential descriptions of experience, 33, 36, 37, 40, 60, 133, 157, 240. *See also* Descriptive Experience Sampling
Myin, Erik, 60

Nabokov, Vladimir, 30, 168
narrative, 3–4, 6, 12, 31, 35–36, 69, 113, 121, 241, 282; narrative comprehension, 28–29, 32, 60, 168, 288, 301; vs. science, 132
narrative theory, 3, 69, 113
Nell, Victor, 39
New Criticism, 65

New York Yankees, 270
Noë, Alva, 60, 95

O'Regan, Kevin, 60

paraphier, 297–99
personal dimension of the book, x, 5, 8, 21, 178, 191–93, 200, 203, 208, 315–16
Phelan, James, 30
phenomena, 36, 51, 79, 84–86, 89, 126–27, 134, 136–37, 144–45, 147–48, 152–54, 156–60, 163–67, 170–75, 178, 183–87, 191–94, 201–3
phenomenological methods, high-resolution vs. low-resolution, 77–79, 84. See also Descriptive Experience Sampling
phenomenology, 69, 173, 189–90, 266, 286; while reading, 11–13, 52, 57–60, 78
The Phenomenology of Everyday Life (Pollio, Henley, and Thompson), 77–78
Pollio, Howard R., 77–78
A Portrait of the Artist as a Young Man (Joyce), 112, 119, 122
presuppositions, vs. tendencies, 118–19, 123–25, 127, 131, 134, 141–42, 149–50. See also bracketing presuppositions

Radvansky, Gabriel A., 28
referential descriptions. See molecular vs. referential descriptions of experience
retrospection, 43, 46, 50–52, 78, 90–91, 101, 253–54, 263, 301–5, 308. See also memory
Richardson, Alan, 31
The Rime of the Ancient Mariner (Coleridge), 121
The Road (McCarthy), 68–73, 79, 90, 97, 104–5, 145, 288

Russian, 133, 139–41, 291
Ryan, Marie-Laure, 39

Saki, 43
Saturday (McEwan), 280–81, 289, 293, 295
scanning (in Marco's experience samples), 223–24, 228, 244–47, 249–52, 257–58, 263, 266
Schiff, András, 236
schizophrenia, 84–85, 95
Schwitzgebel, Eric, ix–xi, 3, 6, 18, 102–3, 115, 161, 164, 204–5, 236, 279
Science and Human Behavior (Skinner), 154
science of experience, 119, 161, 213–15, 264–66, 268; and DES, 178–79, 214, 309; and the pristine vs. broad experience distinction, 108, 126, 176–77
sensory awareness, 48, 117–19, 125, 140, 268–70, 277, 286, 290; definition of, 243–44; and embodied cognition, 238, 283–84, 289; in Marco's experience samples, 218, 244–46, 264–66, 301, 303–5, 310–12
sharing experiences, 16, 18–19, 60, 86, 102–3, 132–34, 189, 214–15, 239, 292; and delusion, 128, 177; in engaging with literature and film, 65, 121, 145, 275–76; and humans' biological makeup, 83, 87, 97, 284. See also individual differences in experience; intersubjectivity
Sherlock Holmes, 252–53, 308
significance. See experience
Sikora, Shelley, 31
Sipprelle, Carl N., 161
skepticism, 37, 89–90, 97–98, 283; vs. affect-laden presuppositions, 219
Skinner, B. F., 17, 154–59, 164–65, 170–72, 204–5, 215

slippery terms, 80
Socrates, 128
solid thought, 258–59
subjunctification, definition of, 255; in Marco's experience samples, 287
suspension of disbelief, 121–22

Tan, Ed S., 288, 294
tendencies. *See* presuppositions
Thompson, Craig J., 77–78
Tim (DES subject), 190–91
Troscianko, Emily, xi, 22, 31
truthiness, 121
Turner, Mark, 288

unsymbolized thinking, 270, 286

validation, 14, 16, 73, 77, 208, 270
Van Leeuwenhoek, Antonie, 122
Van Peer, Willie, 31

visual imagery, ix, 3, 22, 91–92, 142–44, 204, 279; in Marco's experience samples, 223, 229, 301; in the *Metamorphosis* study, 26, 28–29, 32, 39, 43, 46, 48–49; in McCarthy's *The Road*, 69–76; in McEwan's *Saturday*, 280–81, 288–89, 293
Vonnegut, Kurt, 43

The Well-tempered Clavier, 236
"Why I Am Not a Cognitive Psychologist" (Skinner), 154–55
Winawer, Jonathan, 133, 139–42, 270, 291
Woolf, Virginia, 5, 241

Young, William P., 43

Zemeckis, Robert, 93–94, 99, 106
zirconium dioxide, 272–73
Zwaan, Rolf A., 28
Zyngier, Sonia, 31

COGNITIVE APPROACHES TO CULTURE
Frederick Luis Aldama, Patrick Colm Hogan, Lalita Pandit Hogan, and Sue Kim,
Series Editors

This new series takes up cutting edge research in a broad range of cognitive sciences insofar as this research bears on and illuminates cultural phenomena such as literature, film, drama, music, dance, visual art, digital media, and comics, among others. For the purpose of the series, "cognitive science" will be construed broadly to encompass work derived from cognitive and social psychology, neuroscience, cognitive and generative linguistics, affective science, and related areas in anthropology, philosophy, computer science, and elsewhere. Though open to all forms of cognitive analysis, the series is particularly interested in works that explore the social and political consequences of cognitive cultural study.

A Passion for Specificity: Confronting Inner Experience in Literature and Science
    MARCO CARACCIOLO AND RUSSELL T. HURLBURT

www.ingramcontent.com/pod-product-compliance
Lightning Source LLC
Chambersburg PA
CBHW032000220426
43664CB00005B/91